Parched
City

A history of London's public
and private drinking water

Parched City

A history of London's public and private drinking water

Emma M. Jones

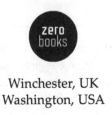

Winchester, UK
Washington, USA

First published by Zero Books, 2013
Zero Books is an imprint of John Hunt Publishing Ltd., Laurel House, Station Approach,
Alresford, Hants, SO24 9JH, UK
office1@jhpbooks.net
www.johnhuntpublishing.com
www.zero-books.net

For distributor details and how to order please visit the 'Ordering' section on our website.

Text copyright: Emma M. Jones 2012

ISBN: 978 1 78099 158 0

A CIP catalogue record for this book is available from the British Library.

Design: Stuart Davies

Printed and bound by CPI Group (UK) Ltd, Croydon, CR0 4YY

We operate a distinctive and ethical publishing philosophy in all
areas of our business, from our global network of authors to
production and worldwide distribution.

CONTENTS

Acknowledgements   vi
Introduction   1

Chapter One   10
Wells, Conduits and Cordial Waters: drinking water
sketches A.D. 43–1800
Chapter Two   34
Private Water and Public Health 1800–1858
Chapter Three   58
Philanthropic Fountains 1852–1875
Chapter Four   83
The Birth of Bacteriology and the Death of
Corporate Water 1866–1899
Chapter Five   105
ChloriNation 1905–1933
Chapter Six   122
Blitz on the Board 1937–1945
Chapter Seven   140
Purity and Poison 1948–1969
Chapter Eight   160
Maggie Thatcher, Jane Fonda and the
Water Cooler 1973–2000
Chapter Nine   196
Wasteland and Council Pop: tracking the
anti-bottled water zeitgeist 2010–11
Chapter Ten   233
21st Century Tap Water 2011–2012

Conclusions and Questions   262
Notes   292

Acknowledgements

Researching this book was possible because of the public learning resources in London that I had free access to and the skilled professionals who assisted me at those institutions. Above all, my thanks go to the staff at the City of London's London Metropolitan Archives where I must pay particular credit to Jane Muncaster, Jeremy Smith and Claire Titley for their sage advice, generously given on many occasions and their patience with numerous queries.

Sincere thanks are also due to The Authors' Foundation and its 2011 panel of assessors who granted me an award to buy some invaluable writing time. Their professional endorsement was a great vote of confidence that boosted me in the middle of this project.

Thanks also to Capital Radio for permission to quote from an interview with the former Metropolitan Water Board engineers Arthur Durling and George Graham.

For the contemporary chapters, my interviewees were extremely generous with their time and professional knowledge. Warm thanks is given, therefore, to Maria Andrews (formerly of Waste Watch), Megan Ashfield (Populous Architects), Ralph Baber and John E. Mills (The Drinking Fountain Association), Victor Callister (City of London Corporation), Professor Jeni Colbourne (Drinking Water Inspectorate), Kath Dalmeny, Christine Haigh and Jackie Schneider (Sustain), Michael Green (tapwater.org), Jenny Hall (formerly of the Museum of London), Guy Jeremiah (Aquatina/Find-A-Fountain), Jarno Stet (Westminster City Council), and Steve White (Thames Water). I am also appreciative of Cory Environmental Services for allowing me to visit its Materials Recovery Facility in Wandsworth and to the Veolia employees in Westminster who sifted the bins from Piccadilly Circus on my behalf.

Respondents to my call for drinking fountain memories were also very generous in their contributions, so many thanks to them and to the local history societies and colleagues in other organisations who took the time to disseminate my request.

I also want to thank Jakob Horstmann at Zed Books for his advice about publishing and Tariq Goddard of Zer0 Books for such an enthusiastic response to my initial proposal.

Friends have been more than generous with their queries about my progress, even when it was painfully slow, and offered much moral support and plenty of welcome distractions. In particular, my thanks go to Sue Baker, Katie Bradbury, Ally Branley, Kevin Brown, David Cross, Kirsty Cunningham, Rose Dawson, Katherine Davey, Alexandra and James Goddard, Julia Griffin, Helen Griffith, Ashley Kelly, Launa Kennet, James Kidd, Torsten Lange, Emma Reynolds, Dinah Roe, Mark Smith, Jason Vir, Julie Watson and Adam Wilkinson.

Eílish and Gerald Chapman (my much-loved in laws) have both been great sources of support. Thanks also to Dr Bruce Stewart, my learned stepfather, and my brother, Nick Stewart who have given me plenty of votes of confidence.

A very warm thanks is reserved for Declan Jones, my father, for his positive feedback on my initial chapter and his firm belief that I could complete the project. His comment that my writing is "muscular" still baffles me, but I accept it. Sigrid Castle, his partner, also offered generous encouragement.

Above all, there are three women without whose support I simply could not have written this book.

Dr Barbara Penner offered continuous encouragement and intellectual inspiration throughout my project. As an editor, her input was invaluable. I still have no idea how she squeezed in reading drafts of chapters and my manuscript whilst writing her own book (actually, two books!), lecturing and mothering, but I am indebted to her for giving me this time. Look out for her forthcoming book, an architectural history of the modern

Bathroom (Reaktion).

Sheila Geraghty, my mother, financially supported my first period of my research, which laid the foundation for the rest of the book to be built upon. For that material help, I am extremely fortunate and very grateful indeed. Her moral support throughout the project was unfaltering.

Grace Chapman, my partner, has been my emotional anchor. She has patiently listened to my various rants about drinking water over the last two and a half years, and occasionally now gets on the anti-bottled-water soapbox herself. Grace's comments on the content of early chapters were both sharply critical and encouraging but, most of all, I thank her for putting up with me during grumpy spells and a long period of meagre income on my part. My resourceful cooking skills possibly have something to do with her tolerance.

Introduction

Water should be treated as a social and cultural good, and not primarily as an economic good. The manner of the realisation of the right to water must also be sustainable, ensuring that the right can be realised for present and future generations.
(United Nations, 2002)[1]

In spring 2012, Londoners had reason to contemplate their tap water less absentmindedly than usual. Drought is an apocalyptic word. Fears about the official state of drought were muted by the measure to combat it. 'Hosepipe ban' has a cosy, suburban twang. This phrase reassures us that, although lawns might turn crispy brown, our drinking water source is not seriously threatened. Since 2007, London's water stress categorisation by the Environment Agency as 'serious' has not translated into a situation where essential water uses are curtailed. Not having drinking water on tap would be unimaginable in this leading world city.

Even if London's tap water supply was temporarily suspended, the city is well served with an alternative, equally reliable drinking water source. Bottled water flows into London, as steadily as the subterranean pipes through which more than two billion litres of premium treated tap water are pumped daily. There is one significant difference; a standard bottled water brand, such as Coca Cola's Schweppes Abbey Well (£1.60 for 500ml), is approximately 2462 times more expensive per litre than tap water (this figure is based on a metered supply).[2] Despite that price gulf, London luxuriates in a twin drinking water system for those who are able, and willing, to pay for both supplies. In the twenty-first century city, therefore, the spectre of prolonged thirst seems unlikely. This reality starkly contrasts with the estimated 780 million people elsewhere in the world who do not have access to a safe, reliable or affordable drinking water supply for their basic hydration or cooking needs.[3] Excessive drinking water choice in this developed world city is yet another example of how we have exceeded the limits of what we need to live well. As the recently updated, seminal, environmental polemic *Limits to Growth* asserts about unsustainable economic growth and modes of production, 'the world is in overshoot mode'.[4] Put simply, we consume and produce more than we need. My real question is how might we change this paradigm, at least for one essential product?

London's drinking water excess is inherently flawed, both environmentally and ethically. Environmentally, sufficient energy; human resources; materials and money are lavished on the treatment of raw water to produce tap water of a quality that both meets and way exceeds our needs. Tap water standards produce the same consumable whether it is poured into one's mouth or down one's toilet, or used to mix cement (for the latter example, apologies to those builders who strive to employ grey water technologies). In 2011, a desalination plant even joined Thames Water's arsenal to quench Londoners' thirst. It performs alchemy on the tidal reaches of the river to produce freshwater.

As we know, this resource is increasingly politicised, globally, in the context of climate change, but freshwater is also a pawn between competing economic ideologies and nations. Such machinations determine how water abstraction is licensed through land ownership, how the aquatic environment is managed, how water is distributed and at what cost. In the case of London, we must remember that the water we drink is a corporate product, mostly served up by Thames Water but also, on the outskirts of Greater London, by the multi-national Veolia, and two smaller concerns (Essex and Suffolk Water, Sutton and East Surrey Water). Reins on these corporations' freedoms exist in the form of the Environment Agency (abstraction and pollution), OFWAT (economic check) and the Drinking Water Inspectorate (product safety) but it is important to note at the outset of this book that the water industry was privatised in 1989, in England and Wales, as part of a particular economic and political ideology. Few would argue, as we will see, that there were not significant problems with the water, and wastewater, industry prior to privatisation. However, those challenges were outsourced.

Despite Thames Water's vast water resources, its move to desalination and its impressive coterie of water scientists (even if they are somewhat anonymous), Londoners seek alternative drinking water products and in extraordinary quantities.

Plastic bottles are mass produced, daily, in locations far away from London, filled with water siphoned from underground resources on private land, then transported vast distances to bring drinking water into the city. In quantity, annual bottled water sales for the whole of the UK tally with London's daily water consumption, as measured by Thames Water (the season does, of course, have an impact). These two billion litres of bottled water equate, however, with extraordinary levels of waste, most of which does not enter the recycling stream, fossil fuel consumption and personal financial waste. Why do the inhabitants of this leading developed world city need bottled water today?

Ethically, the commodification of drinking water for exorbitant profits is at odds with the landmark announcement in 2002 by the United Nations, of the human right to 'affordable' water, specifically for 'consumption, cooking, personal and domestic hygienic requirements' (more recently, the equal recognition of a right to sanitation has joined this revision of the International Covenant on Economic, Social and Cultural Rights).[5] In industrialised nations and cities such as London these basic water rights are largely fulfilled, except notably for the delivery of affordable hydration to public spaces. Of course, consumers have the right to choose whether or not they purchase bottled water but when affordable, or even free, drinking water access is not designed into the city outside our domestic environments, or deliberately designed out, that choice is limited.

Capital-sized gulps of the United Kingdom's bottled water habit are proportionately large due to obvious factors such as population, the capital's heat island effect and tourism, particularly in the summer months. Most of that gulping and sipping takes place outside private homes and outside buildings adequately served with kitchen sinks like places of work where they are obligatory, or drinking fountains in prisons and schools. In the case of the latter, these resources may have been hard fought for as additions to a school building from local council funds or often from charitable donations. Incredibly, drinking fountains are not compulsory in schools.

Bottled water is a convenience product. It provides easy access to fridge-chilled water and a portable package to transport around the city. When we are truly thirsty, little else will satisfy our craving than plain water. The simple craving for thirst relief, when the tap is out of reach, is one reason for London's steady demand for bottled water. Increased awareness about healthy eating also makes water a more culturally popular hydration choice than sugary carbonated drinks. Bottled water's advertising gurus have massaged the healthy hydration choice vigorously in their spin with much success. One international study of consumer attitudes towards bottled water revealed that the product is not necessarily perceived to be safer than tap water, but it is considered by consumers to be healthier and therefore more desirable as part of a lifestyle package.[6] This consumer view is not a new one in London.

Historically, connections between health and drinking water quality have played a significant role in the development of a market for bottled water. Roots of attitudes to, and mythology about, London's drinking water quality run deep, particularly in the fraught nineteenth-century public health debates. A hotly contested topic was whether cholera and typhoid were caused by the foul air, or 'miasma' (think clouds of faecal pollution) emanating from the Thames, or by drinking the river water itself. During that period, public and political imaginations alike dreamed of alternative water sources to the local Metropolitan offer. One grand engineering dream was to siphon supplies from the Welsh mountains in pipes spanning the breadth of the country. This hankering after non-urban and more 'natural' water is echoed by a contemporary penchant for drinking water that originates in the wilderness rather than the city. Evian, for instance, features alpine imagery on its labels to remind us of that water's fifteen-year percolation through the Alps. Of course, stringent scientific tests are performed on that product to ensure that nature has not poisoned it with unsafe levels of naturally occurring chemicals such as arsenic or fluoride. Advertisers have triumphed in focusing our attention on the desirable provenance of 'natural' bottled water, rather than making us think about how their products journeyed from pristine sources to our corner shops. Sell-by dates, stamped subtly on the necks of bottles, often state upwards of a year from their appearance on the shelf. Freshness is guaranteed, but this is clearly not the same as drinking from a cool mountain stream as much as the bottle's label might have us believe.

In comparison to London's generous flow of tap and bottled water, its third drinking water source is paltry.

Public drinking fountains are curiously uncommon, unlike office water coolers. Links between bottled water consumption and a lack of public tap water access surfaced, in the second half of the Millennium's first decade, as a subject of environmentalist and urban management debates about how to reduce levels of plastic waste. A tentative fountain renaissance has been stimulated in some quarters as a result. However, the general absence of these amenities as a common feature of a global city, of London's stature, begs questions about how drinking water access is controlled and managed. How might free public water be offered in a country where the water industry itself has been privatised? Who should bear responsibility for its provision?

The control of urban water supply is an instrument of great power and wealth that evolved with Britain's industrialisation and imperial expansion. London's domestic water pipes were laid by many private corporations and remained in their ownership until 1902.

In Matthew Gandy's account of the role of water engineering and supply in lubricating New York's economic and geographical growth, he asserts: 'The history of cities can be read as a history of water.'[7] Many readings of London's rich, convoluted and controversial water history exist. This book does not aim to retell those civil engineering narratives, which thoroughly document the evolution of how London's water supply is managed and distributed. By amending Gandy's statement slightly to 'the history of cities can be read a history of *drinking* water', we have a finer sieve through which to filter and extract a more specific history of London's water. This both simplifies and complicates the water picture. By inserting drinking before the more generic subject of freshwater, some subjects connected with water appear in a more specific light and other subjects must also be included. Architecture, culture, economics, environmentalism, law, medicine, politics, even religion, and science all have a bearing on this story. As the medical historian Anne Hardy noted about English water histories: 'Although various accounts of the history of water technology, and learned articles on the political and administrative aspects of water supply have been written, the history of water in relation to public health remains largely unexplored.'[8] Benefitting from Hardy's own response to this dearth of research and building on some of her discoveries about the eighteenth and nineteenth centuries, my focus on drinking water places the body, human health and the consumer in the foreground of this tale.

Whether we see drinking water as a commodity or a utility or a basic human right, understanding its nuanced history is vital for informing decisions about how future cities might benefit from referencing lessons of the past. Two scholars of London's nineteenth century water consumer politics, Frank Trentmann and Vanessa Taylor, frame their research in this way: 'Water continues to bring together long-standing issues of citizenship, social exclusion, consumer education and human development alongside more recent concerns about sustainability. Historians and social scientists would do well to reintegrate ordinary goods like water into the study of consumer society.'[9] Considering that 'ordinary' good more specifically as *drinking* water raises some questions more prominently than others. When did concerns about water quality for human consumption first arise in London and how have they altered? Is there any truth in the urban myth that eighteenth and nineteenth century Londoners, even children, consciously chose to drink alcohol instead of water because they believed it to be contaminated? When did packaged water first appear as a product? What caused the bottled water market to grow so dramatically in the 1980s?

Answering these questions would have been impossible without the ground laid by many excellent scholars. In addition to urban water researchers, such as Matthew Gandy, Anne Hardy, Vanessa Taylor and Frank Trentmann, I would particularly cite the social historian John Burnett's chapter on drinking water in his book *Liquid Pleasures*, published in 1999, as an invaluable reference. As he notes 'water remains the principle liquid drunk in Britain', reminding us how physiologically central the substance is to our daily lives.[10] As we know, water forms a large percentage of our matter, a constituent of our very cells, our blood and our vital organs. We can get it from fruit and vegetables and yet we often crave this vital liquid as a sole substance of nourishment.

This story expands on aspects of Britain's drinking water

history that Burnett illuminates in *Liquid Pleasures*, using London as a further anchor to see how the city shapes our relationship with using, and demanding, pure water refreshment.

As an architectural historian employing my drinking water sieve to trawl London's modern history, I want to find out more about how urban spaces were produced in relation to water access, how they were used, how they were experienced and how they have changed over time. This spatial question — private, public and other — is a neglected facet of most existing London water histories. Everyday demands for water in the city have greatly shaped the design, use and experience of our built environment. Built objects and material products such as conduits, pipes, water coolers and sites of water treatment plants can be highly significant in what they tell us about drinking water's role in our culture and society. Consider, for instance, the curious nineteenth century fountains that pockmark London, with their desiccated pipes and litter-filled bowls. Why were they built and for whose use? What caused them to fall into disrepair? And how does the contemporary privatisation and commercialisation of the public realm affect the production of similar civic amenities?

To pursue this new, spatial history of London's drinking water, I have conducted extensive, original primary research. My trawls through London's water-related archives, coupled with voices from some essential scholarly and literary secondary sources have produced the story that follows. That story continued to evolve as this book was being edited. Early in 2012, I talked to protestors from the Occupy movement who confirmed that their drinking water sources were twofold. The first was bottled water donated by visitors to the camp. The second was the loads hand-carted by activists from the City of London's sleek new drinking fountain; an amenity inaugurated in 2010 as the Square Mile's own civic challenge to corporate greed and unsustainable modes of production.

Our tale starts very close to that fountain's location, a few metres below ground, in the remains of Londinium.

Chapter One

Wells, Conduits and Cordial Waters: drinking water sketches A.D. 43–1800

*Your Petitioners doe humbly desire, for that there is great defect
of water, in the said conduits: and that it is a generall grieuance,
to the whole City...*
(Water-Tankerd-Bearers, Citie of London, 1621)[1]

From the Roman City and throughout the incremental introduction of piped domestic water from the late sixteenth until the
mid-nineteenth century, most Londoners' water depended on
vast quantities of daily labour, either expended by them or by
others on their behalf. This chapter draws a historical map of
some of the urban spaces tied closely to water access and traces
when and where the issue of water quality arose. Traversing this
expansive historical terrain, we will briefly dip into larger
subjects, such as the early mineral water market and spa culture,
which other researchers have documented in depth. My aim now
is to set the drinking water scene in pre-modern, early modern
and eighteenth century London. From here, some of the key
themes in the city's modern drinking water story begin to ripple
out.

Londinium

Early Britons' settlements on the river Thames pre-dated the
foundation of the Roman city. This riparian, or riverside,
community had no shortage of running water at its disposal. And
below the ground, former waterholes contain material evidence
of a spiritual culture. Vessels recovered from these underground
pits, dated as early as 1500 B.C. are believed to have been
offerings to the 'netherworld of spirits'.[2] Remnants of decayed

food, tools and weapons found within the watery subsoil played a symbolic role in this community's culture. After A.D. 50, pre-Christian forms of water worship persisted as Roman beliefs mingled with these pagan practices. For the Mediterranean inhabitants of Londinium, some may have viewed the Thames simply as a conduit to the mythological River Styx, a realm of the Gods. For instance, remains of the upper body of a marble sculpture of a male, from circa A.D. 150, are thought to represent a water god who inhabited the liminal space of the river, hovering between life and death.[3] Water's spiritual associations did not, however, displace its practical role in daily life. Plumbing was an important characteristic of Roman civilisation.

Geographically and geologically, ancient London was by no means parched. The Thames was naturally important for transportation; however the tidal river was not a likely freshwater source. Underground water supplies (aquifers) served that need, as well as two other rivers (surface water).[4] Unlike other Roman cities, renowned for their hydro-geological engineering feats; Londinium had no need for aqueducts. The contents of the Chalk, London's vast groundwater source, lay just metres below layers of brick earth, sand and gravel sitting above the impermeable London Clay. Within hours of digging, a task most likely performed by a slave, the water swilling underfoot added to resources from the Fleet and Walbrook rivers. The contours of the city's two hills also meant that, in places, water rose very close to the surface.

Londinium was the only urban centre in Roman Britain with a watercourse running through its city centre, the Walbrook.[5] On a recently revised map of Londinium (by the Museum of London), the Walbrook river and many tributary streams can be seen snaking under the ancient city's walls and between the amphitheatre and the basilica, with the Temple of Mithras situated on its banks just before the river flows into the Thames (near modern-day London Bridge). Archaeologists are certain that Londinium's urban designers were more than aware of the hydrological wonder underground and recent discoveries endorse their view.[6] However saturated the ancient city might have been, were its inhabitants really water drinkers?

Vitruvius, a Roman architect, is the first recorded architectural critic and theorist in the west. He promoted water's centrality to a high standard of living. In fact, he dedicated an entire chapter to the substance in his famous architectural treatise: *Ten Books on Architecture* (circa 20–30 B.C.). Even though Vitruvius wrote long before Londinium was founded and he wrote in balmier Mediterranean climes and drier landscapes than northern Europe, it is thanks to him that we have clear evidence that in Roman culture water use was not confined to the indulgent bathing practices of a leisured elite. They were definitely drinking water.

According to Vitruvius, water was not only consumed as a wine-diluter to keep Bacchus at bay, it was also consumed neat: 'Water, offering endless necessities as well as drink, offers services all the more gratifying because they are gratis' (his interpreters clearly enjoyed his intended pun).[7] For Vitruvius, not all water was equal. He believed that the rainfall of stormy weather was particularly vital as a liquid. The architect's writing offers strong evidence of Roman cultural beliefs that water was a substance of purity and health because of its ability to cleanse the inaccessible inner landscape of the body. Ingesting healthful waters, according to Vitruvius, could even cure defective internal organs. And Athenians apparently distinguished between the water sources from which its citizens could safely drink, and those for external functions such as washing.

Ancient springs were not always thought to be pure and nature's raw bounty was recognised as both blessed and cursed. Environmental pollution caused by poisonous metals such as gold, silver, iron, copper and lead were known to seep into water supplies in certain geological areas. One Persian spring was even reputed to have caused its drinkers' teeth to fall out.[8] Drinking water also had pleasurable associations for Vitruvius. Some springs were thought to make people drunk 'even without wine', whilst other sources were renowned for exciting erotic arousal.[9] Whatever its effect, Vitruvius' sommelier-like description of water endowed the liquid with a flavour spectrum ranging from a touch on the bitter to the outright delicious.

High Street Wells

One beverage that was certainly consumed in the Roman City of London, and in no mean measure, was wine. Barrels were shipped up the Thames' estuary from Germany and Spain, in vast quantities. Those barrels provided the materials for the construction of one system of wells (a second type had square shafts lined with timber). Once the wine had been quaffed, re-using the barrels involved removing their tops and bottoms so that the tightly bound strips of curved wood could be employed to reinforce the earthen walls of the well-holes reaching down into underground sources.[10] Remnants of this system are preserved in the Museum of London, including fragments of a ladder used for descending into these watery shafts. One can easily imagine the staccato rhythms of bodies disappearing and reappearing from a cluster of eighteen wells, near contemporary Queen Victoria Street (it adjoins Mansion House tube station with Blackfriars bridge).[11] Although most of Londinium's wells are thought to have been associated with individual buildings, this cluster formed a definite centre for communal water access. Queues and jostling may also have occurred at this cluster and, no doubt, gruelling journeys with water vessels from the source to homes and places of work. Remains of plumbing infra-structure near some wells also suggest the conduction of fresh-water supplies direct to local buildings. Pipes were constructed from different materials to visually distinguish the flow of fresh, inbound water and used outbound water from the city, with impressive sanitary nous.[12]

Wells were not all used in the service of the greater civic good. Some wells were entirely private and relate directly to the social inequalities embedded in Roman civilisation. Location was everything. The labour cost, in terms of time and energy, for those who had to transport their water from the public source to the point of use can only be imagined. As the classical historian Peter Marsden summarises: 'There were three classes of people in Londinium apart from Roman citizens; the free, the freed and the slaves. The native Britons, who were free but had none of the special rights of a Roman citizen, were known as the Peregreni.'[13] The Peregreni were essentially Londinium's working class.

These inhabitants' daily lives forged a very inner-city experience. They lived in tightly packed timber-frame 'Mediterranean style' houses. At Londinium's height between A.D. 100 to 200, many of the city's population — anywhere from circa 24,000 to 45,000 people — were working iron and leather for a living.[14] This industrial activity was concentrated in the north of the city, close to modern-day Moorgate, on the banks of the Walbrook. Waste from this industry saw vast quantities of materials, such as iron slag and the by-products of tanning, entering the watercourse. Downstream of the tanners and ironmongers, the Walbrook's contents would not have been appetising to dip into, no matter how dehydrated those workers were. Archaeologists have deduced that the underground water-fed wells, constructed a few metres away from the Walbrook, were an important source of drinking water. It seems plausible to imagine that they provided refreshment for these workers and for local residents own freshwater needs (both cooking and drinking).

Whilst the Romans and the Peregreni were in the bacterio-logical dark, we know from Vitruvius's writing that the corre-lation between illness and the consumption of polluted water was understood on some level: 'Deadly types of water can also be found; these, coursing through harmful sap in the earth, acquire a poisonous force in themselves.'[15]

Aqua Superior

Remains of a high-tech well in Londinium, one of two unique to Roman Britain in the city, suggest that effectively filtered water was pumped out of the earth close to the amphitheatre on Gresham Street.[16] Although the engineering ingenuity of this 'water-lifting mechanism' sank to a similar depth to the crude 'barrel' wells, a great quantity and quality of water could be guaranteed thanks to slave labour. Operated by a chain-and-bucket system from above ground, this water would not be muddied by the boots of a person climbing down into the well shaft for instance.[17]

Only discovered in 1988, today one can roam around the amphitheatre's ruins below the Guildhall Yard. Up to 6,000 spectators could be found here baying for blood at gladiatorial spectacles, or participating in less gory religious activities.[18] Either pursuit equalled the production of lots of thirsty spectators. Calculations show that the mechanical wells would have produced two litres of water per second, or seventy-two thousand litres over a ten-hour period. Though the technology's chain-and-bucket system has been praised for its early engineering ingenuity, it has also been noted that constant slave or animal energy was needed to turn its vast wheels.[19] How much of this water was for drinking only cannot be known for certain. For instance, there was a bathhouse just south of Gresham Street that also needed a water supply, but evidence suggests the bathhouse was actually served by cisterns that drew directly from the underground supply.[20] However, a design to extract water at a point of naturally high filtration through sand filtration suggests the organisation of the resource into hierarchies of quality for different uses and users. Possibly, the best drinking water in Londinium was reserved for those in the best seats in the amphitheatre. Labour was essential to the production of both that high quality commodity and water drawn from less high-tech wells. Although Vitruvius wrote that water was gratis, this human cost of hydration was evident in this northern outpost of the Roman Empire.

No association has been made between Londinium's decline and waterborne disease. But decline it did. The ancient city is believed to have been uninhabited after the gradual ebb of Roman occupation, circa A.D. 450, until the first Christian Saxon settlers arrived in the early 600s.[21] During that interlude, dust settled over grand villas and wells alike.

Middle Ages

In that transition period, some minor evidence of early-Saxon presence in the former city has been detected — such as a lost brooch — but these traces were scattered by transient people.[22] New foundation stones were only laid once more when Christian London became the seat of an archbishop in the seventh century. Evidence that water drinking was a common practice beyond London came in the form of bronze cups suspended from posts alongside springs on the 'highway'.[23] These cups were gifts from King Edwin of Northumbria, permitting the traveller to enjoy raw water supplies freely.

Saxons reoccupied London in the sixth century as Britain's new religious culture deepened.[24] St Paul's Cathedral was founded in A.D.604 and during the eighth and ninth-centuries Christian beliefs were further inscribed in churches of a more modest scale inside the boundaries marked by the old Roman walls. Extramurally, Westminster was defined as a community in A.D. 785 for 'the needy people of God' and an order of Benedictine monks settled under the watch of St Dunstan, Bishop of London, in A.D. 960.[25] When Westminster Abbey was completed in A.D. 1065, rudimentary plumbing conducted water for the ritualistic washing practices of the Benedictines. Remains of a tap excavated from the original site are believed to originate from a 'water-filtering system'.[26] No doubt general matter such as leaves and insects had to be strained away, but it is possible that water for cooking and drinking was also treated to some aesthetically superior version of the raw good.

Back inside the walled city, citizens of the City of London were granted a charter outlining their rights under William the Conqueror's administration in 1066. During that century, the only hard water evidence of note in the Museum of London are water-collecting buckets dated from the Norman period, suggesting that new wells had been sunk or rediscovered. By 1215 a government for the Square Mile, with a Mayor and an elected Corporation was in place.[27] Extramurally, parish ward boundaries, such as St Martin-in-the-Fields and St Dunstan, were drawn up during the late tenth and early eleventh centuries. By the end of the twelfth century, Christian London's population was estimated at between 20,000 and 25,000 people, making it the most populous, and wealthiest, city in England.[28]

Twelfth century author William Fitz Stephen wrote of social life at 'special wels in the Suburbs, sweete, wholesome and cleare, amongst which Holywell, Clarkes wel and Clements well, are most famous and frequented by Scholers and youthes of the Citie in sommer evenings, when they walk forth to take the aire'.[29] Two of these wells related to locations of important nunneries founded in this century. Holywell was the site of a major nunnery and Clarkes well was situated just outside the walls of St Mary Clerkenwell, which was founded in 1144 on ten acres of land.[30] Fitz Stephen's reference to the taste of these waters confirms that they were drinking sources. Imbibing 'holy' water was part of Christian culture of this period, in which some wells were associated with the cult of the saints and miracle cures, many with pagan origins. The historian Alexandra Walsham describes how the grounds surrounding certain wells 'became littered with crutches left behind by grateful pilgrims', who presumably believed that they had been cured.[31] External and internal uses of such waters were considered to be equally therapeutic, depending on the ailment.[32]

Fitz Stephen's categorisation of the suburban wells as 'special' suggests that other un-holy wells related to ordinary water uses such as mere thirst relief or cooking. Within the City walls, the supply of ordinary, but sufficient, high quality, freshwater became a quest in the thirteenth century.

Conducting sweete water

Evidence suggests that the plans to convey water from Tybourne 'for the profite of the Citty' began as early as 1236 with donations from 'Marchant Strangers of Cities beyond the Seas'.[33] According to William Fitz Stephen, the City's increasing populace 'were forced to seek sweete waters abroad'.[34] Significantly in this quote, the water's quality ranking as 'sweete' obviously suggests its relationship to human consumption. The project he was referring to resulted in the construction of the City of London's first 'conduit'.

One interpretation of this early form of water engineering, provided by the London water historian H.W. Dickinson, is that the idea for a conduit was inspired by monastic water supplies.[35]

Tybourne was a village in Middlesex, named after the tributary of the Thames on which it was situated near contemporary Marble Arch, some four and a half miles to the west of London. The ambitious project of transporting water from the Tybourne to the City was not completed until 1285, almost fifty years after the donations had been gathered. Lead pipes, also referred to as 'rods', fed the water underground by gravity from the rural west to the urban east. Archaeologists discovered a section of pipe that was destined for the City's conduit two meters underground, with a diameter of almost ten centimetres.[36] Four hundred and eighty-four of these rods were reportedly involved in this ambitious civil engineering enterprise. The early road works must have been quite a labouring and logistical feat (no doubt plenty of medieval travellers were inconvenienced as their thoroughfares were temporarily dug up).[37] Eventually, the receiving 'conduit' for the water rods was built at the junction of Bucklesbury, Cheapside and Poultry, at the heart of the medieval marketplace for food.[38]

The water-engineering historian Hugh Barty-King explains that conduits were simply based on the diversion of an existing watercourse and the employment of gravity. Conduit 'houses' received the diverted water. They consisted of 'a large tank of lead or stone into which the water poured itself, and out of which, by a free-flowing spout or a controllable tap, it poured into a stone basin below'.[39] Architecturally, conduit houses could be modest or monumental.

Cheapside Conduit was the latter. It was a major new civic landmark, as well as a practical resource. The archaeological discovery of the 'long rectangular building' gives us this view of what it consisted of and how the building was used: 'The vault of this building was still intact and the carved greensand quoins and doorway survived at the eastern end. This led to a staircase which would have exited up to the medieval street. Londoners descended into the building to collect their water before climbing the stairs back to street level.'[40] Though there was a practical need to cover the water tank, the scale of the conduit exceeded this function. This excessive mass ensured that the civic and charitable goodwill that had paid for the freshwater bounty could be publicly appreciated.

Did the new water source add to the area's growth and defin-ition as a market and commercial centre? Clearly the quantity of the water was a motivating factor for channelling water in this way, but there is compelling evidence that the quality of this rural water was perceived to be different, 'sweete', and therefore used for specific, dietary-related purposes. John Stow's seminal early-modern urban study, *A Survey of London* (1603), includes this record of the Cheapside Conduit's intended role in medieval water supply: '...for the poore to drinke, and the rich to dresse their meate'.[41] Clearly, the water was considered to be of a dietary quality, though we are left wondering whether the poor drank it only because they could afford no other beverage. One interpretation is that the water was free and publicly available to those on the street, or possibly even to those without a permanent home. However, as we now know, neither the lead leaching from the pipes or the conduit's building materials were good things for human health.

London grew further in the 1300s, with the population doubling by 1340.[42] Perhaps the greater mass of competitors for high quality water was one motivating factor for the Corporation's installation of a Conduit Warden at Cheapside in 1325.[43] Queues for water were likely to be more boisterous than when the Conduits staircase was first used for water seekers forty years previously. There is evidence that the queues were not always socially harmonious. During the 1330s, one group of regular conduit users was criticised because 'the water aforesaid was now so wasted by brewers, and persons keeping brewhouses, and making malt, that in these modern times it will no longer siffice for the rich and middling, or for the poor, to the common loss of the whole community'.[44] The use of water from the conduit to make ale or malt was subsequently banned.

Indoors, medieval Londoners could draw their water from chalk-lined wells within modest houses.[45] Coupled with resourceful home-made guttering devices for rainwater harvesting — sometimes causing neighbourly disputes when they flooded adjacent properties — we know that the conduit was not the only water on offer for washing bodies, or clothes, but were these domestic sources considered to be good enough to cook with or drink?[46] It is hard to know for certain, but they were definitely more readily accessible than the water from the city centre conduit, which could not serve residents living extramu-

rally. So, the Great Conduit, as Cheapside became known, potentially served a number of practical functions including hydration
for those working outdoors, or passing through London
temporarily, and a high quality raw material in the centre of food
production from a source untouched by urban pollution. The
conduit was obviously considered to be successful, or indeed
necessary, as the device was replicated elsewhere the following
century.

'A lusty place, a place of all delytys...'[47]

Just west of Cheapside, lay the other main strip in the medieval
City. On Cornhill, the 'tonne' was adapted into a cistern in 1401,
whilst retaining its penal use on the upper storey of the
structure. On top, rogue bakers, nightwalkers and other 'suspicious persons' could be seen incarcerated in stocks.[48] Conduits
transcended from functional to festive as state pageants or
religious celebrations related to these central features of urban
life. During a 1421 pageant, King Henry the Fifth's wife,
Catherine of Valois, was greeted with high theatricality at the
little Conduit by 'giants of a huge stature ingeniously
constructed to bow at the right moment, lions which could roll
their eyes and...bands of singing girls'.[49] The same account also
recorded how the conduits flowed with wine instead of water
during the pageant.

John Stow, who recorded the rise of conduits before and
during his lifetime, reflected on the disappearance of the natural
environment under the increasingly built-up City and extra-
mural neighbourhoods. He wrote of the demise of the Walbrooke
Stream for instance: 'This water course hauing diuerse bridges,
was afterwards vaulted ouer with bricke, and paued leuell with
the Streetes and Lanes where through it passed, and since that
also houses have beene builded thereon, so that the course of
Walbrooke is now hidden vnder ground, and thereby hardly
knowne.'[50] As water within London submerged from view, Stow

recorded donations for new conduits rising steadily from the late-fifteenth century at the start of the Tudor period and into the Elizabethan period, up until the mid-sixteenth century. Celebrations aside, for many of the City's workforce and residents, the conduits were associated with the gruelling physical task of transporting water. As the historian Mark Jenner has asserted of early modern London (spanning 1500–1725): '…for most households the cost of water lay in the hours spent fetching it…'[51] Energy and time could be displaced, if a household could afford to pay some other body to expend that labour on its behalf.

Collecting water from the conduits created an economy and an official workforce of water-bearers, answerable to the City's Corporation. After 1543, when the City was granted the right 'to exploit all large springs within a five-mile radius' to boost conduit resources, the quantity of work for the water bearers was also boosted and their role in urban water collection provided a much-needed employment opportunity for those teetering on the lower rungs of London's economic ladder.[52] A water bearer appeared as a minor character in Ben Johnson's 1598 play *Every Man In His Humour* in which he was clearly shown to be of a low social rank.[53] Water bearers served wealthy households as dedicated individual servants, or as teams employed by larger companies or institutions. Though water as a raw substance remained free, its transportation to the point of use elicited a charge. Quantity was controlled by the regulated size of tankards that the water bearers had to use. Those standardised tankards bobbing through the Elizabethan street throng, on the shoulders or heads of their carriers, was surely a common sight in early modern London. What exactly the water was used for when it passed from conduit to client is more difficult to ascertain. If the conduits' bounty did indeed remain 'sweete and wholesome' as was intended, then the likelihood of its ingestion is certainly a greater possibility.

We know that people drank at least some pure water in the sixteenth century, because during the Reformation, supping from 'holy' wells was banned as a Catholic practice.[54] The custom, which had continued from medieval times, became associated with anti-Protestant forms of worship such as idolatry, deifying nature and saints as opposed to one God.[55] Waters curative powers were seriously questioned as part of the Reformation's religious revolution. Then in 1542, this time from a secular perspective, more doubt was cast on water's valuable properties. Andrew Boorde, the Duke of Norfolk's physician proclaimed that 'water is not holsome by it selfe for an Englysheman…water is colde, slow and slake of digestion'.[56] Boorde's health 'regyment' also discussed the importance of the use of particular water for dressing meat and baking. He was emphatic that such water must be from a running, rather than a stagnant, source and that for the best results he advised that inferior water should be strained 'through a thick linen cloth'.[57] Boorde seemed to eye the contents of wells with suspicion. Were they stagnant?

By the Elizabethan period, post-Reformation, parish wells had a strong civic function as local domestic water sources and were maintained under the watch of church committees (church vestries became formal governing bodies for parishes from the mid-sixteenth century).[58] The well sources were possibly considered to be inferior to 'rural' grade water from the conduits, as they was not associated with the labour of water bearers. How preoccupied Londoners were with that quality distinction is difficult to know, though no doubt evidence exists somewhere. Mark Jenner has recorded the switch from well to pump as taking place gradually between the early sixteenth to seventeenth centuries.[59] As that low-grade technology evolved, a far more ambitious mode of water supply was also in development.

'A most artificial forcier'[60]

Advances in water engineering were moving beyond the

conduits' gravitational system to the use of wheel-based technologies. Now, water could be transported from a lower gradient to the required point of use, particularly when using the new technology in tandem with the natural power of a tidal river.

The engineer Peter Morris was to push the notion of a convenient water supply into completely new territory. Morris, sometimes appearing as Marsh or Maurice in different historical records, had a nationality as uncertain as his surname. Whether he was Dutch, German or English — all of which have been proposed —the land drainage engineer saw an opportunity to exploit new urban water demand with a massive resource that was currently untapped; the Thames. By the 1570s Morris convinced the Corporation of the City to co-invest in a large-scale experimental waterworks scheme to pump from the river at London Bridge. When construction ran behind schedule, officials were reluctant to part with the second half of the finance but luckily for the entrepreneur, he happened to be in the service of the Lord Chancellor, who had a direct line to Queen Elizabeth I. A state hearing of Morris' predicament, in 1580, concluded that the City Corporation was unfairly withholding monies when the engineer had also personally risked large sums.[61] The next year Morris was granted a 500-year lease for the arch under London Bridge where his giant waterwheel was eventually constructed.[62]

By 1585, water was being pumped from Morris's wheel-based technology directly into the houses of paying clients; London Bridge Waterworks was in business. It was the first mechanically transported water to enter private houses in the capital. The only limitation of the new convenience was the distance that the waterwheel could propel water, so customers had to be resident in the near vicinity of the Thames, and naturally with sufficient income, to enjoy this luxurious supply. John Stow's praise for Morris' enterprise seemed somewhat muted, describing it merely as 'Thames water conueyed into mens houses by pipes of leade from a most artificial forcier'.[63]

London's social stratification of water access had certainly entered a new phase, but what is known of its consumption and use? Though Morris did specify that his machinery was pumping water from the bottom of the river, it is unlikely that the contents of the Thames was considered to be palatable for cooking with or for drinking neat. Also, as he was extracting water from the tidal part of Thames it would have had some measure of salinity. Perhaps his engineers worked with the tides to reduce the salt content? Still, its use for bathing is plausible. Perhaps even a degree of salinity was embraced for that purpose. It could also have been used as a laundry resource, but it is unlikely that river water was consumed as a beverage. Naturally, the river was a dumping ground for all manner of waste and a busy shipping highway but the idea of using it as a source for pressurised piped water had caught on. Bevis Bulmer installed his pumps in 1593 at Broken Wharf, a little further upstream.[64] For wealthy house-holders, pumped water could be used for one set of functions in abundance, whilst water bearers could still be dispatched to fetch superior water from conduits for 'sweeter' water needs.

Morris's civil engineering innovation would become normalised as the convenience and profitability of water's private supply was demonstrated. The next private water entre-preneur borrowed a bit from Morris and mixed it with a dash of the first conduit philosophy, producing convenient domestic water on tap, but of a purer quality and salt free. Work on the New River's construction commenced in 1606.[65]

The New River was a man-made channel conducting water from underground springs in the Hertfordshire countryside north of London to Islington in the expanding suburbs. After many years of development, with funding from City goldsmith Hugh Myddleton, its opening festivities took place in 1613.[66] A statue of the entrepreneur still graces the junction of Upper Street and Essex Road in Islington and a Georgian square is named after him. The New River charter protected the water quality, from which no doubt its profitability could be assured: 'No person to cast into the rover any earth, carrion, nor wash clothes or annoyeth the current, nor convey any sink into the same or lay any pipe to draw off the water, nor dig any ditch, pond, pitt or trench nor plant tress within 5 yards of the river.'[67] If these terms were monitored and upheld, one can imagine that the notion of drinking from this pure new water source might have been entertained more readily than the Thames. Piped, corporate supplies' introduction was followed by more illicit forms of water extraction, which were not appreciated by the London's community of water bearers.

Quills

Undercover, unsanctioned tapping of pipes feeding the conduits was a form of private water supply that mimicked the premise of the new corporate water, but the big difference was that its users had no bill to pay, or a 'fine' as the New River's charge was called.[68] In 1621 the water-bearer 'brotherhood' presented a petition to Parliament, protesting that the appropriation of conduit water for private use was affecting their business, because 'most of the said water is taken, and kept from the said Conduits in London, by many priuate branches and Cockes, cut and taken out of the pipes, which are layed to conuey the same and laid into priuate houses and dwellings, both without and within the City...and many times suffered to runne at waste, to the generall grieuance of all good Citizens'.[69] The brotherhood's frustration was understandable. Some quills tapping the conduit supplies were blatantly illegal, whilst others were sanctioned for the supply of some influential householders, by the Corporation itself.[70] Quoting the law governing the management and use of the conduits, the water bearers believed that this private appropriation of public supply contravened the statute book. In particular, they pointed a collective finger at a plumber on the City's payroll, one Mr Randoll who, 'out of fifteen branches running into private houses' had apparently confessed to laying three of them personally.[71] It sounded as if some palms may have been well greased to extract such favours. Corrupt water siphoning was not the water bearers only problem. Their 'brotherhood' was also unsettled by the arrival of rogue bearers onto London's water scene. They claimed that these imposters were serving single institutions, such as Newgate Prison, and therefore unevenly draining the supplies of certain conduits.

Such petty disputes were eclipsed by the devastation caused by the Great Fire of London in 1666, in which 13,200 homes were decimated. Casualties of London's water infrastructure in the

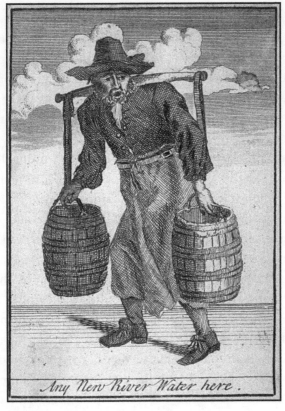

Fresh water seller, ca. 1688. Marcellus Laroon (1653–1702) City of London, London Metropolitan Archives.

1666 fire included Peter Morris's wooden waterwheel and the Great Cheapside Conduit's structure was also gutted. Like all professions, the water bearers and their dependents — a community of four thousand people in total – must have experienced the effects of the fire's devastation on London's social as well as its built fabric. Reconstruction of London Bridge Waterworks soon began and Cheapside was also rebuilt in some form. The illicit practice of quill-laying also resumed. In 1677 Thomas Duncomb swore in an affidavit to the Corporation of the City of London that he did 'dig a trench in the night time' to divert a supply from Lamb's Conduit to a publican's brewhouse.[72]

By 1698, some tensions between the conduit and piped water systems were apparent in a petition issued by Cheapside's residents and water-bearers to the City of London Corporation. The residents claimed that they were in 'great distress for want of water because several of them have their kitchens two and three pairs of stairs high, which is beyond the power of the New River or Thames Water men to raise their water so high'.[73] And the water bearers claimed that if any water was available at the Cheapside Conduit, they could earn a wage and serve the needs of those whom the private water companies were failing. This tension characterised how public and commercial water supplies rubbed against each other in early modern London. Mark Jenner points out how the new water corporations 'individuated and privatised households, reducing their involvement in the hurly-burly of the public water sources, but they were also the first network technologies, binding thousands of households into a common system'.[74]

These shifts in the equality of water access in London had a contemporary resonance with the influential political theories of John Locke. In his *Second Treatise on Civil Government* in 1690, Locke argued that what had been produced by the 'spontaneous hand of nature' was altered when it was mixed with labour.[75] As he elaborated: '...though the water running in the fountain be every one's, yet who can doubt that in the pitcher is his only who drew it out? His labour hath taken out of the hands of Nature where it was common.'[76] Certainly evidence suggests that the conduits' contents were prized on the basis of a quality cooking and drinking product, so in their case labour mixed with the value of a particular grade of water. Maintaining the infra-structure that assured the continual flow of high quality water contributed to its cost as a civic water source.

Cordial and Healthful Waters

From a drinking water perspective specifically, by the end of the seventeenth century an elite commodity entered English culture. The social historian Phyllis Hembry charts how the fashion for hot mineral water bathing enjoyed by Elizabeth I, escalated into the health-related Grand Tour. This activity grew in popularity amongst the gentry between 1585 and 1659. As the historian Alexandra Walsham has argued, the Reformation's suppression of the association between water and healing did not last for long and both the church and the state participated in the culture of reviving a therapeutic water culture.[77] Endorsed by medical men for internal as well as external physical benefits, drinking spa water became a fashionable, healthy habit. Back in England, Hembry explains how in the early sixteenth century a 'shortage of places for bathing led to a movement for drinking cold mineral water'.[78] Bath's famous Pump Room, for instance, started trading drinking water cures in 1706, though its water was thermal.[79] Bottled, English spa waters soon emerged as a new product that could be supped remotely from the spa.

London's coffee houses, well established as centres for social and political discourse by the early eighteenth century, presented themselves as ideal shop fronts for purveyors of bottled water. A roaring trade in both English and Continental spa waters was in motion by the 1730s.[80] Hembry's research mapped London as the centre of bottled water demand. A dozen bottles of mineral water from Bath could be purchased for 7s.6d. (approximately £30, or £2.50 a bottle in modern currency).[81] This new market was clearly highly profitable, so it is not surprising that many miraculously healthy springs were 'discovered' around London later in the century by wily entrepreneurs. Public ownership of natural water sources was fast becoming a quaint old idea.

A whole host of popular entertainment developed around London's own 'spas', for which season tickets could be purchased.[82] Spring water could be enjoyed at the spas themselves but products such as the Hampstead Flask ensured that healthy waters could also be enjoyed remotely from the spas for thruppence (or about £1 today).[83] As Georgian culture segued into the aesthetics of the Regency period, spas morphed into 'pleasure gardens'. Though water drinking was the rasion d'être of these leisurely places, they were by no means alcohol free. Drinking water alone would not have occasioned such festivities for which the London 'Spaws' became renowned. New tastes in alcohol were also being explored.

Eliza Smith's renowned cookbook *The Compleat Housewife*, first published in 1729, contained a panoply of recipes involved, or based on, water. The growth in the popularity of distillation meant that a whole host of 'cordial' waters could be brewed at home. Smith listed recipes galore to cure all manner of ailments, including giddiness of the head and revival from near-death. Her medicinal recipes' ingredients reveal their high alcohol content. Smith's instructions for brewing 'lemon wine', which could pass for 'citron water' if a disguise was required, included a generous two quarts of brandy.[84] 'Plague water' was also infused with a gallon of white wine. As homemade medicines, which were commonly administered by women in the seventeenth and, well into, the eighteenth century,[85] some of the cordial waters were intended as cures for serious maladies such as breast cancer, or to aid labour during stillbirths.[86] Despite the amount of alcohol in the concoctions, Smith specified that spring water should be used as a base. Her specification fitted with the fashion for taking mineral water as a healthy remedy and shows how drinking water's value as a commodity was increasingly tied to its provenance. Spring water consumption by the gentle-womanly and middle class readers of *The Compleat Housewife* was part and parcel of the material comfort their classes enjoyed, but it sounds like a small bottle could have gone a long way. The apparently refined use of distillation, however, was not a practice enjoyed by all Londoners.

'Gin mania', as the social historian John Burnett calls it, gripped London from 1720–51. As he writes: 'The immediate causes of the epidemic were the ease of manufacture by hundreds of small distillers, the low duty of 2d. a gallon, and the absence of any requirement for a retail licence. In 1725 there were a reported 6,187 premises selling spirits in London, excluding the City and Southwark, and in Westminster and St Giles one in every four houses were said to be dram shops.'[87] The inner city neighbourhood of St Giles was portrayed by William Hogarth in *Gin Lane* (1751), as part of a campaign against the spirit's negative social consequences. His engraving famously depicts the debauchery unleashed by the cheap liquor on London's poorer inhabitants. In Hogarth's engraving a mother is shown nodding off with a dreamy, drunken smile on her face, as her baby is falling to the ground from her breast. Other details in the image depict financial ruin-by-gin and death-by-gin, whilst the pawnbroker and undertaker profit.[88]

That decade was also significant in terms of less toxic drinking issues. Medical historian Anne Hardy highlights 1756 as a pivotal year in her pioneering study of London's relationship between water and public health in the eighteenth century.[89] In this year, the medical doctor Charles Lucas' *Essays on Waters* was published. Lucas retaliated against prevailing water snobbery by studying, as he explained 'medicinal quality and uses of simple waters'.[90] Mineral water profiteers cannot have been pleased with this attempt to endow un-bottled water with equally medicinal virtues. The physician examined London's water as part of his project.

Though Charles Lucas siphoned murky water from the Thames, its appearance did not equate with contamination in his eighteenth century eyes. Apparently it was still acceptable in this state for 'drinking or bathing...for dressing of food...making malt and for brewing, for preparing medicines'.[91] Anne Hardy notes that, for this physician, the solid content in the water samples he drew from the river, ponds, pumps and springs — all sources that Londoners were consuming from — was not perceived to present any danger to health. Significantly, the other 1756 event Hardy points to was a publication by another physician warning of 'drinking beer brewed with well water'.[92] Whether it was purported to be good or bad for health, water's drinking quality seemed to be under a new level of scrutiny, in medical-scientific circles at least.

The next significant event in Hardy's account was in the 1790s, when she argues that the emergence of New Chemistry propelled quality analysis forward. New Chemistry was propelled forward by the research of Antoine Lavoisier in France, who reduced chemical substances into a simpler set of elements in a forerunner of the periodic table. Through his experiments, he showed that air could be further defined as oxygen and that water a compound of hydrogen and oxygen.[93] This focus on substances' minutiae brought attention to water's organic contents. Was this a source of impurity? Hardy asserts that such thoughts permeated beyond medical and scientific circles, for example to the architect James Peacock. Peacock patented the theory and hardware for a water filtration system in 1791.[94] His invention pre-dated any use of large-scale filtration technology. In 1793, the designer self-published *A Short Account of a New Method of Filtration by Ascent*. Peacock's aim was to produce a soft water that was not turbid, on the grounds that it was healthier for human consumption than hard water: 'Many are sensible of the indelicacies of turbid soft water; and are thence driven to the use of hard water, although they are not apprized of the probable danger to their health, from the petrifying quality, or from the metallic, or other mineral taints too frequently suspended and concealed therein.'[95] It was certainly an alternative position from the wonders of minerals that the bottlers of spa waters were glorifying. 'Indelicacies', however, were not quite diseases.

James Peacock was promoting his filtration cistern as a domestic product: 'This little apparatus will yield an ample sufficiency of perfectly clear soft water for every necessary use of a small family, of six to eight persons.'[96] The architect envisaged transforming the quality of water in homes by capturing the supply as it entered the service pipe. Peacock's cistern was an elite product intended for those residences that were already plugged into the corporate water network, rather than one designed for water fetched from the parish pump to be poured into. The invention did not make the architect a household name but his notion of filtering water was truly ahead of his time. Sadly for Peacock, he would have enjoyed a more lucrative career a few decades later.

Such technological entrepreneurship in last decade of the eighteenth century was consistent with the age of the industrial revolution that was transforming Britain's economic and social fabric. The growth of cities to fuel the labour for this industrialised society and to transport its products abroad would mean a new demand for water and sanitation facilities.

Consequences for water quality soon became apparent as nineteenth-century London swelled along the banks of the Thames.

Chapter Two

Private Water and Public Health 1800–1858

And so suspicious had several of the great metropolitan brewers
become of Thames water that they had been forced, at vast
expense, to look to wells for their supplies.[1]
(Pollution and Control, Bill Luckin)

The brewers' unease with polluted Thames water described by
the historian Bill Luckin marked the specific shift in public
attitude towards the river that occurred in the 1820s. It was in
that decade that the sharp decline in the river's stock of fish also
had an impact on the fishing economy in central London.[2] The
culprit was obvious. A prohibition on household drainage
connection to public sewers flowing straight into the Thames had
been lifted in 1815.[3] Unfortunately, this coincided with the rise in
purchases of the flush water closet and improved water supplies
to these facilities, at least for those who could afford both
luxuries.

Prior to the 1820s, as James Graham Leigh comments in his
account of London's water companies' machinations, 'water
quality does not seem to have been considered so important'.[4]
Population growth precipitated a rising demand for water for
domestic and industrial uses. More labouring Londoners meant
more call for refreshing beers and, consequently, that all-essential
raw material. Between 1801, the year of Britain's first census, and
1821, central London's population rose from 959,310 to 1,379,543.
A further 200,000 people were counted in Greater London.[5]
Industrial revolution and imperial growth, such as the Act of
Union with Ireland in 1800, created a new flow of migrant labour
into the capital to boost productivity.[6] Many people continued to
rely on the public resource of the parish pump, but as the century

progressed, piped water, even if only to shared communal sources became a standard of modern London life. This chapter explores how notions of water quantity and water quality became contested as Britain's public health movement emerged.

Before 1806, four private companies served piped water to wealthy households, at least those without the convenience of private wells.[7] London Bridge Water Works and the New River companies were still going strong. Also serving homes and businesses north of the river, York Buildings Water Works started pumping supplies at the end of the seventeenth century, followed by the Chelsea Water Works Company in 1723.[8] Early in the nineteenth century competitors to those established water providers surfaced in London's water supply market. West Middlesex Water Works began pumping to homes in the affluent neighbourhoods of Hammersmith, Kensington, Marylebone and Paddington in 1806, whilst in 1807 the East London Water Works Company set its sights on serving the hydration needs of the less well-off side of the city by exploiting the natural resource of London's other river; the Lee.[9] Then, in 1811, the Grand Junction Company promised to supply water of a superior quality from the rivers Colne and Brent to consumers in Oxford Street and Drury Lane.[10] Suburban companies included the Hampstead Water Company, the Shadwell Water Works and, on the south side of the river, the Lambeth Water Works and Borough Water Works.

Areas of supply were ungoverned and unregulated. Consequently, company pipes overlapped in neighbourhoods and those enterprises competed for neighbouring customers. This unsustainable system did not last for long. Between 1815 and 1818, the water companies hammered out agreements to carve London into water supply monopolies. Some corporations did not survive those negotiations.[11] The companies left standing had extraordinary power. As water rates rose steeply in some areas rose following monopolisation, many educated residents were disgruntled.

Anti-Water Monopoly Association

Historians of nineteenth-century water consumerism, Frank Trentmann and Vanessa Taylor point to the mobilisation of residents in 'affluent St Marylebone' under the banner of the Anti-Water Monopoly Association in 1819 as an important, if brief, period of consumer activism. This episode shaped the future of London's public water discussions by igniting 'debate about the rights of householders' of London's middle classes.[12] The minutes of the Anti-Water Monopoly Association's inaugural meeting state that its purpose was 'mutual protection against the arbitrary and oppressive proceedings' of the West Middlesex and Grand Junction water companies.[13] Petitioning about 'supply of this first necessity of life'[14] gained sufficient momentum for a parliamentary select committee enquiry in 1821, however it resolved that the companies' prices were fair.[15]

We cannot say that this water debate was specific to drinking water; however the description of water as a 'first necessity' suggests its role in biology and basic health, along with other uses. Flushing toilets had been entering the homes of the wealthy in larger numbers alongside piped water supplies, however the removal of human waste with water rather than the earth was still a nascent idea, because a waterborne sewage system did not exist.[16] Also, what might have been meant by good quality water at that pre-microbiological point is difficult to discern.

Perceptions of consuming water as a lone substance can be tricky to trace, particularly in terms of its use across the social strata, but the use of mineral water as a medicine was certainly still in vogue in the second decade of the nineteenth century. Mr Lambes Mineral Water Warehouse on fashionable New Bond Street was brimming with competing products, and he had been in business since 1799. One advert prescribing the use of Aluminious Chalybeate Water hints at contemporary thinking about drinking water quality: 'The patient is to begin with one ounce of water, diluted with two ounces of pure rain water.'[17] Specifying the use of rainwater for the ill certainly cast a shadow of doubt over the perceived health merits other sources, such as piped water. Late in the 1820s, any latent doubts Londoners generally might have about whether their water was good, bad or indifferent were awakened when an incendiary pamphlet was published.

The Dolphin & Monster Soup

John Wright claimed that Mr Robson, a former director of the Grand Junction Water Company, had confided in him in 1826 that the source of the company's supply was not from 'the streams of the vale of Ruislip' as its customers had been led to believe.[18] Robson led Wright to the point at the Thames where the Grand Junction was extracting its domestic supply and urged him to expose the company's corruption in his capacity as a writer and publisher. Wright's polemical pamphlet, *The Dolphin, or Grand Junction Nuisance* was published in March 1827, just a couple of months after Robson's death.

The pamphlet's title was a reference to the decorative opening of the Grand Junction Water Company's intake pipe in the Thames. An illustration accompanying the booklet showed the proximity of that pipe to the outfall of sewers. Wright condemned the private water monopolies as an 'unholy alliance' and the Grand Junction Water Company in particular for distributing 'a necessary of life, so loaded with all sorts of impurities, as to be offensive to the sight, disgusting to the imagination, and destructive to health'.[19] Though he was unaware of the precise impact of sewage on drinking water, Wright instinctively knew it was not a good practice for excrement and drinking water to mingle. The author viewed the Company as particularly corrupt because of its misleading adverts to supply 'pure and excellent soft water', when the source was evidently not as pure as the

New River's fairly priced and 'wholesome' water.[20] Wright dramatically exclaimed: 'The very sight of a glass of Grand Dolphin water serves as an excuse for a glass of spirits, to qualify the effects it may have on the stomach.'[21] He also pointed out the capital's water supply inequalities, on the basis that members of the nobility and gentry had private wells attached to their mansions.

The pamphlet's dissemination led to a 'numerously attended' meeting of 'respectable', presumably concerned, people.[22] Sir Frances Burdett raised the water quality exposé in Parliament and soon a *Commission for Inquiry into the Supply of Water* was launched to examine the truth of Wright's claims.[23]

Throughout January 1828 *The Times* published extracts from a document that Wright had furnished the Inquiry with as a supplement to *The Dolphin* pamphlet. The serial was entitled *The Water Question*. This phrase would become synonymous with public and political discourse surrounding London's water until the end of the nineteenth century.

In the first edition of *The Water Question*, Wright records his pleasure that the Dolphin pipe intake 'in the Thames at the foot of Chelsea Hospital...is now almost as well known and as much pointed at, by passengers going up and down the river as the Royal Hospital itself'.[24] He also declared that customers should have been informed about the new point of extraction and supplied with an analysis of the water. His latter point raised the important question of how quality was measured, and by whom?

Passionate as he was about his water pollution position, Wright had no scientific acumen to offer. In the next instalment of *The Water Question*, he claimed: 'The impurity of the water, which so greatly injured the health of inhabitants, arose, not from particles of matter floating in the fluid, but from the quantities of matter held in chymical solution', adding that 'no filtration could remove this species of impurity.'[25] Unlike the eighteenth century water-testing doctor we met in chapter one, Charles Lucas,

Wright saw matter in water as 'impure'. Evidence was needed to back up this position.

Chemists were to become critical figures in the water quality and treatment debate, though the science was still an occupation populated by amateurs.[26] Wright pronounced that one chemist, Dr Paris, agreed that filtration was pointless, however other experts did not concur. Those chemists who publicly defended the filtration solution in the scientific press were, in Wright's mind, trying to extinguish the validity of the government Inquiry. Wright's rhetoric reached fever pitch over this 'doctored', that is filtered, water.[27] For him, consuming filtered water, which masked impurities, might make the English a filthy race and a mockery of the cleanliness-is-next-to-godliness maxim.

Grotesque imaginings of the Thames' contents in this public debate was an irresistible subject for the leading caricaturist of the period, William Heath, or Paul Pry (his pseudonym). Published in 1828, Heath's *Monster Soup* presented Wright's claims with equal doses of humour and horror. The etching's publisher, Thomas McLean, issued daily caricatures of popular political subjects, so it is likely that the image was widely circulated, for instance in coffee or teahouses, or perhaps even the public house, where beer consumers may have been keen to scrutinise the raw materials of their pints more closely.[28] Those who were passed a copy of *Monster Soup* might well have dropped their cup or glass, like the caricature's human subject. Hydras; gorgons and chimeras with razor-like teeth, over-sized eyes, spines and pincers presented an unsettling view of the teeming inhabitants of London's main water source. Of course, it was satire, but was it exaggeration or merely magnification?

A contemporary archivist noticed the caricaturist's final stroke of humour: 'The P.P. of the signature raises his hat to a tiny pump, saying, *Glad to see you hope to meet you in every Parish through London.'*[29] This footnote might well have indicated that

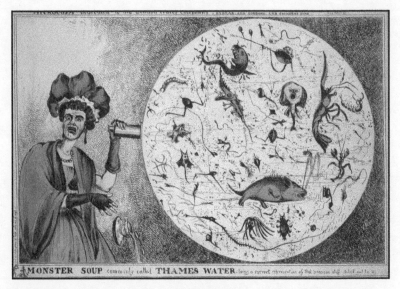

Monster Soup, commonly called Thames Water, 1828. William Heath
(1795–1840) Wellcome Library, London.

Heath, and others, thought pump water to be a safer bet than piped water. That view certainly tallies with Dr Charles Lucas' analysis of London's water sources back in 1756: 'Well or pump water approaches nearest of that of springs or fountanes.'[30] Despite the time lapse between these two pieces of evidence, it certainly points to a differentiation between water sources and therefore drinking water quality made by, at least some of, London's citizens.

Monster Filter

In 1829 Chelsea Waterworks responded to the water confidence crisis by dismissing Wright's negative position on filtration and employed a filtering system invented by James Simpson to treat its supply.[31] We can consider this move to capture the minute or invisible contents of London's raw water as the first step towards modern, industrial water treatment.

John Wright's critique of London water suppliers alluded to

the connection between drinking water and disease, mooted in some medical circles. For instance, he referred to a doctor's report about army troops contracting dysentery as result of their drinking water supply.[32] His question about disease striking London in the context of the water quality inquiry was prescient: 'Although this enormous metropolis may at the present moment be, generally speaking, in a healthy condition, does it therefore follow that it will always remain so?'[33] It was not long before his question was answered. Cholera morbus, also known as malignant diarrhoea, was a disease that had been previously associated only with 'natives' in the east.[34] Cholera's geography changed in 1832.

Caused by the Vibrio Cholerae bacterium, cholera's symptoms were the same then as they are now in countries with poor sanitation or sewage-contaminated water supplies: Severe diarrhoea, followed by rapid dehydration, the malfunctioning of vital organs and then death within days, if untreated.[35] William Marsden, a surgeon at the Free Hospital, founded as a result of the 1832 cholera outbreak, wrote of reactions to the disease's arrival: 'On the first appearance of this unknown disease in London, medical men of every grade, more particularly those in the higher walks of the profession, on viewing the afflicted patient, became terrified and panic-struck; and the public, in consequence of their professional advisers being ignorant of the nature of this malady, were completely bewildered and paralysed...the richly-endowed hospitals of this Metropolis closed their doors against the wretched sufferers, the affluent inhabitants fled, and the great wealthy members of the faculty dared not, or would not, condescend to visit the habitation of the afflicted.'[36] The Free Hospital provided an open door to those who contracted cholera, in an act that was equally humanitarian and medically pioneering because treatments for cholera were still entirely experimental.

Marsden and his colleagues used a saline solution treatment, which involved copious rehydration with water before patients ingested the salty fluid.[37] Presumably the Grand Junction Company's supply was not being used if they were to have any success. Records of the hospital's patients list those treated with the saline therapy as seventy-seven in total. These patients were all discharged. The Free Hospital's experiment was stunningly important, as cholera's treatment today is still the oral administration of water and salts.

From the scant coverage of the epidemic in *The Times*, it is clear that the disease was confined, at that point, to the 'poor, the wretched, the dissipated, and the destitute', as Marsden collectively referred to the victims.[38] The hospital's work certainly made no headlines. However, the subject was deemed worthy of attention by the satirist George Cruikshank. His 1832 illustration of the *Water-King of Southwark* represented Londoners decrying the condition of the Thames, as the source of their piped water. Crowds gather on the banks, with a chorus exclaiming: 'Give us clean water!', 'Give us pure water!', 'We shall all have the cholera.'[39] Cruikshank's representation of a politically vocal public, probably of middle class economic status, was common for satirists at that time and clearly cholera was a current issue. Also in 1832, the first of Britain's parliamentary Reform Acts was passed, widening the electorate to include all (male) property owners. Instinct told Cruikshank, and the public he was representing, that the condition of Thames and the outbreak of cholera was no coincidence. Connecting a particular water company with the disease suggested a relationship between the fatalities from cholera and the geography of the private water supply. Chelsea Waterworks, with its grand new filter, for example, was not satirised.

On her *Promenades Dans Londres* the radical French socialist Flora Tristan noted Chelsea's 'monster filter', designed to produce 'clear' water, as she termed it, for Londoners.[40] She critically observed that good quality water was not available to all citizens. In her *London Journal*, Flora Tristan recorded a lack of 'sumptuous and monumental fountains' like Paris but described the alternative: '...one does encounter iron pumps in many streets. An iron chain is affixed to the post with a dipper...This dipper is the economical goblet offered to the pauper by his lord and master, the rich man.'[41] From Tristan's interaction with London's wealthy inhabitants, she gathered that they were not in the habit of water drinking from the pumps. She quoted the following, possibly from an anonymous source but more likely as a shorthand for their general view: '"...here water costs the people nothing, they may drink at their convenience without going to draw water from the river"'.[42] One gets the impression that what she really felt about the inequity of London's segregated water supply was not uttered in polite conversation: 'In a country where scarcely one person in twenty-five can drink wine, and one in seven drink beer, is it not ironically insulting to offer the people of London water which has been dirtied by all the drains in the city?'[43]

Flora Tristan's account of 1830s London generally documented some of the living conditions that would preoccupy Britain's public health movement. As she wrote about St Giles Parish, which was hidden from the view of genteel eyes down an alleyway off Oxford Street: 'In St Giles one feels asphyxiated by the stench; there is no air to breathe nor daylight to find one's way. The wretched inhabitants must wash their own rags, and they hang them out to dry on poles that stretch from one side of the alley to the other, so that fresh air and sunlight are completely blocked out.'[44] Tristan's visceral account of the ghetto, a place that became increasingly associated with Irish immigrants post-famine, was consistent with the descriptions of urban squalor that the social researcher Edwin Chadwick would horrify, and entertain, middle and upper class readers with in his 1842 book *The Sanitary Condition of the Labouring Population of Great Britain*.

Edwin Chadwick's role in Britain's public health movement is extremely well documented therefore this account only briefly references how his concerns bore on the drinking water debate. Firstly, Chadwick was highly critical of the 'capitalists' who sold water in London.[45] He believed that water provision should be a municipal affair to improve drainage and support the 'promotion of civic, household and personal cleanliness'.[46] Improving standards of hygiene was closely connected in the sanitary reformer's mind with improving standards of morality. Chadwick argued that an abundant water supply was the answer to disease amongst the 'labouring population'. His gaze on water was trained on the quantity needed to wash ones body and home, and drain 'filth' away, rather than a concern about the quality of water that might be ingested for drinking or cooking. Legislation soon followed his unsanitary account.

1844's Metropolitan Buildings Act concurred with the Chadwickian drainage position. All new buildings were to have improved, covered drainage systems but, problematically, waste from properties with water closets was to be drained into the Common Sewer.[47] This drainage legislation preceded an effective sewage system. That issue was not considered more deeply until the members of a Royal Commission met in 1847 to discuss how the health of London's inhabitants might be improved. The same year, the national Towns Improvement Clauses Act was passed, with a clause that would be detrimental to river water. Under its terms, the new Metropolitan Commissioners of Sewers was empowered to ensure that the 'effectual draining' of London was carried out.[48] To achieve that end, these Commissioners were free to enforce the connection of sewers 'to communicate with and empty themselves into the Sea or any public River...'.[49] Whilst a full scheme for achieving that effectual draining was being planned, the move positively encouraged even more raw sewage to flow into the Lee and Thames. It only added to the problem of water closets becoming ever more normal features of middle class London homes. The engineers' task was unenviable and the scale of what had to done and how it could effectively be achieved, would not be resolved overnight. Cholera erupted again in 1849.

In the City of London alone, more than eight hundred people died from the bacterium's violent assault between June and October.[50] The Free Hospital's treatment method was clearly not in use by the doctors who saw these patients, if they received any treatment at all. One reason for this disconnect between 1832 and 1849 was the rise of an idea from the Chadwickian school of public health.

Miasma theory proposed that fatal diseases such as cholera were being transmitted via the air. This belief laid the blame for disease firmly on the doorsteps of the poor. Their dirty environments were producing the filth that was mobilising in air and infecting not just them, but now other classes too. Only one person ventured to posit a different argument during the 1849 cholera outbreak. This doctor was convinced that cholera was being transmitted via drinking water. His name was John Snow.

Though John Snow's evidence supporting his theory of cholera's waterborne transmission was still accruing in 1849, he was moved to publish his work-in-progress, *On the Mode of Communication of Cholera* immediately after the epidemic. He dismissed the 'miasmists' because their view that cholera could be 'inhaled and absorbed by the blood passing through the lungs' necessitated a predisposition for 'a great number to breathe it without injury'.[51] To Snow, this was not plausible because cholera's symptoms did not manifest in the manner of other blood poisoning diseases. He believed the symptoms pointed to its transmission in the alimentary canal and he suspected the disease's form was related to 'the continuity of molecular changes, by which combustion, putrefecation, fermentation, and the various processes in organised beings, are kept up'.[52] His interpretation sounded distinctly microbiological, even though that realm of knowledge was in its infancy. This first published thesis about cholera was drawn from fresh evidence of the 1849 epidemic. Snow believed that it followed the pattern of 1832's outbreak, in which he saw a connection between company water serving east and south London that was drawn from the sewage-contaminated river. Two neighbourhoods where cholera levels were curiously inconsistent in their spread featured in his pamphlet.

The first neighbourhood was a poor community. Thomas Street in Southwark lay opposite the Tower of London, where two courts of modest housing lay adjacent to each other. As Snow wrote: 'Now in Surrey Buildings the cholera has committed fearful devastation, whilst in the adjoining court there has been but one fatal case.'[53] The only difference that Mr Grant, the assistant surveyor of the Commissioners of Sewers noticed in his report, studied by Snow, was that in the courtyard of Surrey Buildings 'the slops of dirty water poured down by the inhabitants into a channel in front of the houses got into the well from which they obtained their water'.[54] The neighbouring courtyards did not share the water source, but clearly the cheek-by-jowl conditions suggested the air quality shared between the residents was the same. Snow's second case, significantly, introduced a neighbourhood that would not have been deemed unsanitary by Chadwickian standards into the equation.

Albion Terrace in Wandsworth, as described by John Snow, consisted of 'genteel suburban dwellings of a number of tradespeople'.[55] The community's twenty fatal cases of cholera were blamed, by Snow, on the contamination of a shared water tank by a leaking cesspool which the surveyor Mr Grant found when the ground was opened up. In fact, Snow wrote that the victims themselves 'attributed their illness to the water', noticing it was impure but consuming it anyway; obviously without the knowledge that it could be fatal.[56] The doctor explained how secondary infection could spread via hands and food once the cholera 'evacuations' had contaminated anything that might be subsequently ingested. He countered Dr Milroy's report to the General Board of Health that Albion Terrace's mortality was caused by an open sewer in Battersea Fields transmitting cholera into the air, by pointing out that the houses surrounding the exclusive water supply of the affected houses, were 'quite free' from cholera.[57] Snow concluded in his pamphlet by a persuasive argument that his theory was more optimistic: 'What is so dismal as the idea of some invisible agent pervading the atmosphere, and spreading over the world?'[58] He proposed that, 'if the writer's opinion be correct, cholera might be checked and kept at bay by simple measure that would not interfere with social or commercial intercourse...'[59] Despite Snow's pragmatic stance, the miasmists were firmly attached to their pessimistic worldview. When cholera vanished again, Chadwick and his colleagues may well have agreed that a storm had simply cleansed the air.

Water became more politicised in London as a result of the epidemic. Educated professional citizens and official sanitary reformers alike sheltered under the umbrella of the Metropolitan Parochial Water Supply Association in 1850. Its concern, liker the Anti-Water Monopoly Association before it, was the control of water by private corporations, rather than the quality of the supply. Publicly controlled water and 'a constant supply at high pressure' was the Association's goal.[60] But in London's scientific community, others were convinced by John Snow's thesis and were consequently preoccupied with the finer constituents of water.

One result of the waterborne movement was that microscopist Arthur Hill-Hassall examined London's corporate water supplies, publishing the results of his study in 1850. He qualified that his experiment was needed because of the public focus on the 'defective condition of the water supply of London'.[61] The physician-cum-microscopist was dissatisfied that the only infor-

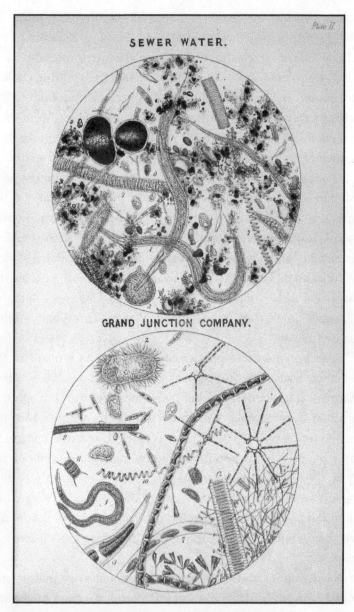

Sewer water and Grand Junction Company, Plate 1
*A microscopic examination of the water supplied to the inhabitants of London
and the suburban districts*, Arthur Hill-Hassall (London: Samuel Highley,
1850) Wellcome Library, London.

mation chemists produced about organic matter referred to 'traces'. What were traces? Like Snow, he thought there was more to the science of water analysis: 'It will become apparent that these traces...are complex in organisation, endowed with life and in many cases possessed of active powers of locomotion.'[62] Also referring to these microscopic inhabitants of London's water supply under their popular title, 'animalcules', Hill-Hassall admitted that nobody knew what they were.

Christopher Hamlin, a historian of nineteenth-century water analysis, pinpointed that the importance of Hill-Hassall's book 'was to make microscopic life a new category of impurity, and a great deal of debate in 1851 and 1852 was concerned with what exactly such creatures signified'.[63] At this point chemists and microscopists were competing in the water analysis sphere, but neither knew how to conclusively explain the significance of the revelations produced under the lenses of their microscopes.

Hill-Hassall's lurid microscopic drawings were presented to Parliament, possibly during the 1851 Metropolis Water Supply Bill's debate when there was much discussion of animalcules.[64] Whether the politicians involved were of the Chadwickian or Snowian schools of thought, the state of London's water was equally problematic. Much of the debate revolved around the provision of more water to purify the slums, or 'disgusting dens' according to one speaker in the House of Commons. Water's cost was also noted: 'Nine different companies distribute water into the houses at exaggerated rates, and the poor people who cannot meet the demands of the companies are often obliged to drink the hard disagreeable water of the wells.'[65] For that speaker, the well water was still not perceived to be unhealthy per se but he was clearly indicating that piped, softer water was more palatable. Quality was important to other debaters. Mr Moffat referred to evidence in the Board of Health's reports which claimed that 'the quality of the water was very objectionable and unwholesome, and that organic and vegetable matter was found in it of a highly prejudicial character'.[66]

Beyond the House of Commons' debating chamber, many an M.P. may have been enjoying a premium glass of drinking water at the Great Exhibition during the summer of 1851. The Exhibition was *the* social event of that year. Over six million people attended, many travelling by train from outside London and internationally. Covering twenty-six acres of Hyde Park a monumental glass structure, known as the Crystal Palace, was designed by the architect Joseph Paxton to showcase the wares of more than one thousand exhibitors from every nook and cranny of the British Empire. At this *Great Exhibition of the Industry of all Nations*, the burgeoning fashion for teetotalism was reflected in the catering specification: 'The contractor at each area must supply fresh filtered water in glasses gratis to visitors, and keep a sufficient supply at each area…no wines, spirits, beer or intoxicating drinks can be sold or admitted by the contractor.'[67] Schweppes was awarded the contract to keep the refreshment rooms supplied with this free water, though its origin was not described. Those who wanted to pay for their water at Schweppes' concession could opt for soda water, an innovation made possible by the company's development of carbonation and the mass production of fizzy soft drinks.[68] A live soda-water aeration performance by one Mr Cox was also reported to be pulling in the Exhibition's crowds, possibly because he gave away free samples.[69] A water purification outfit also exhibited its wares.[70] Teetotalism, otherwise known as temperance, was also present in a guerrilla stunt at the Great Exhibition's centrepiece, the Crystal Fountain, where a mass of teetotallers 'thronged from all parts of England into the metropolis in the pursuance of a half business-like, half-festive "temperance demonstration" '.[71] The demonstrators ritualistic surrounding of the Crystal Fountain — though it was a decorative rather than a drinking fountain — offers a curious insight into water's symbolic potency as public health was becoming increasingly tied to social reform. From a practical perspective, more teetotallers meant a greater demand for quality-assured drinking water.

Back at the House of Commons' debate about the Metropolis Water Bill, a statement by Sir W. Clay drove to the heart of the issue: 'The only question for the House was, what conditions they ought to impose on those to whom the supply of water was entrusted?'[72] In the legislation that followed, London's corporate water supplies were regulated for the first time and public health principles became legally tied to the supply of urban water. Following the vigorous exchanges of medical, public health and political opinions about water during the debate, the Metropolis Water Supply Act became law in 1852. By 1855, companies would be required to 'effectually' filter their water, transport it in covered aqueducts or pipes and provide a constant supply.[73] From a quality perspective, the most significant clause picked up on the argument of Joseph Wright, that the point of abstraction in the Thames was critical: 'No water company after August 31, 1855, should take its supply from the Thames below Teddington Lock.'[74] This point on the river, in west London, was where it ceased to be tidal and therefore where, upstream, the water was entirely free from salt.

A competitor to the water companies' river-derived source, the London (Watford) Spring Water Company promptly saw an opportunity to cash in on public concern about animalcules. The company employed two leading microscopists to dip their test tubes in the Thames above Teddington Lock and analyse the results. They reported that it was 'a water much contaminated with organic matter…one of the last sources to which the Metropolis should look for a supply of pure water'.[75] Watford Spring's contents, on the other hand, were found to 'be free from organic matter as any water can be in its natural state', conveniently for those on the water company's payroll.[76] But before the new abstraction and effectual filtration systems were in place, cholera broke out again in 1854.

This time cholera struck in the heart of John Snow's own cosmopolitan, central London neighbourhood of Soho. In the course of ten days between August and September 1854, cholera bacteria multiplied wildly within a short radius of a water-pump at the junction of Broad Street and Cambridge Street. Snow's claims, in conjunction with the fieldwork of Reverend Whitehead, about the pump's role in dispensing the disease convinced the local vestry to have the handle of the pump removed on the 8th September.[77] Snow's famous cholera map was based on the lives that the epidemic claimed in relation to that Broad Street pump.

His insights into the consuming habits of Soho's residents prove that, despite water's bad press, earlier in the century, its consumption was a widespread practice in daily life. However, as Snow himself reflected about consumption habits: 'The English people, as a general rule, do not drink much unboiled water, except in warm weather.'[78] The outbreak occurred at the height of summer during this outbreak and the range of people ingesting the Broad Street pump's water cold was clearly recorded by John Snow as he mapped the pattern of consumption and cholera contraction. It was consumed in a local coffee house at dinnertime, as a mixer for shops selling sherbet, or to dilute quick nips of brandy or other spirits in nearby pubs.[79] That pump's water quenched the thirst of workers in local percussion-cap and dentistry material manufactories, but plain water consumption was not confined to those who, economically at least, had no other choice.[80] It was enjoyed by an army officer dining in Wardour Street and an 'eminent ornithologist' who lived on Broad Street, though he decided against drinking it after noticing the offensive smell around its vicinity on 2nd September.[81] An ex-Soho resident living in Hampstead was even brought a bottle from the pump by her visitors, as she apparently preferred its taste to her local supply.[82] Snow's record of these consumer habits shows the centrality of the pump to neighbourhood life, despite the availability of piped water. This suggests at least two things. One is that the pump was reliable for a fresh supply given the intermittent nature of the corporate water. Or that the underground supplies were perceived to be more drinkable and tasted noticeably different to river-derived water. The popularity of the pump is mirrored by a detail in 1828's *Monster Soup* caricature in which the stick figure of Paul Pry, who we have already met, doffs his cap to a parish pump.

There is little doubt that some Londoners preferred pumped to piped water. Still, Snow's second tranche of evidence about 1854 also shows that drinking piped company water was habitual. Either way, water drinking was evidently a commonplace way to quench ones thirst and it was not widely associated with disease at that point.

John Snow explained that since cholera had disappeared in 1849, south London's domestic water supply had significantly altered. Southwark and Vauxhall Company and the Lambeth Company were in competition, just like the pre-monopoly era at the beginning of the century. Their pipes ran side-by-side in certain districts. The parallel supply of different water provided an opportunity for Snow to further his thesis about the cholera tragedies recurring in London, and elsewhere. As he wrote: 'Each Company supplies both rich and poor, both large houses and small; there is no difference either in the condition or occupation of the person receiving the water of the different companies...as there is no difference whatever, either in the houses or the people receiving the supply of the two water companies, or in any of the physical conditions with which they are surrounded, it is obvious that no experiment could have been devised which would more thoroughly test the effect of water supply on the progress of cholera...'[83] To aid his research, the Registrar General's office agreed to provide the physician with the addresses of people as they died from cholera in those districts. Snow set about tracking the damage caused by the

Lambeth Company's water, whilst a doctor called John Joseph Whiting volunteered to take on the districts supplied only by the Southwark and Vauxhall Company. Snow recounted: 'Mr Whiting took great pains with his part of the inquiry, which was to ascertain whether the houses where the fatal attacks took place were supplied with the Company's water, or from a pump-well, or some other source.'[84]

One frustration for the duo was that residents often did not even know which company they, or their landlords, were paying. If the dwellers could not find any receipts for bills, Snow had a back up plan. He took a sample of water from each of the cholera-struck properties and performed a chemical test. Results were matched with the average sodium and chloride levels that he had already established in the two companies' supplies. Over the four weeks of the epidemic, three hundred and thirty-four people died from cholera in the area that the two companies supplied. Snow and Whiting established that 286 of the households affected were supplied with water by the Southwark and Vauxhall Company, whilst the Lambeth Company was found to be responsible for only 14 cases of infection.

Steven Johnson, author of a recently-published interpretation of Snow's legacy, *The Ghostmap*, summed up the lukewarm response to the physician's theory in those post-cholera years thus: '...miasma retained its hold over many, and Snow himself was often subjected to derisive treatment by the scientific establishment' (for instance peers writing in *The Lancet* medical journal).[85] The ideological gulf between the two schools of disease transmission continued but one clear decision was made as a result of the Metropolitan Commission of Sewers fieldwork. London's 'filth', quite crudely, its faeces, needed to be removed.

In the same year that Snow's revised, and now seminal, thesis *On the Mode of Communication of Cholera* was published, 1855, the Metropolis Management Act was passed. The Act's implications were seismic. It would institute a governance structure for building the modern world's first citywide underground water-based sewerage system, under the governance of the Metropolitan Board of Works. Painstaking surveying and designing by the Metropolitan sewer commissioners, including Joseph Bazalgette, had translated into a coherent set of plans for radical underground sewage works. New housing would be condemned if water closets failed to be 'furnished...with suitable water supply and water supply apparatus'.[86] Sewage was to be removed from sight, and therefore from contact with the air, and, most critically, it was to be discharged into the Thames in locations far removed from London's population. These locations would also, therefore, be distant from points of water abstraction. Miasma theory was still going strong, but the vast plumbing system was equally instrumental in preventing water-borne disease transmission.

Governance to build London's sewage system was in place, but the essential finances were not. Consequently, the subterranean makeover made a sluggish start. Sewage farms were already in vogue at that point, but any waterborne sewage entering the Thames, pre-1858, was raw. In 1856 the Board of Health's Medical Officer, John Simon, published a report which examined the plausibility of cholera's waterborne transmission, and though he was not entirely convinced about the veracity of John Snow's theories, he admitted that more evidence pointed towards disease transmission via water rather air. On that basis he wrote: 'Whether water can be securely drunk from rivers polluted by urban drainage, interests more or less every part of the country and whatever facts can terminate this doubt, bear upon every plan for the water supply of a population, and upon every plan for the drainage of a town.'[87] In essence, Simon was questioning the natural capacity of a river to recover from sewage pollution. The answer lay in a method for examining water that could offer a definitive ruling on its quality for human consumption, but that science was still floundering.

Plans for sewers to bypass central London were still on the drawing board when the famous 'Great Stink' occurred. As temperatures rose in the summer of 1858, the stench from the Thames wafted into national newspaper headlines. *The Era* vented its disgust by suggesting that the Thames be renamed 'the great sewer of London'.[88] A visceral verse from *The Morning Chronicle* also conveyed the inhaling horror to its readers. Those remote from the Thames certainly got a vicarious whiff:

'Piff, piff-piff! how horrid
Is thy filth, thick as cream,
Baked by Summer's sun torrid,
It reeks with foul steam!'[89]

The excretions of two million people must have been quite a convincing olfactory argument, especially when they were lapping up against the river's north bank at the Houses of Parliament. Promptly, the Government rushed through a bill to unlock funds for the Metropolitan Board of Works to get things flowing, out of central London.[90] The historian Bill Luckin argues that the motivation to clean up the Thames was not only a result of the river's impact on the quality of local life, but because of its secondary role as a symbol of the heart and power of the British Empire.[91] A polluted Thames was a source of international humiliation. As Luckin argued: 'To save the river was to consolidate the new urban-industrial order.'[92]

Within that industrial order, steam engines had by then revolutionised control over water distribution through vast pumping technology and therefore modes of production and consumption in turn. New technological water innovation would also be ushered in with the Local Government Act of 1858, which acknowledged that urban municipalities needed to invest in large-scale infrastructure to treat sewage *before* it entered rivers.[93] On the sewerage front, London's revolutionary sanitary

engineering project led by Joseph Bazalgette transformed underground infrastructure during the 1860s, creating embankments
such as Chelsea to house the pipes. How soon water quality
would be transformed by sewerage and diseases like cholera
extinguished remained to be seen.

Above ground, a minor clause in the 1855 Metropolis
Management Act raised the issue of public water access: 'Every
Vestry and District Board shall have full Power and Authority to
cause any Wells to be dug and sunk in such public Places as they
think proper, and also to erect and fix any Pumps in any public
Places, for the gratuitous Supply of Water to the Inhabitants of
the Parish or District.'[94] What this water might be used for was
not specified, though it seems likely that it was intended largely
for cleansing, of streets for instance, rather than primarily for
drinking. If the sources were imagined for drinking use, it was a
worrying proposal given the Broad Street example. Quite
separately from the dictates of the state's public health administration, public fountains were about to become extremely
fashionable.

Chapter Three

Philanthropic Fountains 1852–1875

'Water is always distributed in the cities of England by companies that would not allow the establishment of street fountains because they would be a serious obstacle to the profits they must derive from their enterprise.'[1]
(*The Public Fountains of the City of Dijon*, Henry Darcy, 1856, trans. 2004)

French hydro-geologist Henry Darcy's acerbic comment was unlikely to have reached the ears or eyes of the people who propelled London's fashion for fountains throughout the remainder of the nineteenth century. He wrote it in a book about public fountains in Dijon — certainly a niche subject — of which the English translation was only published recently. Whether or not his scorn for the commodification of water crossed the English Channel, it most certainly applied to London's tangle of corporate water suppliers in contrast to other English cities' municipal systems. This chapter investigates how Darcy's statement could not have been applied to the drinking water on offer on London's streets just ten years later. The story starts, however, not in London but in the north of England.

A Liverpudlian Gentleman

Like London, Liverpool experienced unprecedented population growth in the early nineteenth-century. As the port for northern manufacturing cities and a departure point for immigrants journeying across the British Empire, ships were constantly sailing into and out of its docks. In 1801 the city had eighty thousand inhabitants, yet by 1841 there were more than a quarter of a million people recorded in the census.[2] Liverpool was a centre for the flow of labour. Karl Marx's analysis of Capitalism's mode of wealth production would soon deduce, human Labour was an essential cog in propelling the economic system's perpetual motion towards profit. Industrialised cities such as Liverpool did not have the built infrastructure for its inhabitants to keep pace with the growth of the human workforce that was needed to sustain the increasing scale of Victorian merchants' profits.

Similarly to London, the consequences of people living without adequately planned sanitary infrastructure in Liverpool endangered lives and threatened to spread infectious diseases. Liverpool pioneered the collective 'cleansing' of the working classes before any other city in Britain of the period, with the opening of Frederick Street baths in 1842.[3]

The bathhouse was a product of concern from prominent citizens, who pressurised the city council that a sanitary overhaul was needed to prevent the recurrence of a cholera epidemic like 1832.[4] Frederick Street bathhouse was considered to be a national model for social improvement and contributed to the passing of the Baths and Washhouses Acts later in the decade.[5] As socially important as Liverpool's bathhouse was, the building was eclipsed by the scale of the city's other civic and industrial architecture. Vast warehouses had been constructed to house cotton, sugar and tobacco at the port's docks, before their dispatch for processing elsewhere. The merchants who owned and controlled these goods had formed a powerful new middle class in the city. Charles Melly was one of these businessmen.

Melly had a Swiss father and the Liverpudlian family remained connected with relatives in Geneva throughout his life. As a boy he visited a Swiss spa, so he had an early introduction to the cult of hydrotherapy, which involved being immersed in, or ingesting, mineral water.[6] When he married, the newlyweds travelled to Geneva as part of their honeymoon tour in 1852. This kind of tourism had become increasingly common to people of his class, with the advent of train connections to Britain's ports. An 1838 guidebook, *Murray's Handbook for Travellers in Switzerland*, pointed out something that became a source of fascination for Melly in Geneva: 'One characteristic and very pleasant feature are the Fountains, the never-failing ornament of every Swiss town and village.'[7]

Though he may have seen such fountains in Switzerland when he was younger, the mature Melly, coming from the working city of Liverpool, was impressed that people had access to a free drinking water supply on the street in Geneva.[8] He later wrote of 'the beautiful stone water fountains which are so abundant in that city, indeed in every town in Switzerland, and on the Continent generally'.[9] Rome's influence on urban design during the Renaissance saw the spread of public water to many European cities as a trope of Baroque architecture.[10] In Switzerland, fountain keepers were appointed in the sixteenth century to supervise public fountain construction and to ensure their maintenance.[11] Caring for these public resources evidently survived as a civic job into the 1850s when Melly was honeymooning.

Melly returned to Liverpool inspired. He conducted interviews around the docks to find out of if public water was needed and observed the way others used the city. The pattern of people's working lives in Liverpool meant that they were out of their homes for long periods of time. The merchant's research concluded that 'the labourers, shipwrights and porters employed in our docks and warehouses live at a considerable distance from their work; often two or three miles...they generally carry their dinner out with them, and only return home after their day's work is done'.[12] Quizzing dockworkers and local policemen, he was satisfied that the quantity of immigrants leaving from the port to America and Australia alone created sufficient demand for drinking water.[13] In 1853 he arranged for two modest public taps to be installed at the docks. Their popularity convinced the merchant that a fully-fledged fountain would be used. The following year, Melly financed the building of Britain's first 'Continental-style' granite drinking fountain on Prince's Dock. Three months after its inauguration, the use of the fountain was surveyed over twelve hours. More than two thousand drinkers were recorded.[14] Judging by an illustration of a Liverpudlian fountain in 1856, the bold sensuality of the baroque fountains Melly viewed on his honeymoon was not replicated in his gift. Its utilitarian design was more no-nonsense English, than romantic European.

Ideologically, there was something radical about Charles Melly's project. He was advocating that drinking water should be free, indignantly exclaiming that '...although Liverpool's domestic water supply was municipally owned and managed, not one drop of it was to be had without paying a water rate'.[15] Melly compared the situation with Geneva: 'There the water is the property of the town authorities, and is distributed by them to the citizens through the means of large public fountains, free of cost.'[16] A capitalist promoting such a view about natural resources and profit making may seem surprising, however he was typical of many merchants for whom economic and religious philosophies ran on parallel tracks. As a Unitarian, Melly had a moral duty to do good deeds. The historian Howard Malchow points out that northern non-conformists, such as those of Unitarian faith, were also culturally wedded to promoting 'cleanliness and sobriety'.[17]

Melly appears to have convinced Liverpool's municipal water supplier of the merits of free water. In just five years, the city was supplying water to forty of the merchant's public fountains.[18] Cities and towns such as Derby, Glasgow and Hull soon followed his lead, however London was still without such civic facilities. In 1858, Melly publicised his hydration achievements to an audience at the National Association for the Promotion of Social Science. At the same event, W.F. Cowper also presented a paper.[19] Cowper was an M.P. who had senior governmental roles in the development of education and health policies. He must have been convinced by the Liverpudlian's arguments because the following year Cowper was instrumental in London's public fountain movement. However, he was not the leader of the ambitious project. That role would fall to his fellow M.P. and personal associate Samuel Gurney.

In 1857, when he was in his early forties, Gurney took his seat for the first time in the Chamber of the House of Commons. Within a year, the civility and comfort of that gentlemanly environ was unsettled by the infamous 'Great Stink'.

A Benevolent Banker

Although Gurney had been elected an M.P., he appeared to be more driven by his religious and moral convictions as a Quaker, rather than his political convictions. His time in Westminster did not cause much of a stir but his impact on the philanthropic sphere would be significant.

The name Gurney is historically associated with both Quakerism and banking. Quakers numbered less than fourteen thousand people in Britain in 1861 yet their influence in business was disproportionate to the size of this community.[20] Without Quaker entrepreneurship, Barclays bank or Cadburys would not exist. Quakers, or the Society of Friends, did not accept the doctrine of the Anglican Church of England. Their belief that God, or the spirit, resides within each person, without the need for an external intermediary was considered to be radical. For one, it challenged the need for powerful male leaders. Quakers were branded, with other Christian minorities, such as Unitarians, as non-conformists. By Samuel Gurney's time, the ban on the open worshipping of the 'peculiar people', as they were also known, had been lifted.

One benefit from the Quakers historical marginalisation was the development of a strong kinship network, which preserved their religious culture. Known amongst themselves as Friends or Cousins, this community embraced members of their own faith through extended family networks, both nationally and internationally.[21] The economic, moral and spiritual flow of support from this social network created a fertile ground for Quaker-run businesses to flourish.[22] Whilst most Quakers were ordinary middle-class folk, a group of highly successful industrial innovators and financiers, of whom Samuel Gurney was one, formed an elite group of Friends. Whilst the mantra of free trade they advocated kept the profits rolling in, a Quaker businessman also had to be involved in good works which were the outward signs of a man's sanctification.[23] The wave of social reform sweeping through Victorian Britain in the mid-nineteenth century provided a perfect vehicle for wealth to be channelled, visibly, into charitable Christian deeds.

Quakers were also active in the temperance movement, through which they participated in a broader social and religious sphere of respectability. Charles Melly's fountains were featured in a popular temperance publication, the *British Workman's Almanac* in 1858. The Almanac provided a calendar of monthly prayer, verse and illustrations to help working people keep themselves on an honest, sober path.[24] In the midst of these pages, a labourer and two male youths were shown drinking from ladles at a fountain in a northern city. The brief accompanying article proclaimed that a metropolitan equivalent was needed.

Literature of this nature was endorsed by London's own network of temperance supporters. In November 1858, a letter by Samuel Gurney was published in the London newspaper, the *Morning Chronicle*. It was penned from number 25 Lombard Street, where his family bill broker firm was based. This lengthy quote from the letter importantly clarifies Gurney's motivations: 'I have long been sensible to the great public want there is of drinking fountains in London. As the case now stands, there is little choice for the wayfaring poor between actual thirst and the quenching of it with beverages supplied at public-houses...In Liverpool, where, through the wisely-directed liberality of Mr Melly, free public drinking fountains have been erected...There can be no reasonable doubt but that drinking fountains, similarly distributed throughout the leading metropolitan thoroughfares, would confer an immense boon on the poorer classes...with a view of commencing the movement in London, I caused a respectful memorial to be addressed to the vestry of St Pancras, requesting permission to erect a public drinking fountain near King's Cross Railway station, at my own expense.'[25]

Gurney then proceeded to vent his frustration at the vestry of St Pancras' subsequent refusal to entertain the idea. He suggested that publicising its opposition would rouse more '"enlightened"' supporters.[26] The philanthropist was already on a mission, but it was obviously one designed to dispense sobriety as opposed to social justice. He announced that he was about to make similar offers to other vestries. The negotiations with the proprietors of the land, where fountains might best serve Gurney's proposed target users, were underway.

If the vestry of St Pancras was not convinced, other prominent people rapidly endorsed his proposal. 'What is good in Liverpool is good in London seems to be the dictate of Mr Gurney's philosophy, and I think most Christian minds will pronounce it to be a sound one', wrote Mr H. Burdett Worthington.[27] Professor Marks of Marylebone announced that his parish colleagues 'would not be doing their duty if they did not... aid this noble project'.[28] Such publicity also aroused the interest of a barrister, Edward Wakefield, who became Gurney's key ally. Fortunately Wakefield was also a talented wordsmith. He penned *A Plea for Free Drinking Fountains* (1859), which was instrumental in attracting the prestigious supporters in the competitive Victorian market for good causes.

Taking up Charles Melly's radical baton, Wakefield argued

that water was a necessity for human life, no less than air. His attack on his own class asserted that 'those who lead sedentary lives, or have always at hand the means of anticipating such wants, know little of the intensity of thirst generated by bodily exertion, especially in hot weather'.[29] He reminded readers of John Snow's discovery of polluted pump water and repeated the popular urban myth that decomposing matter from the bodies in London's graveyards had infected the groundwater. Wakefield argued that fountains could help people to change their consuming habits and eventually cure the great national stigma of intemperance.

On 5th February 1859, *The Morning Post* announced that a highly influential association was being formed around the public drinking water agenda.

A Sobering Mission

That spring, The Metropolitan Free Drinking Fountains Association was inaugurated with a ceremony in the Willis' Rooms in the heart of political and gentlemanly clubland on St James Street; the prime social centre for Liberal politics and the place where the Liberal Party was founded just months later.[30] The Earl of Carlisle took the helm as Chairman and addressed the gathering of Liberal-leaning politicians; Gurney, Cowper and the press, with evident enthusiasm for the project. He was shortly to become the Lord Lieutenant of Ireland, so the endorsement of this particular social reforming mission by someone of his status reflected the group's level of influence. Carlisle pointed out that, despite the vigour of London's many social reform groups, 'this was certainly the first meeting that has been held in London in connection with public drinking fountains'.[31]

Charles Melly attended as an honorary guest. The Chair praised his inspirational work, lamenting London's slow response to his example. Carlisle then announced with great gusto that the first metropolitan fountain, funded by Samuel Gurney, would soon be unveiled. It is likely that he was aware of the public scrutiny that would follow the meeting, so he diplomatically explained how the Association's ambitions might be gradually realised. Parishes could not be assumed to take a proactive lead on the project; however he suggested that larger organisations, such as the City of London Corporation and the Crown's Woods and Parks might be willing partners.

Temperance was on his agenda but, like Wakefield, he admitted that the fountains might not immediately dispel the proletariat's fondness for ale, or gin. The Earl of Albermarle was more optimistic. He had incredible hopes that the fountains might 'check those habits of intemperance which caused nine-tenths of the pauperism, three-fourths of the crime, one half of the disease, one third of the insanity, one-third of the suicide, three-fourths of the general depravity and one-third of the shipwrecks that annually occurred'.[32] Returning to practical considerations, Carlisle revealed that the fountain designs would be led by functional concerns: '...no prudent person would dream of throwing away money unnecessarily upon embellishment and ornament.'[33] He did concede that an inscription or two might not be considered excessive. This was an important selling point for would-be donors listening in the audience, who may have been wondering how a gift to this organisation might reflect on their social standing.

Lord Ashley took to the podium too. His participation, as one of the architects of the Metropolis Water Supply Act 1852, lent public health gravitas to the occasion. Ashley's participation reassured donors, and the public, about the intended water supply. His description of the water from existing street pumps as slow poison generated a sense of urgency about why this alternative water source was needed on the street. Underground water could not be trusted. These future fountains would issue water from private company sources (now regulated to a degree), drawn beyond the reach of the polluted metropolitan environment. John Snow's findings had not caused a closure of all parish-pumps, and, as we know, London's underground sewage system was yet to be constructed. Contaminated or not, it is clear that the fountains were not primarily intended for the Association's own members or prospective donors' use but for the benefit of those who might be dissuaded on the street from squandering their wages on alcoholic refreshments.

Alongside this patrician moral stance for temperance, a more humane sense of social justice in providing free, safe drinking water was also present. This was apparent in statements, though they were typically overloaded with sentiment, such as this: 'The streets of London are continually crowded with human beings who amid the heat and dust and excitement, are peculiarly subject to the sensation of thirst...porters toiling under heavy burdens, messengers hastening on their errands, mechanics going to and fro from their work, cabmen, carmen, itinerant vendors of fruit and vegetables, flower girls, and multitudes of others whose occupation lies almost entirely out of doors.'[34] These depictions of daily life's physical strain backed up Melly's thesis that the labouring class needed water outdoors because, for many of them, that was their primary place of work.

Fountain Fever

Following the rousing speeches and publicity generated during its first meeting, enquiries to the Association's small administration came flooding in. Just two weeks after the Association's inaugural meeting, Gurney's own fountain was due to be unveiled in the wall of St Sepulchre's Church in the City of London. The location was resonant for him, as it lay opposite Newgate Prison where his Aunt, Elizabeth Fry (née Gurney), had carried out radical penal reform.

On 20th April 1859, the fountain's ceremonial opening took place. The *Illustrated London News* depicted, with a likely dash of artistic licence, a raucous crowd surrounding the dignitaries who presided over the blessing.

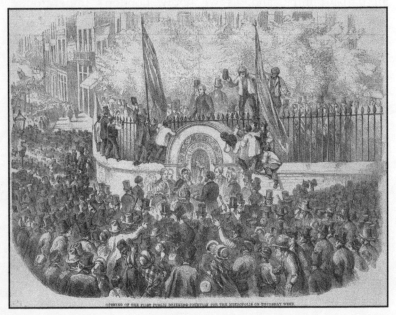

Drinking-Fountains. Illustrated London News, Saturday 30th April 1859, p. 432, Issue 971. City of London, London Metropolitan Archives.

The structure itself was modest, apart from the detail of a scallop shell fanned coquettishly above the waterspout. A wide granite bowl was set into the railings of the church with the inscription 'The Gift of Sam Gurney M.P.' and written below, the polite request, to 'Replace the Cup'. Metal cups were permanently attached to the fountain by chains. This feature was a reminder that germ theory was yet to be discovered.

Though the Association appointed Dr Lankester as its Medical Referee to attest to the quality of the water supply and filtration, the possibility of people passing diseases to each other either orally or via unwashed hands was not considered. Lankester's letter of support for the Association stated his hope that fountains would displace the need for people to use wells but, as an enthusiastic microscopist, he advocated the use of filters inside the plumbing to strain off impurities.[35] St Sepulchre's fountain was inscribed 'Filtered water from the New River Company'. Drawn from its rural Hertfordshire spring, distinguishing this supply from the brew in public wells was a unique selling point of the new fountain.

The Lady Newspaper announced plans for the forthcoming fountains and, in its view, the positive addition they would make to London by 'providing an alternative to the public house and the low company found in those establishments'.[36] The publication's editors approved of Gurney's association with plans of social progress and reform such as 'reclamation of the criminal, freedom for the slave, instruction for the ignorant, [and] homes for the outcast'.[36] Observing the opening day's proceedings, the *Lady's* reporter claimed that a drinking fountain was an 'unmistakably feminine' device, and therefore fitting that female lips should quaff the first draught.[37]

Mrs Wilson, the Archbishop of Canterbury's daughter, was the one who quaffed. Before she did so, she was assured that fountain trials in other English cities had proved to be safe for health. After Mrs Wilson's first suspenseful sip, the *Illustrated London News* reported that she it to taste excellent.[38] A final announcement declared that the fountain was for the special use of the working classes and was committed to their care.

After St Sepulchre, the Association pushed to get as many fountains installed as possible in London's busiest thoroughfares.[39] A slew of adverts were placed in newspapers to generate further support. At £25 for a mural (wall) fountain and £50 for a standard (free-standing) fountain, these price tags needed to be explained before donors reached for their chequebooks (the figures translate approximately into contemporary currency as £1,000 and £2,000 respectively).

Edward Wakefield defended the high cost of the fountains for several critical reasons in *The Times*.[40] Medical advisers had stipulated that despite the overhaul of London's water supply, additional filtration was needed at the point of consumption. Carbon, in the form of loose animal charcoal, would be fitted inside each fountain. And granite was needed to keep supplies cool. Iron was cheaper, but it conducted heat and would therefore produce tepid water. Wakefield also pointed out that London's lack of available walls for mural fountains meant more freestanding installations would be inevitable. They simply cost more to manufacture. As the Association intended for these objects to appear across London's busiest thoroughfares, aesthetic considerations were also paramount to the fountains relationship to existing buildings and street furniture. They needed to be of a high architectural quality. Wakefield reassured prospective donors that all of these stipulations could be compatible with judicious economy. The Association's architect Robert Keirle, who came up with the design templates, was working in the popular Gothic Revival style. His involvement ensured that a good dose of Christian morality would be encased in the proposed structures. Gender-wise, the fountains were tinged with a male sensibility. Though The Lady's Newspaper had described the fountains as innately feminine, it was common for the objects to be referred to as 'handsome' by members of the Association.[41] Apart from the fleeting figure of Mrs Wilson, its cast was all male. At the outset, the 'masculine' standard fountains were rolled out around the city. One anomaly was a Water Lily design for the daughter of the famous British tea and coffee merchant, Thomas Twining who was another high profile member of the group.[42]

The Art of Persuasion, and Persistence

A major challenge the Association faced was the carved-up management and ownership of London's public spaces. Bureaucratic barriers came in the form of parish vestry committees, the Corporation of London and the Metropolitan

Board of Works. The fundamental change the latter wrought was bringing together representatives from the City and the vestries to co-operatively work towards improving drainage, paving and lighting in their respective areas. One would think that all plumbing matters would fall under this collective command but, somewhat ludicrously and inconveniently, the vestries remained in charge of decisions about altering any mains supplies or pipes in their parishes. Given that there were fifty-four parishes, communicating with them all and reaching consensus with any, let alone all of them, was some task.

On top of this challenge, engineers from each private water company had to be consulted about every installation. Translating fountains from the drawing board to locations and, finally, functioning objects was complex. The process revealed much about the workings of the Victorian city. Some of the issues were petty and painfully parochial. Concerns ranged from the possibility of the fountains becoming a gathering place for unsavoury characters, to parishioners having their Sunday Best splashed by overflows.[43] Certain vestries saw the scheme as an opportunity for generating some cash and charged the Association to use their ground.[44] Where there was benevolence, there was also business.

The fountains also fell outside the official state mandate for London's sanitary overhaul, so members of the Association had to convince officials, probably already harangued by their public duties, time and time again of their value. Unless these individuals were evangelically waving temperance flags, or avowed campaigners for equitable drinking water access, co-operation was unlikely. At least in the Square Mile Gurney's status as a banker appeared to ease negotiations at least with its management.

In summer 1865, after six years of work, the Association measured its impact during a twenty-four hour survey. Conducted in July, the figures certainly testified to the popular use of the fountains. At St Sepulchre's, 2647 drinkers were recorded; at London Bridge there were more than 3,000 people quaffing that day and in Bishopsgate, 6,666 people were chalked up as they rehydrated.[45] Either temperance had been taken to with amazing zeal, or these amenities proved that there had been a gaping chasm in public water sources, at least those deemed to be safe.

Free Water?

The notion of the private, corporate water flowing freely outdoors was novel. At that point, people could still be prosecuted for giving away, or selling domestic water, such was the value of having a safe supply on tap. For the Association, the problem was that the fountain water was not free. Who was going to pay for a continuous, daily supply of water to hundreds of fountains in perpetuity? Individual donors had signed up to purchase a tangible object but to pay for the liquid was a more abstract gift. Representing donors in water was rather more challenging than in stone and possibly less appealing to potential supporters.

One pragmatic voice had raised the water cost issue at the inaugural meeting but his tentative words were lost in the excitement of the occasion. W.F. Cowper had emphasised Melly's point about free water: 'It is desirable the water rates should be paid by local bodies, the association only erecting, or contributing to the erection of, and maintaining the mechanical appliances of the fountain.'[46] Whilst Cowper's point was astute, what he was suggesting was more complex in London than in Liverpool. In Melly's city, one body controlled its water supply. In London, the pipes of the eight different private companies were snaking around under the streets. Wherever these pipes pierced the ground for a new fountain, that patch of public thoroughfare could be under the jurisdiction of one of many organisations. In whose interest was it to foot the bill? It was unlikely that any of the Association's members could have forgotten about the cost of water, when they all had to pay for a supply to be piped into their own homes. But the outlay for private water versus public water was a very different affair.

Some vestries were convinced of the fountain's local benefits and committed to the whole cost of the water supply. Other vestries agreed to pay a share, and some refused to contribute to any of the project's costs at all. In the City of London, Gurney must have wooed the Commissioners of Sewers and Highways. The body agreed to pay the full cost for a number, though not all, of the fountains on its territory. No organisation was bound by law to embrace the Association's charitable scheme. Even where agreement was secured, pro-fountain committees inevitably changed membership over time. Whilst the granite remained fixed in place, there was no guarantee that the water supply would flow without the consistent willpower of some party or other. In the Association's 1867 report, donors were reminded that, of the capital's 100,000,000 gallon daily supply, 'every drop in this vast store is the property of water companies, who require to be paid for all they deliver...enabled by steam power and engineering skill to supply the wants of their customers by forcing their water into every house in London'.[47]

Obsolete fountains would not look impressive. To ensure that donated fountains did not run dry, the Association either had to pay for the water supply itself, or convince water companies to become donors. This angle had the advantage of good public relations for the corporations. Even in homes equipped with plumbing, the supplies purchased from the companies were notoriously intermittent. Taps often ran only once a day, during which time householders filled up as many storage containers as possible and used the resource gradually.[48] In the competitive water marketplace, having a company's name etched into public space, as the New River Company's had been on Gurney's first fountain, could not have been bad for business.

The New River Company donated ten guineas per annum to the scheme in 1861, though whether that money was for water alone was not stated.[49] Certainly by 1867, it granted a free supply along with Grand Junction and Vauxhall Water Companies.[50] The annual cost for each fountain had been calculated at about five pounds, so Chelsea Water Company's subsidised 'two-pounds per annum' rate reflected a decent donation (about £100, in 2011). Before its first decade was out, the term 'free' had become such a misnomer that it was evident why the charity dropped the word when it elongated its name to the Metropolitan Drinking Fountain and Cattle Trough Association to embrace public water provision for animals (troughs can be seen across contemporary London today, often operating as flowerbeds).[51]

Fountain water was not free, so wasting it was also controversial. Some companies stipulated that the quantity of water should be controlled by the installation of a tap to prevent waste. The Association found maintaining this system impractical because of the 'rough usage to which it [the tap] must always be exposed at a street drinking fountain'.[52] This surprising operational fact reveals that, without a tap, the fountains ran continuously day and night, despite the furore about the expense of water. The Association quoted from the fountain gospel of Charles Melly once more, to justify the need for a constant flow of water. Melly advocated that the sight of running water was attractive; it naturally cleansed dust from clogging up the apparatus; fountains were perceived as operational and reliable; the water could be heard at night and more drinkers would be served rapidly during busy spells because a tap would not have to be turned on and off each time somebody drank.[53]

The West Middlesex Water Company did not want the function of its public supply to supplant the need for domestic water. The company wrote a letter of complaint to the Association about water being carried home from a fountain in Chiswick for private use and threatened to cut off its supply unless a tap was installed.[54] Unsurprisingly, that company was not a free water donor to the Association.

Relationships with the companies were uneven. By 1873, the East London and New River Companies both retracted commitments of a free supply and began to charge for a metered rate, Chelsea stuck to the subsidy system, whilst Lambeth charged the full rate.[55] Only Southwark and Vauxhall offered an entirely free water supply, along with Kent Water Company.[56] The Association was at the mercy of the whims of corporate water culture.

The Long Haul

Water supply was a necessity but maintaining each object was also critical to ensuring they were the great 'boon' to London that the Association had claimed. Once the idealism of the early years abated, the organisation's improvised operations had to enter into some nuts and bolts pragmatism. For instance, in order to manage a programme of maintenance, the Association had to be informed about instances of damage. There was also the inevitable wear and tear to installations as the first decade took its toll.

A concern that arose only months into the Association's operations was the weather.[57] As autumn turned into winter, temperatures plummeted and pipes threatened to freeze and crack. Problems also came when water over-spilling from the constant flow caused a hazardous, frozen surface to form around the fountains and the possibility of turning London's streets into an impromptu ice ballet was not entertained.[58] The Association's committee decided that the fountains needed to be turned off during frosty weather. After that first winter, operations revolved around the 'season'.[59] For those people who had come to rely on the free water source, losing it during these months must have affected their daily consumption. Horrifyingly for the temperance supporter, perhaps the thirsty returned to the comfort of the public house?

Maintenance needs increased with the volume of fountains. Fittingly, Gurney's own installation was the first casualty, with the loss of a few bricks. Some parishes that had agreed to participate in fountain upkeep reneged on this commitment. After a couple of years, the fountains in Mile End and St Mary's, Islington, were said to be in a disgraceful state.[60] Deliberate vandalism, such as stolen cups, was common — one man was even imprisoned for fountain vandalism[61] — but accidents were also inevitable. Consequently, an ad hoc programme of maintenance was supplanted with a bi-weekly inspection and cleaning routine for each installation, swelling the presence of the Association's maintenance staff amongst the array of street workers.

By the mid-1860s, neighbourhoods across central London had fountains dotted along their arterial routes. Poor neighbourhoods such as St Giles, Mile End and Whitechapel all had provision to cure drunkenness, with mural fountains installed outside workhouses. Many fountains were also located in strategic proximity to public houses. Copycat fountains also began sprouting up without the involvement of the Association. Perhaps fearing that neglected objects, built under the baton of others would tarnish its name, the Secretary was instructed to write to the daily newspapers in 1866 urging corporate bodies and private individuals to place all dry and dilapidated fountains under the care of the Association at once.[62] Soon it took responsibility for ensuring the water supply and maintenance of all London's fountains (whether or not they were under the Metropolitan Fountain Association's official banner). Commitment to a high quality service was fuelled by the extraordinary calculation that up to 400,000 drinkers a day were using these amenities in 1867.[63] If it was exaggerated, the fountains must certainly have been busy enough for readers of the Annual Report to credit this kind of figure. Such use conveys a sense of how significant a part of daily life the fountains had become.

Charitable Brewers

Temperance was still in fashion. Zealous claims were made in the Association's literature that the fates of the thousands who are now ruined in body and soul, the occupants of lunatic asylums and prisons might have been saved by drinking from water fountains.[64] The National Temperance League and the Vulcan Temperance Society were donors and Gurney also promoted his cause at the Band of Hope's annual meetings.[65] The latter's objective was to divert young people from parental alcoholic paths. Meetings took place at Exeter Hall on the Strand, a building at the centre of London's evangelical Christian world. It was also a venue where middle-class brewers could go and salve their beer-soaked consciences.[66]

The Quaker name Hanbury was synonymous with brewing and yet it appeared repeatedly in the Association's list of donors. As the historian Vanessa Taylor stresses: 'Drink traders were to be found at all levels in the Association: as executive committee members, vice-presidents, trustees, regular subscribers and occasional donors. Most were members of Samuel Gurney Junior's family network, which remained central to the Association from 1859 into the twentieth century. Apart from the Gurneys, this comprised members of the Fry, Hanbury, Hoare, Buxton, Barclay, Bevan, Bell, Birkbeck and Pelly families.'[67] Such outright hypocrisy was tied up with Victorian class relations and moral politics in which brewers were keen to profit whilst remaining respectable.

In John Stuart Mill's 1859 book *On Liberty*, the political philosopher criticised temperance culture by decrying how 'the limitation in number, for instance, of beer and spirit houses, for the express purpose of rendering them more difficult of access and diminishing the occasions of temptation, not only exposes all to an inconvenience because there are some by whom this facility would be abused, but it is suited only to a state of society in which the labouring classes are avowedly treated as children or savages'.[68] One can imagine Mill furiously penning this statement from a cosy nook of a heaving Victorian pub. During the national debate over pubs closing on Sundays in 1864, a left-wing professor of political economy also went on the offensive. He raged: 'The poor man's Sunday dinner is to be spoilt, while the gentleman or tradesman who keeps a cellar may enjoy himself...The working man will not stand this sort of legislation. Every sober and respectable man who has been accustomed all his life to fetch his beer for his Sunday dinner from the public-house round the corner, will feel himself personally insulted when he finds the shutters up, and the law tells him that men of his class cannot be trusted with intoxicating liquors.'[69]

Voices of the fountain users are conspicuously absent from the Association's records. Members were evidently convinced that they knew what was best for the population at large. A brief glimpse of a fountain user's view arrived in a letter from one Mr Day. He requested permission for boys to sell lemonade powder at the fountains. A cold response was recorded in the minute book: 'The Committee decided that it would not be advisable to adopt Mr Day's suggestion.'[70] Sticky hands spoiling donor fountains might have aroused disdain. Newgate Market butchers also wrote a sarcastic note to Samuel Gurney, published in the *City Press*, praising him for his great temperance reform.[71] One gets the impression that they got their refreshment elsewhere. Listings for publicans in a contemporary business directory filled more than ten pages (in a very small typeface), so the clash of cultures was not insignificant. Fountains were often situated in close proximity to licensed premises. Some of the great names in British brewing found emblazoned on public houses were also neatly listed in the Association's annual reports. Social status could be accrued by donating drinking water whilst raking in beer profits.

Bombastic Benevolence

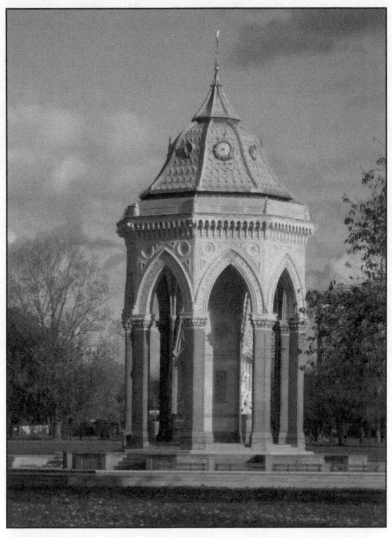

Victoria Fountain (restored), Victoria Park, London, November 2012.
Author's own photograph.

High society figures were attracted to the Association's work. Angela Burdett-Coutts, the wealthiest heiress in Britain at the time, donated a fountain to Victoria Park in East London in 1862.

With its 'rus in urbe' design, the park embodied the contemporary spirit of environmentally led social reform. Under the watch of the government's Commissioner of Works, who happened to be W.F. Cowper, Victoria Park was a high profile urban reform project. However, this donation was not to be credited to the Association. Angela Burdett-Coutts was the only name to be connected with the gift.

Named the Victoria Fountain, her sixteen-metre high and twelve-metre wide canopied edifice, replete with Gothic Revival arches and cherubs, cost the equivalent of £250,000.[73] Burdett-Coutts favourite architect, H.A. Darbishire, was the designer. Drinkers could be sheltered under the canopy as they refreshed themselves, from cups inscribed 'Temperance is a Bridle of Gold'. If the spectacle of Connemara marble from the west of Ireland and pink marble was not theatrical enough, the fountain's unveiling on a summer's day was equally audacious. The unveiling was a major social occasion, at which two brass bands played and some 10,000 spectators were in attendance according to *The Times'* reporter. Local newspaper coverage heaped praise on the benefactress, gushing that the gift showed her Christian love, and that 'she knew the wants of her fellow-creatures'.[74] Burdett-Coutt's over-the-top gift reflected the Association's success for tapping into the environmental and moral reform zeitgeist in the highest of social echelons. She set the precedent for flamboyant fountains.

The M.P. Charles Buxton, who was also a member of the Association, followed her extravagant lead; however his fountain had a less egotistical function. It was produced at arms-length from the association, perhaps because it was an intensely personal project, as its inscription suggested: 'This fountain is intended as a memorial to those members of Parliament who, with Mr Wilberforce, advocated the abolition of the British slave trade, achieved in 1807; and of those members of Parliament who, with Sir T. Fowell Buxton, advocated the emancipation of the slaves throughout the British dominion, achieved in 1834.'[75]

This was Buxton's memorial to his father. With a budget of £1200 the architect S.S.Teulon, a rebel interpreter of the Gothic Revival's principles, was let loose. The fountain was sited in Parliament Square and unveiled in March 1866.[76] Solemn, yet ornate, the object's arched octagonal structure with an eight-metre spire. In its original state, the fountain was surrounded with bronze figures, each one representing a British ruler from Londinium through to Pax Britannica. The modern innovation of brightly-coloured enamel overlaid on its iron surfaces, as a technological buffer to the effects of air pollution, was applauded by critics.

In the summer of 1866, however, cholera revisited London. One week's death toll, as recorded by the Registrar General, was 2,661 people.[77] Those victims were concentrated in East London. Just a few years earlier, at the other end of the social spectrum, Queen Victoria's husband Albert had died suddenly from typhoid fever[78] (now known to be a bacterial disease transmitted via faeces or urine).[79, 80] Bad drainage at Windsor was blamed, but precisely how it was transmitted was contested.[81]

During the ensuing resurgence of political and public debates over sanitation, water and disease in the late 1860s, the subject of public drinking fountains did not arise. As we have noted, they were peripheral to the official sanitary revolution that was underway. As the state was fast creating a template for modern sanitation, the notion of water access on the street perhaps evoked a somewhat retrogressive step towards the medieval city of conduits, rather than a plumbed-in metropolis as the flagship civilisation of the British Empire. Still, in the margins of the Victorian city's sanitary upheavals, sufficient donations enabled the Metropolitan Drinking Fountain and Cattle Trough Association to continue its charitable work.

London's 1875 drinking water map showed that it had built 276 fountains across the capital, financed by a plethora of

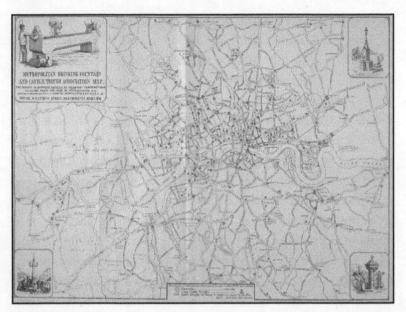

Metropolitan Drinking Fountain and Cattle Trough Association Map, 1875. City of London, London Metropolitan Archives. Courtesy of The Drinking Fountain Association.

donors.[82] But the infamous 'water question' was still far from being resolved.

Whether water was being pumped into drinking fountains or domestic cisterns, the public health furore over the role of this 'basic good' in epidemics was still being contested. How water could be scientifically determined as being conclusively good or bad for human health was to transform by the end of the century. But the process of that transformation was by no means smooth.

Chapter Four

The Birth of Bacteriology and the Death of Corporate Water 1866–1899

'...the Londoner may go to bed at home in full confidence that he could hardly find a town in the country so free from the dangers of the tap.'[1]
(*The London Water Supply*, Arthur Shadwell, 1899)

The tap water quality guarantee that Dr Arthur Shadwell proclaimed all Londoners could enjoy by this point may have been debated by his readership.[2] As a medical professional, who had reported in 1892 from the front line of cholera epidemics in Germany and Russia, he was more than aware of the dangers the tap could dispense. His confident statement demonstrates that, by that point, drinking water had divided into two clear categories: either it was safe or unsafe for human consumption. This chapter investigates how, by the close of the century, it was science rather than social reform that led drinking water and sanitation standards into the twentieth century.

Testing the Waters

Post the 1866 cholera epidemic, those who were already convinced about the theory of water-borne disease transmission had good reason to view the tap with suspicion. The disease's recurrence posed at least three questions. First, could water companies be breaching the Metropolis Water Act's requirement that water should only be abstracted from above Teddington Lock? Second, were filtration methods failing to remove the cause of disease? Third, was the ongoing construction of London's subterranean plumbing still permitting sewage to leak into mains water pipes? As the sleuthing carried out by John

Snow had demonstrated, cholera's presence could be traced to a particular company pipe, but what test could detect water's contamination *before* it was transmitted to the consumer? Preventing epidemics required an accurate method of water testing, which scientists struggled to devise because of the yawning gap between theory and practice. Essentially, scientists were not sure what they were looking for under the microscope.

One French researcher was suggesting a new view of organic matter's presence in liquids. We can thank France's love affair with wine for driving Louis Pasteur's research. His advances in microbiology — though the science did not yet have that disciplinary title — were focused on preventing the unidentified diseases that destroyed vats of profitable wine. Pasteur built on research conducted in the 1830s that proved the involvement of living, organised beings in both making and spoiling alcohol.[3] His experiments in 1864 endorsed that nascent theory by demonstrating how these tiny life-forms could be starved of life by heating wine to a precise temperature for a minimum duration.[4] Despite the evidence of life shown by Pasteur, the infusoria (as these unexplained agents were named) remained in the realm of chemistry.[5] His discoveries did not cause an immediate link to the contemporary understanding of water quality, however, it is significant that microbiology's gradual emergence was mirrored by the struggle to conclusively analyse water quality in Britain.

As mentioned in chapter two, London's water analysts were divided into two camps. Microscopists remained at large in the second half of the nineteenth century, but chemists won the prestigious contracts for advising the government.[6] London was centre stage in the profession's development.[7] Though public health was a national campaign, the scale of London's social problems, married with its status as the national and imperial capital, made disease prevention an imperative there.

With the Metropolis Management Act of 1855, Medical Officer of Health posts were created in 1856 to keep a local eye on diseases and their potential causes.[8] Officers were part of a developing public health administration as the pendulum of the water question swung from quantity to quality. Other experts were needed to decide whether new sewage removal and treatment methods were improving water quality. The professional status of a 'water analyst' was relatively obscure in the late 1850s, when this post was created within the offices of the Registrar General. William Farr was also still based in that office.[9] As we learned in chapter two, the statistician worked with Snow during his groundbreaking research in 1854.[10] Farr evidently had a more than cursory interest and faith in the connection between drinking water and disease. As his *Oxford Dictionary of National Biography* entry states, he 'used many of his reports to demonstrate the waste of human life caused by preventable diseases'.[11] When the celebrated chemist Dr Edward Frankland was appointed as the department's water analyst in 1865, in Farr he had at least one sympathetic and learned colleague in situ.[12] The urgency of Frankland's task was soon augmented by the new cholera outbreak in the summer of 1866, in East London. Statistics from the Registrar-General's office, for late July and early August, recorded circa 1,000 deaths a week from the disease.[13] *The Times* report of the latest figures poignantly noted: 'It is remarkable how large a number of the victims are very young children.'[14] This comment included London's weekly toll of around 300 deaths from diarrhoea, showing the extent of the waterborne and sanitation issues.

At that point, Frankland's method of water analysis failed to detect a source of cholera but later that year, as historian Christopher Hamlin points out, he began to read the water patterns differently.[15] The chemist began to separate water's microscopic constituents into two identifiable groups; decay and life. His growing expertise led to his enlistment as a consultant to the government's *Royal Commission on Water Supply*, which was first launched in 1866. From that point, there was a serious focus on water examination.

Tests on various corporate water supplies for the commission produced hard data to show that filtration's efficacy was patchy.[16] Success or failure was measured in degrees of clarity or turbidity. Frankland found that only the New River and West Middlesex companies had achieved a consistently clear water standard. 'Very turbid' water was recorded in supplies produced by Chelsea, Lambeth, and, with its grand double-barrel title, Southwark and Vauxhall companies.[17] In 1869, a local Medical Officer also recorded that Southwark and Vauxhall's product still left much to be desired, when he likened a sample to 'diluted pea-soup or to a yellow November fog'.[18]

Evidently, the clause of 1852's Metropolis Water Act stipulating that companies must achieve 'effectual filtration' was not being satisfied in that corporation. This is not surprising when engineering techniques were open to interpretation and no company was being put on trial for failing to meet these standards. In response to hard evidence of water quality disparities, the government's Privy Council dispatched a recently appointed Sanitary Inspector, Mr J. Netten Radcliffe (a sympathiser with John Snow's theories), to inspect how various company filtration regimes and technologies differed.

Wading through Mr Netten Radcliffe's in-depth 1869 report, the *Turbidity of Water of Certain London Companies*, graphic details about water treatment practices, including Southwark and Vauxhall's filtration method are available. Prior to filtration, that company allowed water to subside in reservoirs before transferring it to filter beds. These beds were constructed from layers of sand and gravel of varying coarseness, forming a total depth of six feet, six inches.[19] In general, vast spaces were required to hold the quantity of water to be poured into these enormous sieves. In East London, for instance, the Middlesex Filter Beds occupied ten acres (today, the beds are preserved as a wildlife sanctuary in suburbia).[20] Between the Southwark and Vauxhall, and West

Middlesex, companies the former's pea soup appearance and the latter's crystal clear product were found to be the result of subtle variations in the thoroughness of subsidence and differing ratios of water-quantity-to-filtration surface area.[21] West Middlesex's subsidence technique was extremely thorough and its ratio of water-quantity-to-filtration surface was low. Southwark's was the reverse. However, a third company — Grand Junction — with a similar profile to Southwark and Vauxhall in terms of subsidence and filtration method produced water that was only 'occasionally' turbid. In the end, the factor unique to Southwark and Vauxhall's infrastructure and procedures was found to be its complete lack of 'storage or service reservoirs for filtered water'.[22] Post filtration, this company's water was transferred directly out of the filtration system into the engine wells and pumped into the mains. This infrastructural gap was thought to cause the fluctuations in filtration speed, which in turn produced a negative effect on water quality. Still, the value of such detailed inspections was restrained by the use of the naked eye to read water quality as simply clear or turbid.

For Frankland, the invisible was becoming more pertinent to his view on determining drinking water quality. One interpretation of the chemist's view of water pollution was offered by the Chief Medical Officer, John Simon, as a 'skeleton of sewage'.[23] It was certainly an evocative, if repulsive, phrase. But pollution was not the *Royal Commission of Water Supply's* only concern.

The *Royal Commission on Water Supply's* other objective was to explore the 'practicability of obtaining large supplies of water from the mountainous districts of England and Wales'.[24] There was a prevailing sense in the public health establishment that London's water sources could never be wholesome, with or without effective analysis. That view of water's literal dirt was paralleled by an ethical critique of its corporate ownership, control and governance.[25] A statement from the Registrar General's office in the Commission's 1869 report clarified its anti-corporate-water position: 'There seems to be no efficient means of enforcing an observance of this provision of the Act [Metropolis Water Supply Act 1852], and the neglect of the companies to comply with it...shows the necessity for some change in the system of supervision to which the supply of the Metropolis is subjected.'[26] A House of Commons committee reached the same conclusion.

Within the din of these arguments, it was the overriding desire for a *constant* water supply that became the most audible cry for a change in London's water management (not achieved since the 1852 Act). A description of the intermittent supply to one neighbourhood was used as evidence of this great need: 'Smaller service pipes, into which the water is "turned on", as it is called, during only one to two hours each day, the consumers receiving during this short time the whole quantity required for the day's consumption, and storing it for use in cisterns provided by themselves. On Sundays, as a general rule, no supply is given but exceptions are made by many of the companies in poor neighbourhoods where the receptacles are insufficient.'[27] These storage arrangements were deemed to be responsible for the proliferation of diseases in poor areas, whilst in wealthier homes the cisterns were considered to be inconvenient because of the cost of their maintenance and repair.

A stunning suggestion was emerging from the Commission's 1869 report that was finally given voice in the conclusion, that 'a sufficiency of water is too important a matter to all classes of the community to be made dependent on the profits of an association'.[28] The report suggested that London's water be managed municipally, like Dublin, Glasgow, Liverpool or Manchester. John Simon, Medical Officer to the Privy Council, passionately endorsed this conclusion in his own public health report of the following year, writing that the water companies' 'colossal power of life and death is something for which till recently there has been no precedent in the history of the world; and such a power, in whatever hands it is vested, ought most sedulously to be guarded against abuse'.[29] Simon also pointed out that no water company had yet been sued for negligence. There was certainly no shortage of data to support any claims against the water suppliers.

Despite the swell of anti-corporate sentiment, the public versus private water ownership argument was parked for a couple more decades. Legislation consolidating the Commission's findings still ensured radical changes to meet the daily water needs of Londoners.

1871's Metropolis Water Act enforced the demand for a constant water supply. For the first time, Londoners might enjoy running water on Sundays.[30] All the companies had to comply with the act swiftly; within eight months. Not only was the supply to be regular; but its distribution had to be engineered to reach the top storey of any building in London, no matter how high.[31] Co-operation from property owners was mandatory. Providing and maintaining plumbing for pressurised mains water to be conducted through their buildings became a legal duty. The protocol for transferring to the new regime was strict. A water company had to announce, in the press, its intention to switch to providing constant supply in a particular district, after which landlords had two months to deliver their ends of the bargain. If the landlord failed to comply, premises were categorised as unfit for human habitation. Essentially, a new standard of living, in water terms at least, was set. Significant clauses concerning quality also appeared in the Act. A Water Examiner post was created within the Board of Trade, with the authority to 'inspect water quality'.[32] The terms of those inspections mutated as the discipline of bacteriology gained notoriety.

Germ Theory and Table Water

When Dr Robert Koch's observations of bacteria's reproduction on slices of potato led to his 'germ theory' of disease being reported in the early 1880s, the theory was met with scepticism in some sanitary circles. A report from the 1884 *International Congress of Hygiene* in The Hague referred to the 'supposed germ of cholera' and, the following year, a journalist attending the Annual Sanitary Institute Congress in Leicester reminded his readers of the doubt which shrouded the German doctor's analyses: '...even if the germ theory of cholera were accepted to be true.'[33] But, as one science historian claims: 'The development of solidified culture media by Koch was without a doubt the most important single development in the history of microbiology after the perfection of sterilisation techniques.'[34] Germs were still the preserve of scientific professionals for a few years, as the discipline of bacteriology became more widely practised in London's laboratories and was applied to water analysis.

In the domestic sphere, a drinking water filter from the first half of the 1880s and the appearance of a new drinking water product by the end of that decade shows how germs entered the public domain.

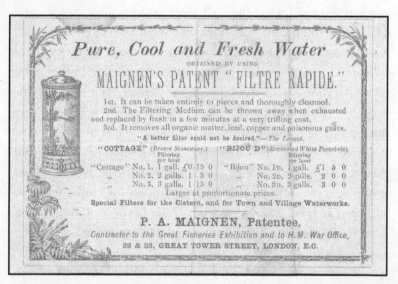

Advertisement for Maignen's Patent Filter Rapide, 1883. Wellcome Library, London.

An 1883 advertisement for a dining room filter for the London-based purveyors of the *Maignen's Patent Filtre Rapide* assured would-be customers that 'it removes all organic matter, lead, copper and poisonous gases'.[35] Germs were not mentioned. Customers could opt for a plain brown Cottage Filter or a Bijou Filter; the latter was decorative white porcelain. Whatever ones aesthetic preference might be, from a functional point of view the size was commensurate with the rate of filtration. The most expensive filter, at £1 15d. was said to produce three gallons of filtered water an hour. Maignen's filter was apparently superior to other brands on the market (at least according to its promoter) because it 'is so easily cleaned and renewed'.[36] Other filters, claimed a chemist vouching for the product, were feared to do more harm than good to health because they gathered dirt.

By 1889, the negative publicity about germs relationship to public water supply opened up the market for new drinking

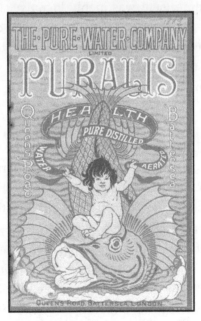

Advertisement of the Pure Water Company, Battersea, ca. 1889.
Wellcome Library, London.

water products, such as *Puralis* by the Pure Water Company.[37] A reporter from the *Pall Mall Gazette* visited its producer's premises in Battersea the same year. There, 'pure' water was being produced through distillation, for use as 'table water' and even for a luxurious, lime-free bath as a beauty treatment for ladies.[38]

The Pure Water Company's proprietor pronounced to the Gazette's reporter 'we cater for the masses' and his sales testified to a successful product, with figures doubling in ten years from 10,000 to 20,000.[39] Not all of these purchases were for the London market. Mr Hartley's product was also being shipped to Egypt and South America, where the gospel of temperance had spread. His advertisement's claim that distilled water was the only reliably pure water was backed up with a quote from Professor Frankland, no less, reminding consumers that boiling water was not a guarantee against germs. Perhaps Frankland did not trust the general public to sufficiently boil their water. Either that, or his product endorsement was highly lucrative. The Pure Water Company was also conscious of the need to differentiate its product from mineral water brands: 'It is well to bear in mind that aerated distilled water, not being a mineral water, does not lower the system. It can be drunk daily.'[40]

The Balfour Commission

The same year that the Pure Water Company was touting its wares (1889), the London County Council was formed. It was not long before the infamous London water question arose as a governance issue for the Council.[41] Should it be the controller of London's water supply? That question was central to the proceedings of the Balfour Commission (named after its Chairman Lord Balfour), or the *Royal Commission to Inquire into the Water Supply of the Metropolis*, which held its first session in Charing Cross, on a spring day in 1892.[42] Discussion of depleted water supplies dominated the Commission, amidst fears that London's water was running out.

A contributor to the Commission's enquiry, Mr William Booth Bryan, engineer to the East London Water Company, blamed people rather than the hydrological cycle for the low reserves. In Booth Bryan's view, shortages were the result of 'the carelessness of the poorer class of their customers. The alien immigration in the east of London had especially caused an immense amount of waste'.[43] He cited clothes washing techniques by the 'aliens' as one cause of lavish water use and the engineer relayed to the commission how he had personally observed taps that had been left running from a train (it must have been slow-moving for Booth Bryan to catch such details). East London's growing demand, with population growth, did raise the topic of where water might come from other than the Lee River. Drawing from The Chalk aquifer beneath London was one option but there were concerns that its use might deplete the New River's sources for middle and upper class homes in Islington.

Such tensions over future water resources and their distribution between different corporate providers, and their diverse customers, renewed the question of municipalising London's water supply. Within the debate on that subject, one pro-municipalisation representative from the London County Council voiced his concern that the Council might be obliged to supply public fountains for free.[44] This reference to drinking fountains is a rare mention of the public sources in official sanitation discourse, but it suggests their prominence in daily life at that point. Despite the fears germ theory unleashed in some London circles, 16,452 people were recorded drinking from three fountains maintained by the Metropolitan Drinking Fountains Association, over twenty-four hours at Clapham Common, Bishopsgate Church and London Bridge in 1891.[45] The Association's drinking fountains count in the capital was 690 in 1892.[46] If the London County Council official read the organisation's latest report then he may have known that it was struggling to cover the costs of building, maintaining and supplying the fountains with water. In fact, the Association was refusing to construct any more because of financial restraints. It may seem like a minor issue in the vast urban water network, but the drinking fountains were a highly visible public emblem of Victorian London's water politics. If water supply moved to state governance and ownership, then should free drinking water be a public service rather than the work of a charity? Free drinking water was an issue far removed from the quantity of supply that concerned the engineers contributing to the deliberations of the Royal Commission.

An engineer from East London Waterworks was convinced that the River Lee's capacity should be boosted 'by means of a system of storage reservoirs'.[47] Other engineers agreed about similar proposals for west London. Mr C.J. More, engineer to the Conservators of the Thames proposed that 'the storage of water in reservoirs at the upper end of the Thames basin would be the most beneficial arrangement which could be adopted for the river generally'.[48] In the Commission's report, storage reservoirs were also recommended for abstractions from both the rivers Lee and Thames, with a combined capacity of 352,000,000 litres but the need for reservoir construction was not immediately enforced on the water companies by law (the significance of this stasis will become apparent in the next chapter). Quality issues also featured strongly in the Commission's final report. On the municipalisation question, the jury was still out.

The Balfour Commission's 1893 report acknowledged that the science of water quality for human consumption had 'passed from the domain of chemistry into that of biology'.[49] Pathogenic bacteria were now accepted as an official threat to drinking water's safety. The report concluded that London's water quality was excellent and pure, citing the lack of Asiatic cholera as one reflection of the supply standard.[50] Even so, recommendations for quality assurance were made: 'In order to preserve the wholesomeness of the water as delivered to the consumer and in order further to meet the not unnatural sentiment against drinking water, which, though wholesome, has been polluted at an earlier stage, all possible vigilance should be exercised to prevent unnecessary contamination of the Thames and Lea and their respective tributaries, to ensure the thorough treatment of all sewage, before it is allowed to pass into the rivers, by the most efficacious methods that science and experience may dictate, and to enforce the adequate storage and filtration of such water as is abstracted at the intakes.'[51] Filtration regulations were also to be stepped up and enforced by the Public Water Examiner.

A new understanding of the interdependence of drinking water quality and sanitation was becoming integrated into environmental and urban policy decisions. 1894's Thames Conservancy Act legalised the Commission's recommendations and instituted the prevention of pollution in the river's catchment area, specifically for the protection of water for 'domestic supply'.[52] For the first time in its history, London's primary water source became a conservation area.

The Franklands

Also in 1894, a seminal text that applied germ theory to water quality was published. One of the authors of *Micro-Organisms in Water* was Edward Frankland's son, Percy. Initially he followed in his father's footsteps as a chemist, but was seduced by the modern lure of bacteriology. The book's second author was Percy Frankland's talented research colleague. She was his wife.

Grace Frankland was a scientist, a writer and an illustrator. When the husband-and-wife team's book hit the international science shelves, her drawings of bacilli showed the frail intricacies of the world she routinely viewed through her microscope.

The rational style of her translation of bacillus from the lens to the page shows how the era of sensationalist animalcules had evolved with the establishment of microbiology as an official

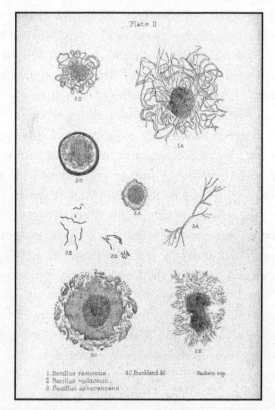

Grace Frankland's sketches of bacilli, Plate 2. *Micro-Organisms in Water*, Percy Frankland and Mrs Percy Frankland (London: Longmans and Green, 1894). Wellcome Library, London.

science. The Franklands' research was groundbreaking in applying bacteriology, as a branch of microbiology, to drinking water. This explained how they realised that after Koch's 'the possibility was at once opened up of approaching the solution of problems connected with water-supply which had long been matters of dispute and speculation amongst hygienic authorities'.[53] In practice, they had already been working on developing solutions in the context of London's water supply.

Percy Frankland was employed to apply bacteriological analysis to the Lee and the Thames for the first time in history, between 1885 and 1888.[54] His tests revealed seasonal variations in the microbial population such as that in the wetter months the rivers became increasingly laden with agricultural effluent from land upstream. How could water be treated to offer protection from the pathological microbes such material, or other effluent, carried?

Micro-Organisms in Water reflected on the outcome of tests that the Franklands had conducted on different water companies' filtration results. Their analyses of slow-sand filtration practices showed surprising results. Generally, the technique reduced the presence of microbial life effectively.[55] Variations in filtration methods across the companies provided data about which techniques caused the most potent levels of bactericide. Quirks in London's treatments, rather than standards, furnished the scientists with rich bacteriological evidence about water treatment. They noted how these variables were innately beneficial to progressing their discipline: '...in no two of them is the process at the present time carried on under precisely similar conditions.'[56] Filtration's success in removing bacteria, good or bad, was naturally not known when the Chelsea Waterworks Company invested in London's first 'monster' filter, as Flora Tristan christened it in the 1830s.

The efficacy of domestic water filtration, in bacteriological terms, also concerned the Franklands: '...suspicion has fallen upon filters as a class', they reported.[57] Filters were clearly a lay device thought to improve the quality of water to a wholesome category, suggesting generally safe use after filtration for drinking and cooking. But by the time the Franklands published their book in 1894, they assessed the contemporary fashion for filtration, remarking that 'it is becoming not an uncommon practice with many to boil suspicious water intended for drinking, and thus to dispense with filters, or, at most, to use them only for aerating the water after boiling, and so remove the flat and vapid taste possessed by boiled water'.[58] Boiling was also in vogue on the other side of the Atlantic. The Franklands cited an 1890 *New York Medical Record* article, which explained the devastation caused to water's microbial population when it was boiled for five minutes at one hundred degrees centigrade.[59] This method for sterilising water was only just percolating from the scientific community to other literate publics.

Another accidentally beneficial factor in the production of healthy water, documented by the Franklands, would be highly significant in the future of modern water treatment. During their experiments, the bacteriologists discovered that the containment of water before it was filtered caused organisms to die off rapidly: '...a process of starvation may go on, for the organisms present in the impounded water find themselves imprisoned with a limited amount of sustenance...'[60] They suggested that the relationship between water's storage and bacteriology needed further research, in London and internationally.

The scientific gauntlet they threw down would be picked up, but not until the next century. By then, Grace Frankland had been elected a 'Fellow' of the Royal Microscopical Society when she was forty-two; a high honour for a female scientist (her application to the Chemical Society was rejected).[61] Before that Fellow accolade was bestowed on her in 1900, London's century-long water question drama had a fraught closing act.

A series of 'water famines', as they became popularly known, turned the possibility of water shortages, raised as a concern during the Balfour Commission, into a live issue.[62] Strangely, these shortages were not called droughts but 'famines', perhaps more aptly given drinking water's dietary necessity. Consequently, the pitfalls of a disjointed system of water management and ownership re-entered the public and political spotlight.

1895's harsh winter caused widespread damage to mains pipes. Customers in Lambeth and riverside residents from Kew to Rotherhithe (served by Southwark and Vauxhall Water

Company) lost supplies temporarily, or completely. The Lambeth Water Company unleashed seven hundred men to repair pipes.[63] In the districts where supplies were entirely lost; the company dispatched other staff with water carts for dehydrated households. In spite of these measures, there was a public backlash against the water companies. One critic blamed the impact of the natural disaster on the companies' failure to lay their pipes at sufficient depths to withstand the effects of the frost.[64]

Just months after the havoc wrought by 1895's cold weather, a hot summer severely depleted the River Lee's reserves. East London inhabitants suffered. According to *The Times'* Special Correspondent 'the most numerous and indignant complaints have come from Hackney', where the 'very poor' and 'middle-class population' were both reduced to three hours of running water instead of a constant supply.[65] In Hackney Wick, categorised as very poor, stagnating sewage was blamed for fatal cases of diarrhoea.[66] Shortages recurred in 1896.

Notices were posted by the East London Waterworks Company in July stating that supplies would be restricted to six hours a day.[67] Furthermore, 'consumers are advised to fill any available vessels while the water is on, to use it strictly for domestic purposes, and beyond all things to avoid WASTE in any form. Persons are especially cautioned against using water for gardening or other similar purposes'.[68] Another company notice warned that 'WILFULLY or NEGLIGENTLY' wasting water would lead to penalties of £5, with re-offenders risking their supplies being deliberately severed.[69] A blame game unfolded, with the public accusing the companies of exacerbating natural causes by poor operational control, whilst the East London Waterworks Company's management was convinced that consumers were wasteful. Casting doubt on the behaviour of the poor was a familiar dynamic in the paternalistic culture of the water companies and public health reformers, but this power dynamic was being unsettled by the increasing enfranchisement

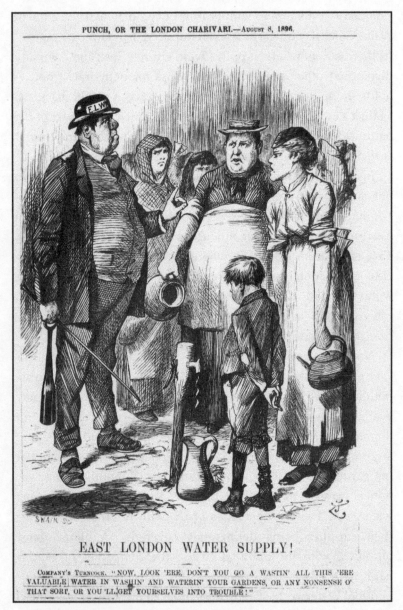

East London Water Supply. Punch or the London Charivari, 8th August 1896. City of London, London Metropolitan Archives. Courtesy of Thames Water.

of the (male) public.

In *Punch's* satire depicting the social outfall of the water shortages in East London, it is hardly likely that the women featured could have washed many pairs of socks or watered many plants with the vessels they were being berated for using.[70]

Drought did not strike East London again in 1897 but its recurrence in 1898 brought public outrage to a head. Again, supplies ceased to be constant and householders could only turn on their taps for three hours each in the morning and evening.[71] Notices with instructions in Hebrew reflected the impact on East London's Jewish residents.[72] Whether English speaking or not, consumers were vocal. Frank Trentmann and Vanessa Taylor's research exposes how the water famines revitalised Water Consumer Defence Leagues born in the 1880s after a high profile court case when a barrister successfully challenged the inequity of corporate water rates.[73] The East London Water Consumers Defence Association, for instance, was pro-municipilization and threatened to boycott payments to its water supplier in lieu of periods when supply waned.[74] These disgruntled consumer experiences echoed decades of jibes against corporate water ownership and management from state public health officials, medical professionals and, in this final decade of the century, the London County Council. Trentmann and Taylor have established how this period forged consumer empowerment in London specifically because of the ongoing water question. Their argument ties this new consumer consciousness more broadly to citizen entitlements in the modern city, due to water's core value in defining and providing a civilised standard of urban life.[74]

The case of London was indeed complex but more fuel was added to the water question's finale by events some forty miles away from the city.

Typhoid started claiming lives in Maidstone in September 1897. By the 8th of October, *The Times* reported that 1,457 people in the town had been diagnosed with the fever. The same article mentioned that a company had donated 3,600 bottles of soda water to the sick, reflecting the knowledge that all was not well with the piped water supply. Progress in water science was officially evident from the engagement of a bacteriologist, Dr Sims Woodhead, to advise Maidstone's water company.[75] He proposed using a chemical measure usually only employed to treat sewage; 'chloride of lime', or bleaching powder.

Chemical sewage treatment commenced commercially in the late 1840s alongside the development of land-based treatment (sewage farms), due to public health legislation and the commercial opportunities associated from re-using the human waste that had to be removed from public sight.[76] By the late 1850s sewage treatment became industrialised and 'cream of lime' was routinely added to deodorise and disinfect sewage.[77] Then, disinfection was not understood in the context of germs. But by 1897, a disinfectant meant something very different to bacteriologists. Even so, Sims Woodhead's solution for Maidstone was maverick. Rather than merely filter water or analyse its chemical and bacteriological constituents, this scientist wanted to *treat* water. Adding ingredients into water was novel.

Maidstone's radical water treatment solution was covered in *The Times*, as part of an ongoing series of articles about the epidemic. Though it was by no means headline news, the procedure was described in some detail: 'About ten tons of lime were mixed in the reservoir with 200,000 gallons of water, and afterwards the mains throughout the town were charged at full pressure with the solution.'[78] The article conveyed Dr Sims Woodhead's view that new cases of typhoid were likely to be secondary and, therefore, that his move to disinfect the water was a reassuring precaution. Apart from an experiment in Worthing with quicklime, the bacteriologist said that he was unaware of any other trial with chloride of lime in public water supplies, in the country.[79] A week later, the success of the treatment appeared to be vindicated in the latest article covering the epidemic. Its author noted that only one new case had been identified in the preceding twenty-four hours.[80] The flushing of the mains with chloride of lime most likely involved about thirty per cent active chlorine in the solution, as a one-off emergency measure. There was no suggestion that such a chemical treatment should be continuous.

Back in London, a new Royal Commission on London's water supply proceeded before the close of 1897.[81] Debating the water companies' future and the viability of a municipal alternative was the Commission's central purpose; the former point was clearly shaky post-famine and the latter was being pushed by the London County Council (it had presented two bills to parliament, unsuccessfully, in 1895 and this very year). A subsidiary issue was whether London's water supply could be brought from elsewhere, on the model of other cities, such as Glasgow. Siphoning the virgin waters of Wales' pristine mountain lakes might solve both the quality and quantity questions.

On this proposal to lay one hundred and fifty miles of pipes from Wales to London, the writer Arthur Shadwell wryly commented: 'What is to prevent an Irish American from blowing up the aqueduct at some point and leaving London without half its water…?'[82] He argued in his populist fin de siècle review of the London water question that the subject had become a 'political question' since the formation of the London County Council.[83] Anti-corporate-water sentiment was being expressed, wrote Shadwell in an 'orgy of vituperation' in which 'good manners' and the 'amenities of civilised life are thrown to the winds'.[84] He defended the companies' reputations on the basis that water had been disease-free for thirty years.

Shadwell was stretching the statistical truth and also displaying yet another example of the time lag between scientific and lay knowledge. For instance, infant mortality statistics from diarrhoea did not figure in his equation even though the disease was still prevalent.[85] Diarrhoea contracted from sewage-infected water was an ongoing symptom of the malaise running through the second half of the nineteenth century's sanitation debate. In short, sewage and drinking water should never mix. Following germ theory's absorption into public health research and practice, bacteriologists were looking into alternative forms of sewage treatment. Public Analysts, as they became professionalised, were pivotal for the resolution of drinking water analysis and treatment, and sewage treatment, by bacteriological means.[86] One public analyst in particular would revolutionise drinking water science in the first two decades of the twentieth century.

Before that could happen, the ownership and governance of water supply radically altered. As the sun set on London's nineteenth century water questions, the era of private water was also fading fast.

Chapter Five

ChloriNation 1905–1933

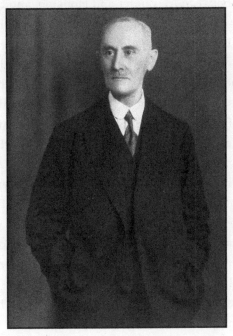

Sir Alexander Cruikshank Houston (undated). Photograph by
Whitlock & Sons. Wellcome Library, London.

*At the time of his death and for many years previously he was
generally recognised as the greatest and most progressive
authority of water purification not only in England, but in the
British Empire, and probably in the world.*
(Obituary Notice for Sir Alexander Cruikshank Houston,
1933)[1]

Google 'Alexander Houston' and the results lead with the
Wikipedia entry for the American heavyweight boxer, followed
by his Facebook profile.[2] In the next page of results, a restaurant

review for J. Alexander's in Houston (Texas) appears. Add 'Dr' before the name and a mere five results appear. Of those five, only one relates to Britain's leading exponent of modern drinking water analysis and treatment of the twentieth century. Insert 'Cruikshank' between Alexander and Houston, and the bacteriologist does surface. However, these results only list his own books, or contributions he made to seminal water treatment texts of the early twentieth century. Little is written about him by other authors of popular history and his mention in the academic sphere is also scant.[3] Even a search in the online archival catalogue of Britain's national Science Museum draws a blank.[4] Fortunately, records of his work during the early twentieth century are held at the London Metropolitan Archives — courtesy of Thames Water's deposits for its predecessors — and the opening quote from his obituary is preserved in the library of the Wellcome Trust.

In this chapter, these existing wisps of evidence about the work of Alexander Cruikshank Houston are thickened up with fresh archival research to resurrect a scientist who should be a household name, at least anywhere in the world where citizens enjoy a safe supply of drinking water on tap.

Wanted: A Director of Water Examination

1902's Metropolis Water Act changed the ownership and governance of London's water supply to a municipal body. The Act included a critical clause that instituted the principle of public health in water's management for the first time. 'Chemical and bacteriological examinations of and experiments as to the condition of the water supplied' had to be conducted by the new Metropolitan Water Board.[5] 'Buildings, apparatus and plant' to conduct these examinations and experiments were to be supplied by the Board.[6] Periodical reports about water quality also had to be published for the water examiner of the Water Board who had to be hosted by the Metropolitan Water Board, at the drop of an

Edwardian bowler hat.[7]

Essentially, the 1902 Act legislated for institutions to monitor water quality, overhauling the shortcomings of its legal predecessors (the Metropolis Water Acts of 1852 and 1871).[8] Now, water quality would be systematically investigated *within* and *without* the water supplier. This transformation did not happen overnight. There was a period of transition when the London water company directors were paid off, their brands dissolved and assets transferred to the Metropolitan Water Board.

The Board started its operations in 1903. Two years later, the structure for the examination of water quality was still being moulded. And in 1905, a stark reminder of the havoc caused by undetected pathogens in urban water supplies was provided by another English city.

Lincoln, the cathedral city in the north east of England, was hit by a typhoid epidemic. On 9th February 1905, the *Daily Mirror* reported that the death toll was already 500. As the newspaper's correspondent wrote: 'A general feeling of alarm pervades the city. Restaurant-keepers and mineral-water manufacturers endeavour to reassure their patrons by advertising that they are not using corporation water.'[9] The report reveals how far lay understanding of waterborne disease had progressed, and also that mineral water was still fashionable amongst some consumers. The arrival of an 'eminent bacteriologist' in Lincoln the previous day was also announced; one Dr Houston.

Alexander Cruikshank Houston was born in 1865, in the colonial city of Mysore, India, where his father was the Surgeon-General. He returned to Britain to study medicine at Edinburgh University, graduating in 1892 with a doctorate in Public Health and Forensic Medicine.[10] From the outset of his career in water research, his interest in the subject was entirely related to its role in public health, namely drinking water. Houston's first assignment was in the north of England, where he spent several years refining his water analysis skills by testing samples in moorland bogs. In the late 1890s Dr Houston joined the water science elite in London. He worked as a researcher in the Local Government Board's laboratory at St Bartholomew's Hospital alongside the internationally acclaimed bacteriologist Dr E.E. Klein. There he realised the scale of research needed to progress his discipline's relationship with sewage and water analysis for safeguarding public health.[11]

In 1898 Houston researched the waste end of the water spectrum when he was enlisted by the London County Council to study an experimental treatment of sewage in bacteria beds at Barking and Crossness, where Bazalgette's pipes deposited their cargoes. Houston must have had a strong stomach. He later reflected on this period: 'At the time when this enquiry was commenced, hardly anything was known of the biological composition of effluents from bacteria beds.'[12] By 1903 he concluded that bacterial sewage treatment should eventually replace chemical treatments for effluents entering the Thames; only on the grounds that the lower portion of the river was not used for abstracting any water destined for drinking. Characteristically, Houston qualified his recommendation with a caution that years of research were still needed by many 'competent workers' before a full understanding of the process of bacterial sewage treatment could be reached.[13] As a personality as well as a scientist, he was notoriously cautious about making grand claims about positive experimental outcomes. During the late 1890s, the Doctor. was also a consultant to some of London's water companies and in this period he perfected a method for measuring levels of sewage pollution (technically the presence of bacterial coliforms, known as b.coli), in water.[14] The standard he established for determining whether water was bacteriologically pure or not was the absence or presence of b.coli per one hundred cubic centimetres of water. His technique was well advanced by the time his services were called on to address

Lincoln's typhoid crisis.

Dr Houston made a rapid analysis of the city's water supply and issued a prescription. *The Times* announced that the bacteriologist and his colleague, Dr MacGowan, 'recommended treatment with hypochlorite of soda'.[15] Retrospectively, Dr Houston recalled how the pair tensely observed 'the behaviour of a certain goldfish in a tank to which a specimen of the chlorinated water was admitted before it passed on to the town'.[16] Evidently the goldfish thrived, because the hypochlorite of soda proceeded until further notice. Following Maidstone's lead in using chloride of lime to sterilise its mains pipes after 1897's typhoid epidemic, this was credited as 'the first systematic use of chlorine in water disinfection' by the water scientist Joseph Race when he penned a history of the radical chemical in 1918.[17] This procedure's distinction from Sims-Woodhead's trial in Maidstone was twofold. The chemical compound had advanced and it was applied as a continuous measure, not just one-off sterilisation.

Chlorine was 'discovered' in the eighteenth century. Swedish chemist Carl Wilhelm Scheele identified an obstinately persistent substance whilst tinkering with magnesium in 1774 but it was only in 1810 that the highly toxic gas joined the periodic table.[18] As an industrial product, the chemical was patented as 'chloride of lime' at the turn of the eighteenth century.[19] In this form, chlorine's toxicity was muted within the substance of slaked lime. Cream of lime's seemingly miraculous power of draining the colour out of any material it came in contact with was of great interest to the Scottish linen industry for instance.[20]

Prior to chloride of lime's use in sewage treatment in the midnineteenth century, one prescient observation about chlorine's biomedical effect appeared in the Lancet medical journal. A Bristol-based doctor, Mr Lansdown, wrote to the Lancet in 1834. He was having some success treating cholera with a medicine called calomel. The doctor shared the confusion he had experienced when he realised that his administration of calomel for its 'purgative' properties was causing a 'remedial' impact.[21] Reflecting on this medical puzzle, the doctor wrote: 'I then thought of the chlorine which it contained, upon which I determined to try the chlorine with another base.'[22] Cholera also abated with this brew. What Mr Lansdown had deduced, pre-bacteriology, was chlorine's bactericidal properties. Some seventy years later, Dr Houston understood precisely why a medicine with significant chlorine content had successfully extinguished cholera. The chemical killed the cholera vibrio bacterium. The concentration of chemical in Lincoln's water had to be precise to balance the need to purge typhoid bacteria and for the water to be drinkable as a new ingredient of the daily municipal supply.

The Times' Special Correspondent in Lincoln, who must have sampled the treated water relayed that it had a 'marked mineral taste and smell'.[23] His scepticism about the merits of the chemical's use was supported by the view of a health professional who believed that it was responsible for causing an increase in colic, irritation of the skin, mucous membrane and eczema, in Lincoln's population. The journalist concluded his article uneasily: '...no one can say what may be the effect of chlorinated water, however dilute, as an article of diet.'[24] When *The Times'* reporter returned to Lincoln city a month later, he remained sceptical about the efficacy of chlorination. He claimed that drinking water was being brought into the town from elsewhere because nobody would drink what was on tap. Apparently the tea made from the public water supply was 'excessively strong and bitter, as if stewed'.[25] He did not dispute the fact that there were no new cases of typhoid, apart from secondary infections. All bacteria, including the offensive typhoid bacillus, in Lincoln's water supply were extinguished at the hands of Drs. Houston and MacGowan. Back in London, the Metropolitan Water Board could not risk a public health disaster like Lincoln's befalling the capital.

In spring 1905, the Board advertised for its first Director of

Water Examination. Dr Alexander Cruikshank Houston applied for the post. He defeated competitors and was unanimously appointed on the 21st of July, 1905.[26] At the age of 39 the bacteriologist was responsible for ensuring that the safety of London's entire drinking water supply, to 6,700,000 people could be successfully proclaimed and attained.[27]

Time and Space

Though critical headway in water analysis had been made by the Frankland family there was still no system in place for the bacteriological and chemical examination of London's water. In fact, the Metropolitan Water Board's Department of Water Examination was the first of its kind in the world. As a public health advocate, Houston's profession fitted with the shift in water supply from private customers to municipal consumers. Health ideals at the laboratory were pursued with pragmatic scientific rigour. Time, patience, and therefore human resources, were needed.

Britain's first metropolitan water examination laboratory was staffed by two chemists, two bacteriologists, two laboratory assistants, six sample collectors and three laboratory boys; all under Houston's direction.[28] The team worked in a four-storey building equipped for the 'Chemical and Bacteriological Examination of Water' on Nottingham Place, just south of Regent's Park.

In the first of Houston's monthly reports, he recorded that his team had examined one thousand samples of London's water chemically and bacteriologically.[29] In this and all subsequent reports he would remind his readership that his work was entirely dependent on his team of experts. As if to underscore why the testing regime was so critical, at the end of the report he included the Registrar-General's tally of monthly deaths, in London, from typhoid fever (23) and diarrhoea (72).[30] The latter was a notoriously common cause of death for the under-fives, at almost ten percent of the total death rates for this age bracket; in 1909, for instance, the annual figure for diarrhoeal-related deaths of under-fives in England and Wales was 5485 children.[31] This goes some way to explaining how important bacteriological research on water was in transforming future public health statistics, in partnership with improving sanitation and hygiene education, such as hand-washing after defecation. Although the sanitary revolution was well in motion, those on the lowest rungs of London's economic ladder may have been using an outdoor privy rather than a private, flushing water closet.[32] Consequently, toileting arrangements in some backstreets were likely to have remained pretty rudimentary and possibly knowledge of dangerous germs.

Alongside its daily water-testing regime, the laboratory carried out extensive research. This science project would influence water treatment across Europe and America, largely through the dialogue its findings generated in professional journals. For instance, when Berlin-based bacteriologist Rudolf Abel published *A Laboratory Handbook of Bacteriology* in 1907, Houston authored the section on water analysis as *the* world expert.[33]

The laboratory's first research project, documented in 1908, tackled a subject that had preoccupied Dr Houston for some time, which was the effect of storage on water quality.[34] His interest stemmed from the Franklands' comment on its neglect as a topic of bacteriological research. From Houston's direct allusion to their observation, it is obviously something he was itching to gain more evidence of, whether of positive significance to water safety or not.[35] Like all science, the process of elimination was a critical part of developing theories. First under the microscope were samples injected with cultures of typhoid bacillus, to test their lifespan during storage. Such samples were often extracted from a 'freshly removed' human spleen.[36] The researchers found that the decline of the deadly bacillus was rapid during the first week of storage and, over eighteen experiments, the data proved that storage was unfavourable to typhoid's survival. Houston concluded that storage dramatically reduced the total number of bacteria and 'the number of microbes capable of growing at blood-heat'.[37] In the published results, his excitement about this sphere of enquiry is palpable. It was fortuitous that a storage system devised for functional reasons had significant implications, he wrote, for 'the ultimate death of the microbes causing epidemic disease'.[38]

Houston thus proposed that the system of storage across the Board's reservoirs be standardised. Parliamentary powers were obtained for the construction of massive new reservoirs.[39] He noted that the Board's arbitrarily unequal complement of storage facilities was a legacy from the private companies. They merely used reservoirs to store turbid river water until it looked bright and clear i.e. to the naked eye. To the bacteriological mind, this was irrational, even ridiculous.

Time was also a critical factor in the storage-equals-safety hypothesis. The bacilli did not expire immediately, though most did die off in the first week, but the optimum period for storage was still unknown.[40] Initially Houston thought that a one-to-two month storage period was needed for 'raw' river water prior to filtering. In the thorough procedures under Houston's watch, no other element of the established treatment process, such as filtration, was to be altered until more convincing evidence of the new system's use had been accrued. For instance, the laboratory conditions that caused the use of artificially bred 'naked' bacilli were somewhat different from what Houston called typhoid bacilli in 'their pathological clothing' i.e. fresh from the excreta of someone with the infection.[41] As with all of the department's reports, reams of charts detailing the experiments' results were published. In later years, it was claimed that he personally drank multiple samples of typhoid-infused water after the proposed safe storage period, to demonstrate his own faith in the efficacy of the measure.[42]

Cholera was the next bacilli in line for the storage test. In 1909 cholera plagued Russia and there were fears that the disease might reach British shores.[43] Cultures of cholera vibrios were securely transported to the London water examination department from Russian victims. Under the lens, Houston resembled their 'darting motility' to 'a swarm of gnats'.[44] Similarly to typhoid, the bacilli obligingly perished in the storage tanks. Not one could be detected after three weeks.

In the laboratory's 1909 report, Dr Houston underscored the difference in abstracted and storage-treated water when he wrote that Londoners were not 'really drinking raw river water but river water, most of which has undergone a remarkable transformation in storage reservoirs'.[45] During storage nothing was added to the water, or taken away, apart from an all-important ingredient. Time, quite simply, was that ingredient. The leap of faith required to believe that fatal diseases disappeared of their own accord now had scientific proof. Without the investment in a specialist institution for water examination, such time-dependent research could never have been conducted and therefore such significant evidence amassed.

Four years into his tenure as Director of Water Examination, Houston believed that the Board's policy should be to achieve 'epidemiologically sterile' water, even before it reached the final filtration stage. He explained this category as follows: 'I mean water which has undergone such a transformation in the storage reservoirs, as judged by b. coli death rate, that the survival in it of any of the microbes associated with epidemic water-borne disease is almost, if not quite, inconceivable.'[46] But there were fresh scientific discoveries from other researchers to factor into the water treatment and safety equation. The discovery in 1910 that typhoid could be 'carried', following the case in America of Mary Mallon, or 'Typhoid Mary', who infected others without displaying any symptoms of the disease herself, raised new questions.[47] An employee working at the purification and distribution works could be such a carrier. Despite the importance of this possibility, Dr Houston took some comfort from the fact that he had yet to find any typhoid bacilli in the Thames.[48]

Proof of the typhoid-carrier phenomena raised the spectre of uncertainty about how it, or other unknown behaviours of waterborne diseases, might render public water at risk. Dr Houston had no doubt that sufficient storage could prevent any vulnerability from pathogenic bacteria, however he was not advocating that river water known to be of poor quality should be abstracted, just because storage would eventually make it safe to drink. Given that storage depended on time, he needed to reduce the risk of any water entering supplies that had not been adequately stored. Adding something other than time to drinking water therefore had to be entertained.

When Houston wrote about his laboratory's experiments with using chloride of lime in the water treatment process, in 1912, he was quick to point out to his readers that the method was not being explored because of the weight of popular opinion about the ill effects of London's hard water on health — not to mention the unsatisfactory soap suds it produced — but because of chloride of lime's germicidal properties.[49] Houston dismissed claims that hard or soft water had any impact on health. He reassured his readers with the following explanation about perceptions of different watery tastes: 'The first thing that occurs when a water is softened is the neutralisation of the free carbonic acid dissolved in the water, which reputedly gives the water its "bite" and flavour. Thus a softened water, in the opinion of many persons, has a mawkish and flat taste. On the other hand, people accustomed to drink a softened water are apt to consider that a hard water has a sharp, almost "steely" taste. The truth is that people get so easily and rapidly accustomed to the change in the taste of a water, produced by its softening that the matter soon ceases to attract any attention.'[50] He clearly had a finely-tuned water tasting palate by this stage.

An 'excess lime method' was developed by the laboratory to maximise sterilisation impact whilst minimising chlorine's lingering after-taste. Houston commented that the method presented a solution to the considerable challenges with water quality in urban wells, which suggested that they were still a presence in some parts of the city.[51] A problem with the lime technique, however, was the substantial cost of the equipment and maintenance. On the other hand, Houston argued that it reduced the need for building new, expensive storage reservoirs. His ninth research report ended with an evangelical statement in favour of the excess lime method: 'Its complete fulfilment would raise the purity of the Metropolitan Water Supply to a pitch of perfection never before attained, if ever seriously contemplated as possible, by any water-works authority in the world, dealing with sources of supply comparable to London.'[52]

Public Water under threat

World War One disrupted the methodological pace of the laboratory's work. Houston had two fears about the war's effect on water security. The first was the greater mobility of international pathogens in an increased quantity of people moving to and from London.[53] His second concern was the likelihood of reduced funding for advancing purification techniques. In 1915, Parliament approved the excess lime treatment to commence in addition to the Metropolitan Water Board's armoury of water treatment along with 'storage for seven days and filtration at double the ordinary rate'.[54] These plans were stalled by the economic impact of the war on the price of coal. The fuel was essential for all pumping, including transferring stored water out of reservoirs and back into supply.

Chemicals had never been systematically added to London's public water supply before, but the war forced the pace of progress. Houston's review of 1916 documented: 'In these circumstances, the Staines chlorination experiments started on 1st May 1916 and they have been continued without intermission up to the date of writing this report (October 1916).'[55]

Varying chloride of lime doses were poured directly into the aqueduct at Staines, bypassing the need to pump water from out of the plant's reservoir, until a quantity of '15lbs of chloride of lime per million gallons of water' was settled upon.[56] Trials transitioned to treatment in June 1916.[57] Houston was satisfied that the level of chlorine saturation could not be detected, when reporting 'nor was a single complaint received from the consumers of the treated water'.[58] This was not an insignificant result, considering the supply was serving approximately 2,000,000 homes. If Houston and his colleagues tested copiously from the Staines supply before that momentous release, he did not reveal what went on behind-the-scenes in his report.

Despite chlorination's success, something made Houston uneasy about the need to opt for chemical treatment and he acknowledged that it could be seen as a 'retrograde step'.[59] His ambivalence about chlorination was understandable, given his progress with developing methods that harnessed nature's own processes of purification. He reassured his readers about the reasons for the move to chlorination because of the exceptional wartime circumstances in 1916: 'In times of great prosperity, this view would (rightly or wrongly) have many advocates. Under war conditions, sentiment ought to give way to expediency.'[60] Amidst the war's profound social upheavals chlorination was not a headline-grabbing story. A brief article in *The Times* in November 1916, *Sterilising Thames Water*, reported an 'inexpensive and innocuous substance' was being trialled to improve water quality and reduce the Metropolitan Water Board's expenditure (by £30 a day).[61] Chlorine was not mentioned in the article. The chemical's title might have been deliberately obscured by editors in the interests of national security, given the unsavoury associations with chlorine's other use as a weapon of chemical warfare in its more lethal, gaseous form. Treatment at Staines was rapidly followed by the introduction of the chemical at waterworks in East London, Kempton Park, Hampton and Kew, and West Middlesex.[62] This swift move to chlorination would never have happened outside the economic climate of war and the profound change in the treatment of London's public water supply caused no furore, largely because it went unnoticed outside the professional water sphere. People were, understandably, focused on the more tragic consequences of the war. Like many large, young and male workforces, the Metropolitan Water Board suffered its own losses as Houston sombrely recorded in a post-war report.

Whilst on the war's frontline, the Chairman of the United Alkali Company claimed that his corporation's supply of thousands of tons of chloride of lime for disinfecting water for British troops on the front had contributed greatly to the low losses of life from waterborne disease. This was remarkable for a product that had apparently been 'barely remunerative' before the war.[63]

Chlorination of Water, by the Canadian bacteriologist and chemist Joseph Race, was published in the last year of World War One. The book was dedicated to Alexander Houston in recognition of his world leadership in water treatment. Two American chlorination pioneers were also credited by Race, but the dedication clearly singled Houston out.[64] Notably, it was addressed to *Sir* Alexander Houston. In 1918 he had been knighted by King George V so at least his work did receive recognition during his lifetime.[65]

Joseph Race noted chlorine's controversy in his experience of leading water treatment policy for the city of Ottawa. Typical complaints were that the chemical killed fish and birds, destroyed plants and flowers, and that animals' refusal to drink it proved that the substance was not to be trusted.[66] To counter these charges, Race kept a tank of minnows in chlorinated water over a period of months and announced that none of them died (perhaps he had read about Houston's goldfish tests before flooding Lincoln with chlorinated water).[67] Race was convinced that chlorine was an agent of health rather than harm. To counter the public concentration of chlorine in public water supplies, the Canadian made a pioneering move of his own when he discovered that adding ammonia prior to chlorination did wonders for the tell-tale after taste of the chemical. Race's method was adopted in London, in an example of how dialogue about water treatment was leading to the creation of internationally recognised practices and standards in the western world.[68]

Post-war, Houston was wholly convinced about the merits of chlorination. However, he acknowledged negative public opinion about the use of chemicals in water in his 1921 report when he wrote: '...there is no doubt that the addition of chemicals to drinking water is repugnant to many persons. It is not desirable to ride rough-shod over sentiment in this matter. Far better it is to admit that there are two sides to every question, and to express the hope that time and experience will modify the opinion of the present-day opponent.'[69] Houston defended chlorination on aesthetic grounds, arguing that any trace of its taste was extinguished before drinking, but it was primarily from a public health perspective that he believed in the use of the bactericide: '...the treatment confers absolute, not merely relative, protection against epidemic water-borne disease.'[70] As the Metropolitan Water Board's Director of Water Examination, he was not about to reverse his decision to chlorinate London's supplies. The holy grail of epidemiological sterility had been discovered.

In 1922, Houston further expounded on the merits of chlorination. Countering claims that chlorinated water was "doped", Houston's rejoinder was not gentle. 'Logically, these people should drink only deep well water and water from virgin moorland, or upland, sources of supply ...There is absolutely no convincing evidence that a properly chlorinated water is in any way injurious to health.'[71] His view was pragmatically situated in the reality of the complex urban environment, where nature was inevitably corrupted. Environmental protection legislation was no guarantee that polluting accidents would not occur accidentally, or even covertly.[72]

Chlorination had started as a lifesaving principle in 1905; it had become an economic necessity in 1916 and by the early 1920s the treatment was accepted as an indispensable aspect of modern water supply in industrialised societies. Public health officials from Cuba, Germany, Norway, Russia and the U.S.A. were sent to the Water Examiner in 1924, as representatives of the League of Nations.[73] Mentioning those visitors in his annual report that year, Dr Houston stressed that 'all year round, engineers, chemists and bacteriologists from home and all the four corners of the globe are constantly visiting the Board's Works and Laboratories, and are given every facility for pursuing their investigations. We certainly learn much from their visits by interchange of ideas, exchanges of reports and so forth...'[74] London was evidently at the epicentre of disseminating intelligence about public drinking water quality standards.

Reportedly a very modest man, as a scientist Alexander Cruikshank Houston was clearly something of a celebrity in his field in the inter-war period. In the latter years of his career, more clues about Houston as a person outside the laboratory filtered through his reports, when he indulged in a quirky addition to their scientific subject matter.

Diaries of rambles he took through London's watery hinterlands formed an appendix to these official reports, with hand-sketched maps to illustrate his rambles.[75] The diarist's literary style was unpretentious and freely mixed local history references with contemporary observations. In one ramble he paid tribute to Hugh Myddleton's legacy as he traced the New River from

Hertfordshire to Islington, pausing mid-route to contemplate his surroundings over a pint of ale at a public house.[76] One irreverent recollection he relayed in these diaries was an unusual working day he spent with his colleagues in 1905, when a vast quantity of fluorescein was added to the New River. In order to determine if water being pumped out of adjacent spring wells into the river might have already naturally seeped into it in the first place, they collected samples from the wells along its course, examining them for any sign of a green hue. The results were negative but Houston remembered 'no more fascinating sight than the New River presented on that occasion — like a glorious wide ribbon of shimmering green extending for miles and miles towards London'.[77] He noted public reactions to be 'impressed', 'startled' and 'puzzled', with a child even exclaiming, '"Doesn't the river look lovely mummy?"'[78] The tale concluded on this cliff-hanger: '...the writer was beginning to wonder if his calculations, that the colour could not reach as far as London, were based on sound premises.'[79] If domestic taps in Islington momentarily flowed green, Houston did not disclose.

The Royal Society1933 obituary that opened this chapter paid appropriate homage to the achievements of Alexander Houston. Since then, his name has sunken into obscurity as surely as the public drinking water revolution he masterminded has become taken for granted. One, perhaps unconscious, tribute to his legacy was the birth of the bubble jet fountain, in the decade of his death. The trust in a safe public water supply that this modernist design celebrates was only possible because of the research Alexander Houston masterminded. By the end of the 1930s, the innocent civic pleasure of sipping from the watery arc of a bubble jet fountain was under threat in London.

Chapter Six

Blitz on the Board 1937–1945

No. No way you would have got me into one of those.[1]
(George Billingham, Engineer, Metropolitan Water Board)

'Those', in the above quote, referred to air raid shelters. George Billingham's memories of working as a water engineer before, and during, World War Two are recorded in a rare interview about London's water supply during the war. During civil defence preparations, the engineer personally studied hundreds of proposals from local authorities suggesting air raid shelter locations. As underground buildings, water engineers needed to advise local authorities about the proximity of mains pipes to suggested sites. Billingham maintained that some of his department's recommendations for relocating sites for proposed shelters were dismissed: 'I didn't like the look of where many of these were going, to be quite candid.'[2] He imagined scenarios of shelters flooding with water. For the duration of the Blitz, the engineer refused to enter an air raid shelter despite the subterranean nature of his profession. As Billingham's recollection confirmed, the nightmare he imagined was realised in one air raid shelter in Stoke Newington in northeast London. He does not elaborate on the scale of the tragedy in the interview but, fortunately, he also does not mention any other similar events.

This chapter reveals how imagining the worst was critically important for the defence of London's drinking water supply during the crisis of war. Preparation for the imagined war and its lived experience are filtered through records revealing the efforts to both protect and maintain a constant flow of potable water to the city during the conflict.

Imagining the Blitz

Air Raid Precautions were drawn up at the Metropolitan Water Board long before war was declared. By the end of 1937 conflict was highly likely, if not imminent, and that London would be targeted as the administrative and economic capital of Britain was inevitable.

Commander Blackwell, the Board's Air Raid Precautions Officer, issued a secret document in December 1937 about his plans. In the document, he acknowledged to its select readership the monumental challenge of defending infrastructure that lay below every street and building likely to be bombed. To focus his strategy, Blackwell identified what would cause the most 'serious dislocation of the system of water supply'.[3] Logically, the mains pipes were his primary concern because of their centrality to the supply network that fed all of London's homes and businesses. The Commander was confident, he declared, that sections of mains pipes could be dug out and replaced in forty-eight hours. 'Fouled mains' also had to be considered.[4] Colonel MacKenzie — the Director of Water Examination who replaced Alexander Houston — had been consulted on this point and proposed that portable gas chlorination units were needed for swift responses to mains pipe casualties. The Board's strategists could not ignore the fact that if clean water pipes could be ruptured, sewage pipes were equally vulnerable to damage and, consequently, sanitary mayhem. At that point, sewerage was under the management of the London County Council.[5] To defend London's potable water supply from external and internal threats, the Board mounted its wartime strategy on two main fronts: engineering and examination.

The Chief Engineer issued an outline of his plans to protect the Metropolitan Water Board's infrastructure in 1938. He was concerned about how the source of the supply itself might be damaged. What would happen if aerial assaults contaminated the main waterworks or stopped their supplies flowing? To reduce the possibility of the plants becoming sitting ducks, the windows of Engine Houses were to be fitted with blackout blinds and wire netting.[6] For East London, the mains pipe visibly crossing the River Lee was noted as being particularly 'open to sabotage', so it was proposed that members of the Home Guard patrolled that area in the event of emergency.[7] As the Board's staff did not usually linger in that vicinity, the Chief Engineer pointed out a practical, and somewhat ironic point: 'There is no water laid on at these works for sanitary purposes.'[8] A temporary convenience would be installed. Later in the war, kits for detecting poison in reservoirs were also doled out to each waterworks for the possibility of deliberate acts of contamination.[9]

Before the war broke out, in June 1939 the Metropolitan Water Board issued warnings about how domestic water supplies might be affected in a bulletin issued to householders. *Air Raid Precautions: Advice to Consumers* writ large the reminder that all indoor pipes were the responsibility of householders.[10] The Board would only deal with outdoor, public pipes i.e. those in the sphere of municipal water. Consumers were advised to familiarise themselves with the stopcock's location to turn off supply when necessary to prevent flooding amongst other damage. Domestic cisterns were to be kept clean for reserve supplies in the event of the loss of mains water. Water from cisterns was to be boiled before use. The document contained a recurrent wartime water theme. 'Consumers should do their utmost to economise in the use of water as large quantities will probably be required for fire fighting.' Water's social and economic value was being reassessed.

Phoney War

On 31st August 1939, the Board's Emergency Committee met to plan for the imminent state of emergency. Key men who were on annual leave, such as the Director of Water Examination, were recalled to their posts.[11] Just three days later on 3rd September, the Prime Minister, Neville Chamberlain, broadcast live from Downing Street declaring that Britain was at war with Germany.[12]

For some time the so-called 'phoney war' ensued before London saw any bombing raids, but social upheavals were already in motion. The prospect of the Board losing its youngest and fittest men prompted a representation to the Ministry for Health and Labour about the consequences of a severely depleted workforce.[13] Employee representatives, the National Union of Water Works, offered to come to the Board's staffing rescue, but another solution was soon ratified to redress the imminent labour shortage, for a complement of temporary assistants.

Those assistants were only to 'be women, or men not liable to be called up for service with H.M. Forces'.[14] The move was as novel in the water industry as for the many professional spheres where women replaced men for the first time. These female recruits included Mrs Gardiner, who took up an unspecified senior post in the laboratories, and Miss E.A. Flint (MSc), who became a 'temporary technical assistant in the Water Examination Department at a salary of £400 per annum'.[15] Such opportunities for women in the water workforce presented themselves because of the extreme conditions of the war. However, over its course, seven thousand volunteers were also trained to assist core staff, though the gender of these recruits is not mentioned in the records. Another human resources precaution the Board took in 1939 was compulsory blood testing. Any employees testing positively for pathogenic bacteria were removed from direct contact with the water supply. This ban extended to employees 'suffering from any intestinal upset associated with looseness of the bowels'.[16] Civil defence was also, therefore, mounted on a biomedical front.

As the likelihood of air raids on London increased, Finsbury Borough Council (now Islington) requested that the Board open its air raid shelters and basement to the public.[17] Permission was granted, at least temporarily. Such arrangements, and their use, show how boundaries between work and home life, private and public space blurred, as unprecedented levels of social cooperation was required.

By August 1940, the war's phoney phase was drawing to a close. Mobilising defence operations, Colonel MacKenzie performed a radio broadcast on the 13th of August to teach Londoners about sterilising their water at home. If supplies were pronounced to be unsafe following an air raid, the sterilising method he described was to be used immediately. MacKenzie encouraged listeners to transcribe his instructions: 'Keep in your house a bottle of chlorinated soda solution. Your chemist can supply you with it... Add ten drops of chlorine disinfectant — I will spell that — CHLORINE — to one pint of water. Stir and allow to stand for five minutes or longer. Then add a crystal of Hypo — HYPO. Dissolve this and you may then drink the water.'[18] The last ingredient was intended to neutralise the flavour of chlorine. Hopefully householders faithfully transcribed MacKenzie's lecture and stuck his sterilisation lesson up in their kitchens or bathrooms. The Colonel claimed that only two brands of disinfectants would safely do the job. Those brands were Milton or Chlor-San. London's chemists must have stocked up to the gills after his high-profile announcement. Milton promptly launched its own advertising campaign, for this essential wartime household accessory.

In MacKenzie's message to Londoners and numerous other drinking water missives that would follow over the next couple of years, the same brands were advocated. Milton and Chlor-san cornered a lucrative market, so anybody with shares in the companies was assured of an undiluted stream of profit with bottles going from between six pence to eight-pence (the equivalent of seventy-five pence to a pound in modern currency).[19] For four and a half pence, a slim-line 'emergency flask' of Milton

In war-time emergencies

Keep this for reference.

MAKE YOUR WATER SUPPLY ABSOLUTELY SAFE

If there are raids with damage to roads, waterworks, etc., or other hostilities occur in this country, it is possible that, in some areas at least, the public water supplies will be contaminated.

If this happens the local water authorities will no doubt warn you, but in any case it will be wise to take your own precautions.

Remember that *all* water can be sterilized for drinking and cooking, and the dangers of water-borne diseases eliminated by adding a minute quantity of Milton.

WHAT TO DO IN EMERGENCY

1. If you have been told or suspect that the main water supply is not up to standard add a teaspoonful of Milton to each gallon of water (4 drops to a tumbler or 10 drops to a pint).
2. If the water comes from sources probably contaminated even in normal times, *e.g.*, ponds, water butts, wells, add a tablespoonful of Milton to each gallon of water (16 drops to a tumbler).
3. If the water is *visibly* impure strain through clean handkerchief and then add a tablespoonful of Milton to each gallon of water.

P.T.O.

4. If the main water supply fails (usually first noticed at the kitchen cold or drinking water tap), draw the boiler or hot water fire and keep the storage tank water for drinking and cooking *only*, adding a teaspoonful of Milton to each gallon of water drawn.

N.B.—*If, after adding Milton to the water, the solution is allowed to stand for five minutes, all taste of Milton will, for the average person, disappear.*

Remember—MILTON

recommended* for

water sterilization

★ *Milton is recognized by leading and independent authorities on water sterilization as the best sterilizer for general use, and has recently been recommended publicly for this purpose.*

A.R.P. For grazes, scratches, cuts and wounds, burns and scalds (*for serious wounds and burns a doctor should of course be called*) Milton is the ideal antiseptic —stable and of standard strength, non-caustic and non-irritant.

8d., 1/4, 1/11½, 3/4 per bottle. EMERGENCY FLASK (for pocket or handbag) 4½d.
INCLUDING PURCHASE TAX.

P.T.O. Printed for Milton Proprietary Ltd., London, N.7, by Waterlow & Sons Ltd., London, E.C.2

Advertisement for Milton, 1940. Wellcome Library, London. Reproduced with kind permission from Milton Pharmaceutical Company.

could also be purchased, for slipping into one's pocket or handbag.[20] Handsome sales of Hypo were also guaranteed assuming that the Colonel's safe drinking water drill was obeyed. It was to be enacted when a notice printed in red ink, was delivered through one's letterbox.[21] When the threat was deemed to have passed, a second notice, printed in green ink, gave the all clear. A leap of faith was required to view the tap's contents as dangerous one moment and innocuous the next. Even those who might have been partial to Schweppes' 'table water' before the war, could not have reverted to that option (unless they had a secret stash), as the product was suspended under the Ministry of Food's rationing protocol.[22] Schweppes brand of soda water was still being produced, so perhaps some who could afford it kept a few bottles of that tucked away for emergencies. This seems to be a petty concern in the wake of what followed.

The Blitz

Blitzkrieg, as the German army's lightning bombing policy was named, was launched on 7th September 1940 over London, in daylight.[23] Fifty-seven consecutive nights of bombing followed.[24] On the ground, the Board's operations were directed from a control room in shifts, twenty-four hours a day, seven days a week.[25] Regular shift patterns were replaced by emergency responses. For staff like George Billingham and his fellow engineer Arthur Durling, there were three-day stretches without sleep as they attempted to repair and restore mains pipes.[26] Billingham acknowledged the Board's preparedness for the Blitz in terms of infrastructure but the chaos unleashed by the bombing of London presented an equal crisis in managing scarce human resources. As he reflected: 'The notion that everything could be controlled centrally at the height of the Blitz wasn't possible.'[27] Districts had to focus on local crises.

Effective communication was decimated by the air raids. The telephone system was often down, or inaccessible. For instance the all-important turncocks, who had the equipment and know-how for switching off supplies to mains pipes had to take shelter from the air raids, just like other civilians. Alternative communications came in the form of a 130-person strong fleet of human messengers on bicycles. They worked in shifts around the clock relaying messages between district foremen and turncocks. A mid-war report from the Board recorded the organisation's delight with the usefulness of the 350 pedal cycles that it had purchased before the war.[28] Arthur Durling, Billingham's colleague, remembered travelling to Plaistow on one of those bicycles after a particularly heavy air raid to determine why the pressure gauges in his district had plummeted to zero.[29] He detoured past areas where unexploded bombs were cordoned off, stopping to peer into open fire hydrants. When he saw that air was being sucked into the mains through the hydrants, part of the reason for pressure loss was explained. As he approached Plaistow high street, Durling saw the other reason. A large bomb crater in the middle of the road was filled with water. The engineer vividly remembered that scene: 'The main had been fractured and there were women with kettles from the houses that hadn't been bombed coming out and they were getting their water from out of the crater, and I suggested to them that they'd better not do this because it was probably contaminated.'[30] It follows that the supply these households had lost, or would imminently lose, made any water precious whether it came from a polluted crater or not. For Durling, the contamination of most concern was effluent from sewer pipes also punctured by the bomb.

This collision between the water expert and laypeople highlighted a lack of common knowledge about sanitation. For Londoners who had become accustomed to drinking from the tap without questioning its safety for more than two generations, water contamination was possibly hard to imagine. But the war was exposing the very infrastructure they unconsciously relied on. What normally lay invisibly functioning below the streets was quite literally exposed as streets and roads were wrenched open.

Maintaining acceptable standards of water quality for drinking and quantity for sanitation was becoming increasingly fraught.

The likelihood of poisonous wastewater entering potable water pipes preoccupied Colonel MacKenzie, but some of his colleagues were sceptical about the danger this presented to public health. In their minds, chlorinating water at source was sufficient for cleansing any contamination further down the line. Fortunately, American research concurred with MacKenzie's doubt that such contamination could be removed remotely. The American experiments proved that intensive chlorination, for prolonged and repeated periods was needed to pronounce pipes that had come into contact with raw sewage to be rendered absolutely germ free.[31] MacKenzie pointed out that one could often smell sewage in craters even if it was not visible. He suspected that the more silent culprits were minor stoneware drains from houses. Materially, they were more vulnerable to the effects of bombardment and even small leakages might prove fatal for the spread of pathogenic bacteria.[32] MacKenzie's policy for sterilising all damaged mains pipes after their repair was enacted, albeit in a mode compromised by the conditions of the war.

Arthur Durling recalled how staff worked from charts instructing them on the ratio of chlorine powder to water needed for the diameter of a given pipe.[33] The correct proportions were mixed into a paste and simply poured from a bucket into the hydrants beside the valves where pipes were reconnected to the main water supply. When Durling recounted the procedure, Billingham laughed on the radio recording at the mention of the familiar bleach product — Stabichlor — which was apparently used rather more lavishly than the charts dictated. 'Usually the fellows who were doing it would err on the side of putting rather more in than perhaps the charts said', confided Durling.[34] Humour aside, the engineer proudly concluded: 'We got away with it and there were no cases of typhoid in London during the Blitz and I think that's quite a record because it was a serious problem... if there had been any waterborne disease in London, well it could have done more damage than the whole of the Blitz had done. At least to people.'[35] According to the bacteriological tests, the staff were achieving outstanding results, but the Director of Water Examination was worried about a solution he perceived to be expedient rather than efficient.[36]

When it came to the decontamination of trunk mains (major arterial pipes) mobile chlorinators were dispatched on lorries. Under MacKenzie's instruction 'a fleet of vehicles and drivers for the sole purpose of towing the chlorinators was on stand by'.[37] Chlorination Supervisors were allocated two mobile chlorinators apiece, each with their own Chlorine Attendant. The supervisors saw that the cargo of gas was pumped into pipes at a high dosage of ten-parts-per-million. Though the plan was to flush any trace of the intense chemical dose out of a pipe before putting it back into service, this did not always happen. On this matter of chlorine lingering in public supplies, Colonel MacKenzie reassured the Board: 'There is widespread realisation that a chlorinous taste spells safety, and complaints have been few.'[38] Success rates were convincing. From seven hundred water samples taken from repaired mains after mobile chlorination, only three were found to have traces of faecal contamination. During periods of heavy bombardment, such essential work was hampered by a lack of available vehicles (and presumably sometimes roads) to tow the trailers into position. The possibility of chlorination failing to counter the effects of sewage contamination may have given the Director of Water Examination sleepless nights, even in air raid shelters. By 1941, chlorination philosophy inside the treatment works had also changed. Pre-chlorination was introduced as a 'fourth line of defence', in addition to 'storage, filtration and terminal chlorination'.[39] As the term suggests, pre-chlorination was a process in which stored water was flooded with chlorine before, rather than after, filtration. The measure was a bacteriological insurance policy. Reinforced buildings were constructed to shield the specialist chlorination technology.[40]

When mains supplies were lost, once the bottles of tap water householders had been advised to stash away had been drained and the contents of cisterns emptied, two potential water sources were left.[41] Standpipes were one source. These devices were a form of temporary plumbing, which involved makeshift vertical pipes poking out of the mains onto the street and fitted with taps. Mobile tanks were the second source, complete with a plumbing system that created a row of queue-reducing taps. In both cases, water access reverted to the pre-modern mode of carting supplies from source to the point of use.

Unsanitary City

On the matter of mobile tanks, the Board stated: 'Attempts have been made to distribute both drinking water and "not drinking water", 'the latter being untreated water stored in former oil tanks to be used for sanitary purposes' (effectively, a grey water solution to sustaining water supplies).[42] It was found, though, that drinking water was favoured because people struggled to find sufficient containers to store separate supplies. 'Sanitary purposes' was simply a euphemism for toilet flushing. London's much lauded, internationally replicated, sewerage system was highly dependent on one thing: a constant supply of water. Without it, the civilised City of London was fast becoming an unsanitary place. No alternative sewage disposal system could be mounted without running water. That fact was evident to tenants and office workers in the City of London during May 1941.

Between the 10th and 11th of May, the most widespread

damage to London's water infrastructure occurred, during the final stage of the Blitzkrieg bombing campaign. 605 mains pipes were damaged alongside the dreadful human casualties and deaths.[43] Other water authorities were drafted in to help, from as far afield as Glasgow. Almost three weeks later, the effects were still being felt in the City of London where the water pipes were bone dry. Gerald G. Caney, a solicitor, pleaded that 'the question of lavatories is getting very serious' in his letter to the local Medical Officer of Health.[44] Another City tenant, the director of Oriental Carpet Importers, was also pining for running water to return to his offices, 'particularly for toilet purposes'.[45] The City's Medical Officer offered his reassurance that standpipes would be erected near their premises, although on the proviso that property owners supplied buckets to transport the supply. Given that a period of three weeks after the serious bomb damage had elapsed since Caney's letter and almost two months by the time the carpet importer wrote, the Metropolitan Water Board was evidently under severe strain.

Obviously desperate to secure alternative supplies, City workers persuaded the fire brigade to pump water from its storage tanks into buildings for toilet flushing.[46] Huge containers of water were located in particular streets for fire fighting. One building that received the fire brigade water was the Avenue Telephone Exchange, just north of the Thames in the City. Staff symptoms soon indicated that the untreated water was being used for drinking as well as toilet flushing. In June, the Ministry of Health enquired about reports of an outbreak of gastroenteritis at the Telephone Exchange, potentially caused by contaminated water. Dr Charles F. White, a City doctor, verified 'seventy cases of diarrhoea and vomiting amongst the telephone girls but added that he was disinclined to discourage altogether the practice of using the firemen's water from static water dams in the streets' because of the equally serious health consequences of leaving toilets unflushed.[47] This case shows the difficult balancing act of maintaining safe water for drinking and sufficient water for sanitation, each critical for the protection of public health.

Following the outfall from the May bombings, the national *War Emergency Water Committee* re-evaluated policy. In future attacks on a similar scale, public announcements were to be made via vehicle-mounted loudspeakers to advertise the loss of supplies and dangers of impure water consumption. Stock requests were to be broadcast, such as 'please use as little as possible and help one another' or 'the water in this district is impure. Until further notice it should not be used for drinking or in the kitchen unless boiled or sterilised'.[48]

As the Metropolitan Water Board stepped up its plans for alternative methods of supply to the mains, other water sources also had to be considered in the event of chemical attack. If mustard gas, for instance, was unleashed close to rivers or reservoirs, they could not be used. Planning for this scenario led to a secret census of private wells to elicit the support of their owners for back up supplies.[49] Any doubt about this water's purity would be extinguished by dosing it with chlorine gas whilst private supplies were sucked from underground and transferred to tanks mounted on vehicles. In 1941, The Board's Chief Engineer Mr Cronin was concerned about the cost of these private resources: 'Arrangements for paying the private well owners are still very nebulous and it would be well if this matter were settled before the event...'[50] One problem was that most of these private wells relied on modern electrical pumps; they would be useless if power went down.

Water for Feeding

London County Council was also interested in the results of the well census remaining covert. Its Londoners' Meals Service was set up a year after the war broke out to feed those whose kitchens had been destroyed in the Blitz, or for whom cooking had become unmanageable.[51] Meals were heavily subsidised, or free, to those who met the conditions. The papers of Mr L.J. Dillon, an employee of the Meals Service show how reliant the operation was on a pure water supply. The Council worked with schools and charities to mount the programme of 170 meal centres, including Mrs Franklin's War Time Kitchen in Paddington for Air Raid Precautions personnel and Post Office workers, unemployed women and refugees. Older unemployed people could opt for the Over Thirty Association, located on Shaftesbury Avenue.[52] Blitz Stew was one meal the communal kitchens offered. A vat of 120 portions required eight and a half gallons of drinking water to combine its other ingredients, which were as follows:

'42lbs root vegetables, preferably half to be carrots, cut small
12lbs of potatoes
4lbs medium or coarse oatmeal
5oz. Plantox or Marmite
8 oz. salt
4 teaspoonfuls pepper
2 tbsp mixed herbs
Gravy browning to colour
6 tins of evaporated milk
9lbs pulse vegetables
10lbs fresh meat'[53]

One could not be too choosy about the distinctive flavour of Marmite or the sweetness of evaporated milk, and vegetarians were in trouble, but the stew sounded nourishing. Superintendents were instructed by the London County Council 'to make it routine before leaving the centres in the evenings to fill all suitable receptacles with water and cover the vessels to keep the water from contamination' i.e. gas attack.[54] Additionally, superintendents were reminded not to use any water 'for drinking purposes (including cleaning of teeth) unless a) it has been well boiled or b) effectively chlorinated'.[55] A consistent demand for this service precipitated a conference in July 1941 about *Emergency Water Supplies for Meals Services*. The Council reported that the Metropolitan Water Board's Chief Engineer had 'prepared for us a list of private wells'.[56] As an essential food supplier, this service was given priority for well water. The conference report also noted that large cisterns were salvaged from debris clearance dumps and sterilised for water storage at Meals Service centres. One such salvage centre was Hyde Park. Footage of the park in Rosie Newman's documentary film *Britain at War* shows cisterns stacked high beside orderly piles of household doors and rows of baths.[57]

Imagining Invasion

Although the Blitz ceased after May 1941, the desire to secure access to private groundwater sources was further bolstered in 1942 by preparations for invasion.[58] The Metropolitan Water Board issued permits to ensure that only a limited number of authorised personnel entered water works plants. Quantities of barbed wire on perimeter fences increased and steel doors were fitted at the mouths of tunnels leading to the mains.[59] The *Invasion Defence Scheme for London* instructed that emergency water supplies must be established, in the event that municipal control of water sources and distribution was lost. Strategists envisaged parachute troops descending into waterworks and sabotaging plant machinery. Imagined simultaneously with an air offensive, sparking demand for fire-fighting supplies, the scenarios were pretty apocalyptic.

In the event of land invasion 'water points' were to be set up with an allocation of drinking water 'on the basis of two gallons per head per day'.[60] At these points, well water would be pumped into a tanker, promptly sterilised and doled out in a similar way to the existing emergency tanker drill.[61] Given the deluge of people anticipated at these points, if mains water was lost across London, a test was carried out at John Barker and Company's well source on 28th November 1942, just off Kensington High Street.[62] An orderly diagram recorded how the flow of people, and water, could be managed. These well-served water points were never needed, as land invasion did not occur, but some Londoners possibly accessed water from neighbours' wells when supplies were scarce.

'O For the Water They Waste in Britain'[63]

The above statement was emblazoned across a poster featuring a lone soldier marching through deserted terrain. A giant domestic tap floated surreally in the foreground of the poster, juxtaposing domestic comfort with the harsh reality of life on the front line. Conserving water for both unknown emergencies and the unknown duration of the war was a recurrent theme of the Metropolitan Water Board's public relations campaign during the war. Remnants of the Board's campaign point to a sustained volley of reminders to Londoners about their duty to value water. The sight of untold quantities of water being used to fight fires during the Blitz created a dangerous perception that supplies were bottomless. The Board's Chairman Henry Berry issued a New Year greeting in 1942, suggesting Londoners resolve '**not to fill** the hand basin when washing but to make it a point of honour to reduce my consumption of water to the absolute minimum in this period of national emergency'.[64] Like Dr Houston in the previous war, Berry's wanted to conserve the coal that kept the water pumping into filtration systems and supply pipes.

A sustained possibility of invasion precipitated a national plan to ration the personal use of water to two gallons a day 'for *all* purposes'.[65] Toilet flushing with freshwater was to be supplanted by the use of wastewater. Successfully instilling such behaviour change presented another challenge.

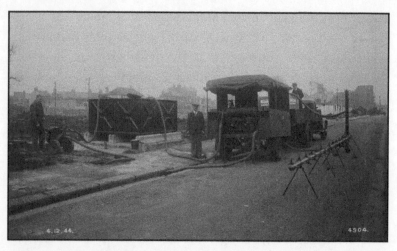

Emergency Supplies, Edward Street, Canning Town, E16, 4th December 1944. City of London, London Metropolitan Archives. Reproduced with kind permission from Thames Water.

Ironically, it was a natural rather than a manmade emergency that caused water rations to be imposed in 1944. A severe lack of rainfall the year before in the London region had affected reserves and sparked fears of shortages. Food could be neatly rationed into packets, tins and weighed in pounds by the Ministry for Food but measuring free-flowing water was more challenging. Commercial water users, such as breweries, had meters but domestic consumers were still charged on the rateable basis calculated by property value (no doubt a value grossly altered by the war and poverty for many Londoners). Between January and May 1944, reports in the national press increasingly highlighted the seriousness of the drought as the summer drew closer.[66] All defects in fittings and leaky taps were to be reported to the Metropolitan Water Board's distribution engineer and the use of hosepipes to water gardens or cars was banned. The need for a Minister for Water was even mooted. The period of water scarcity, amidst the existing wartime austerity was prolonged. In August 1944 London's water scarcity only made a minor news item, despite the fact that the flow of the Thames was 'still one of the lowest on record'.[67]

Some emergency need was still evident from the effects of war and the natural drought in December 1944. A photograph of a mobile emergency drinking water tanker serving Canning Town in East London documented an apparently uncommon sight (mains repair was on the whole reportedly swift and successful).[68] The photograph poignantly conveys the disruption of convenience and comfort through the strange sight of domestic taps relocation outdoors, juxtaposed with gutted buildings and a rubble-strewn landscape.

It is incredible that no waterborne health epidemic erupted in London between 1939–45, despite damage to over 6000 pipes in London's water distribution network.[69] Colonel MacKenzie published an essay in 1945 about his department's measures to safeguard water purity. He proudly quoted a statement from the British Medical Journal, penned in January of that year: 'One of the outstanding public health achievements of the war had been the protection of London's water supply.'[70] MacKenzie's pride about the prevention of waterborne disease was understandable in the context of a city scarred by the loss of 29,890 people during the war.[71] Over 50,000 people were also left with disabling injuries caused by the bombing campaign.[72]

Patriotic pride in London's municipal water protection during the Blitz may have been one factor stoking the controversy that broke out in the 1950s, when a novel new water treatment philosophy from America made its way across the Atlantic.

Chapter Seven

Purity and Poison: 1948–1969

'Fluoridation is undoubtedly the thin edge of a totalitarian wedge.'[1]
(London Anti-Fluoridation Campaign, 1966)

Visions for the post-war landscape were drafted even before the conflict had ended. The London County Council published the first version of its *County of London Plan* in 1943. Housing was naturally central to restoring the stock depleted during the Blitz, however there was also a striking emphasis on the value of outdoor space and how principles of health could be embedded in those designs. As the plan's authors believed: 'Adequate open space for both recreation and rest is a vital factor in maintaining and improving the health of the people.'[2] Other post-war optimists were The Metropolitan Drinking Fountain and Cattle Trough Association, still in business, which announced to supporters in its 1945 report: 'We are looking forward to a future of great activity in replacing structures destroyed in the raids and supplying new ones to the many Playing Fields and Open Spaces that are now being planned by Local Authorities.'[3] The charity was not disappointed. 63 fountains were ordered in 1948 which was the highest number in a single year that the charity had ever installed.[4]

Creating healthy public spaces in that year was an apt expression of a new, socialist medical era. Britain's National Health Service was born in 1948. Concern for public health was paramount to the ideals of the new Labour Government's nascent welfare state, in which free access to healthcare represented an economic commitment to the principle of social justice and equality. Enshrined in the National Health Service Act was the ideal of preventing, as well as curing, illness.[5] This chapter investigates how drinking water became a focal point in the debate over how to deliver this health philosophy of prevention and social equality in a mode that some people were not willing to swallow, under any circumstances.

Visions of Sparkling Teeth

It was in America that the notion of engineering public water to actively improve a population's health first gained ground. News was coming from health professionals across the Atlantic of research and then, in 1945, a trial of chemically enhancing tap water's nutrients with a naturally-occurring ingredient: fluoride.[6] By 1950 American dentists were optimistic about the test results: 'The fluoridation of public water supplies as a partial protection against tooth decay is a tremendous step forward in the profession's fight against dental decay.'[7] The subject of fluoridation entered international public health discourse. Though it was a national issue in Britain, London's experience was contoured by its symbolism as the capital, and also by the complexity of the city's local government structures. Records of the Metropolitan Water Board's (MWB) involvement in the national and local fluoridation debate reveal a period of high emotion, characterised by clashing ideologies about drinking water as an instrument of public health.

MacKenzie remained the MWB's Director of Water Examination after the war. His title was de-militarised by the 1950s from Colonel to plain E.F.W. MacKenzie. The decade had already seen London's post-war austerity relieved during 1951's Festival of Britain celebrations, when the South Bank was transformed into a twenty-seven acre site celebrating 'British achievement in science, technology and industrial design'.[8] If MacKenzie had taken a night-time stroll along the river during the festival, as one of the eight million people who visited, he would have shared the popular sight of a light spectacle illuminating iconic Thames-side buildings, light-based artworks projected into the sky, and even onto fountains and pavements.[9] Whether or not MacKenzie enjoyed this sight, the scientist certainly appeared to share the Festival's curatorial vision that the cross pollination of science and technology could enlighten the future of humanity through new innovations.

In spring 1952 MacKenzie gave a lecture at the Westminster Hospital Medical School. Its subject was fluoridation. His lecture took place midway through the trip of a team that had been dispatched by the British Government to research that very issue. The team had a grand title: The United Kingdom Mission on the Fluoridation of Domestic Water Supplies in North America. Before MacKenzie knew the outcome of that Mission's findings, he was already convinced about the benefits fluoridation could bestow on the teeth of young Londoners, not to mention its effectiveness in cutting the National Health Service's 43 million pound dental bill. This water examiner seemed at ease with his potential role in dispensing an improvement in London's public health. For him it was merely a 'daily supplementation of the fluorine intake in areas where it was known to be insufficient' (fluorine is the name of the chemical in its pure, gaseous form).[10] Importantly to the debate that would ensue, MacKenzie explained that fluoride was already present in all water, but at inconsistent levels. In some parts of America, fluoride levels were naturally higher than others. The effect this had on locals' teeth was a visible mottling of the enamel. Research, initially prompted by this discolouration issue exposed fluoride's agency both as a preventer of dental caries and as the culprit for mottling. When consumed via water, different concentrations of the naturally occurring chemical produced vastly different results.

MacKenzie relayed to the Medical School audience that extensive American-based research into fluorine during the 1930s and 40s had moved to water treatment in some States. America's fluoride research had revealed how precise levels of the added chemical needed to be, in order to achieve the desired effect. As the Director explained from the conclusions of American scientists: '…reduction of caries' incidence in school children might be expected from concentrations of fluorine of between 1.0 and 1.5 p.p.m.' and critically that 'no further appreciable benefit was obtained by a higher fluoride content.'[11] Research underway in the United Kingdom, in the few places where fluorine was at high enough levels to compare with the American studies, was corroborating this view.

Equalising the natural substance involved using an artificial compound: sodium fluoride. Injecting the water supply with fluoride, according to MacKenzie, should not cause any controversy in Britain because of precedents demonstrated by other dietary supplements: 'The ethics of so-called mass medication had been satisfactorily settled in such matters as improvement of flour by calcium, addition of vitamins to margarine or of iodine to salt.'[12] One note of uncertainty that MacKenzie did sound was about the 'possible harmful effects' of fluorine.[13] But there was no doubt from his speech that he was vociferously pro-fluoridation. In his closing words, he posed the American Public Health Association's question about the un-fluoridated States: '"What are the rest of us waiting for?"'[14] 'The same question might well be asked, and indeed is being asked, in this country today', Mackenzie concluded.[15] During his sales-pitch, the Director of Water Examination neglected to mention one critical piece of information. Some segments of the American public were firmly opposed to mandatory fluoridation.

The tale of America's *Fluoride Wars* interprets public response to the first artificial dose of fluoride in Michigan neatly: 'For most, it was another blessing bestowed on us by modern science. But for some, it was one chemical too many.'[16] Members of the United Kingdom's fluoridation mission to the U.S. were well aware of the controversy the subject had ignited there. The visit coincided with the deliberations of a U.S. Government Select

Committee, appointed to *Investigate the Use of Chemicals in Foods and Cosmetics*.[17] In media coverage of the Committee's proceedings, opponents to fluoridation were prominent as the national fluoridation debate ramped up. The U.K. investigators also felt the formidable force of local pressure groups, whose members engaged in public deliberations about the merits of fluoridation. Anti-fluoridation lobbyists in Seattle held enough sway to swing the pendulum completely against the proposed additive.[18]

Tampering with the Tap

Within the MWB's records, the first murmur of opposition to fluoridation in London came from the manager of the *Housewives Today* publication, the mouthpiece of the British Housewives League. In January 1953, a letter sent to the Board, penned by Mr H.F. Marfleet from Stepney Green in East London (clearly not a housewife himself), raised this concern: 'I've heard a rumour that the water supply of the metropolitan area is to be treated with fluorine, which is supposed by some people to be a preventative of dental caries.'[19] Marfleet wanted to reassure *Housewives Today's* readers that the rumour had no basis. The Board's response left the rumour open to further speculation: 'There are no regulations regarding the amount or quality of any substance that may be added to the water. The possibility can, however, be envisaged of the Ministry making regulations in such matters.'[20] It was quite a revelation that additions to the water supply were, in fact, totally unregulated. Chlorine was simply accepted as a necessity.

Four months later, Mr Marfleet issued a complaint: 'As a consumer of Metropolitan Water, I write to register my strong disapproval, and respectfully to ask you to represent this opinion to the Board.'[21] Marfleet feared 'mass medication' would soon be pouring out of his kitchen tap. The same year, the U.K. fluoridation mission to America published its report, which MacKenzie shared with his water examination committee.

Fluoridation's positive impact on dental health was endorsed, as a health measure to top up levels of the substance in areas where it was deficient. MacKenzie acknowledged that public suspicion had to be addressed because of the 'flood of propaganda leaflets and articles' opposing the measure.[22] So despite the endorsement of America's fluoridation policy, the U.K. Mission and the Government remained cautious.

Examples of public opposition in America were cited as grounds for the suggestion that Britain needed its own trials, to supply British-based evidence. A flicker of scientific doubt was also expressed in the U.K. Mission's report: '...evidence of harmlessness is so strong as to be almost conclusive.'[23] Almost harmless was clearly not the same as absolutely harmless. The state's line was to encourage more research about the long-term health effects of 'low levels of fluoride'.[24]

The Times reported from the House of Commons in December 1953 that the Minister for Health, Mr MacLeod, had announced that 'selected communities' would soon experience fluoridation trials. Later on, Norwich was revealed to be one of those trial communities. However, the motion to commence the experiment there was defeated by Norwich City Council in June 1954. 'City refuses to be Guinea-Pig' ran the Manchester Guardian's banner headline.[25] Fifty complaint letters had been received by the Council and none of them were positive about the fluoridation plans.

Four other trials were imminent: Anglesey (North Wales), Kilmarnock (Western Scotland), Andover (Hampshire) and Watford (Hertfordshire).[26] London remained exempt, as Watford lay beyond the MWB's boundaries. Before the trials began, in July 1955 the Ministry of Health issued a 'reference note' to equip health, local governments and water authority officials to defend the virtues of fluoridation.[27] State rhetoric was pitched against increasingly public anti-fluoridation sentiment, encapsulated by one emotive *Picture Post* article entitled 'Hands Off Our Drinking

Water'. Could fluoride enter foetuses or infect breast milk, asked its author?[28]

Language was carefully employed in the Ministry of Health's Reference Note to neutralise the polarised debate. Controlled 'demonstrations' rather than 'experiments' were to take place.[29]

Emotional anti-fluoridation arguments were also addressed in the note, including the belief that fluoridation was poisonous. The Ministry's experts argued that only 'exceedingly high concentrations of fluoride' i.e. of the kind used in industrial processes were known to cause any harm to the human skeleton.[30] It also reassured readers that most fluoride would be excreted in bodily fluids or absorbed as a natural component of the bones. The point that fluoride *naturally* occurred in all water supplies, and therefore *already* entered the human body was driven home: '**What is proposed is to make good a deficiency in those water supplies which lack this beneficial element...**' [publication's bold].[31] Fear was also tackled by the assurance that the fluoride compound to be used in the demonstrations was 'indistinguishable from the naturally-occurring fluoride ion'.[32] Highlighting the chemical composition of water in its raw state ruptured the notion of purity to which anti-fluoridationists clung. What was pure drinking water? The Ministry of Health's answer was crystal clear: 'If it is argued that the addition of fluoride to water affects the "purity" of the water, it can be answered that water in nature is never chemically pure and that most waters have to be treated chemically before they are suitable for supply, about thirty chemicals being used in water works to produce clear and wholesome water suitable for domestic and industrial purposes.'[33] (This was quite an admission.) Of those chemicals, chlorine was paraded as a precedent for why adding substances to raw water, as well as taking them away, could be so beneficial to public health. Like chlorine's prevention of bacterial havoc, the experts argued, fluoride was an equally preventative measure for the health of future generations.

Fluoridation in Andover officially commenced after the trials in 1956 but was arrested by summer 1958 due to public pressure and local councillors failing to be re-elected over this single issue.[34] In Darlington, the Council's decision to try out fluoridation was reversed before trials even began, inspiring other fluoridation opponents to keep campaigning, such as the British Housewives League.[35] In 1959, the League published a pamphlet entitled *Fluoridation — Why and How to Stop It*. The focus of its opposition was now focused on enforcing fluoridation without individual consent: 'The "doctoring" of the public water supply with a substance intended to affect the human body without consent and contrary to the wishes of many consumers, is a violation of such a [human] right.'[36]

Whilst the Housewives League pamphlet was circulating, unbeknownst to its authors, the MWB had commenced fluoridation tests.[37] An internal report divulged that some trials had been made on live works but that the water had not been released into supply. These decisions were under the watch of a new Director of Water Examination, Edwin Windle Taylor. His perspective on fluoridation was less gung-ho than MacKenzie's, but it was evident that he was poised to flick the fluoridation switch if the other English trials were evaluated as successful.

Before those results came through, in 1960 H.F. Marfleet had resumed correspondence with the Board and was told that a decision about fluoridation had been suspended until the results of the trials were made public, due in 1961.[38] Seemingly unsatisfied by this assurance, Marfleet changed tack. A further letter demanded that he be supplied with a list of the 88 names and addresses of each Board member. Anticipating the deluge, the Board's Clerk primed members with a missive about the unfriendly post they might receive. If Mr Marfleet did indeed hammer 88 letters out on his typewriter, copies have not been preserved for posterity in the MWB's archives. Also in 1960, the anti-fluoridation movement consolidated under the umbrella of the National Pure Water Association and the battle marched, with more troops, into a new decade.[39]

In 1962, the long-awaited report on the United Kingdom's fluoridation trials was delivered.[40] The Director of Water Examination reported to his team that the results wholly endorsed American research and that, in the trial areas, five-year-olds' instances of caries had halved since 1955–56.[41] Windle Taylor also wrote that 'no information was received from doctors practising in the areas indicating any harm arising out of fluoridation'.[42] A decision was due on whether the Board would fluoridate London, or not. The legal-technical structural problem this presented mobilised the British Waterworks Association, the national umbrella body for the waterworks industry, of which the MWB was a member. In October 1962, it called for Parliament to act on the matter, on the grounds that fluoridation extended water providers' remit beyond providing wholesome water.[43] The Association argued that legislation was needed '...before any water authority can accept responsibility for the addition of fluoride to the public water supply'.[44]

On 10th December 1962 the Minister of Health, then Enoch Powell, announced to Parliament that, under Section 28 of the National Health Service Act, he was approving 'proposals from the local health authorities to make arrangements with water undertakers for the addition of fluoride to water supplies which are deficient in it naturally'.[45] In the House of Lords, Lord Douglas of Barloch was clearly outraged by the decision, when he spoke: '...may I ask the noble Lord whether consideration has been given to the problem of whether it is legal to add medicines or drugs to public water supply? May I also ask why fluoride should be forced down the throats of everybody, whether they have teeth or not?'[46]

Within days the MWB received a letter from the Ministry of Health permitting it to commence fluoridation, reassuring the Board that local authorities and water undertakings would both

be indemnified against any Court proceedings post-fluori-
dation.[47]

However, that year a question mark hovered over the MWB's
future as legislation was being fine-tuned for a major restructuring of London's governance.[48] In 1963, the London County
Council was abolished and replaced with the Greater London
Council, which would function alongside 32 local borough
councils.[49] From 1965, London's geography would be defined by
610 rather than 117 square miles. This political restructuring
embedded health within the new borough councils, which
would also function as local health authorities.[50] These authorities would therefore decide whether to fluoridate, or not.
Around this vast conurbation, the MWB would still serve up the
vast majority of the population's water (apart from some
peripheral areas) irrespective of borough boundaries. Perhaps
anticipating that fluoridation would prove to be an emotive topic
in local politics, in May 1963 the Board clarified an important
practical point about the prospect of London moving to fluoridation. Internally, the Water Examination Committee's Clerk
declared: 'I am informed by the Chief Engineer that if the Board
decide to adopt a policy of fluoridation, there is little or no possibility of keeping the supply to any particular area free from
fluoride. In other words, none of the local health authorities
could opt out of the scheme.'[51]

Just days later this private statement became public policy.
The MWB would not be 'required to make a decision on the
compulsory administration of fluoride to 2,500,000 people'
without the unanimous approval of London's health authorities.[52] Doubts about transcending its duty as a supplier of pure
water rationalised the decision, along with examples of international controversy. Of these, America's legal battles were cited
along with opposition from medical professionals in Australia.
The latter was an important example of anti-fluoridation opinion
within the peer-reviewed sphere of the scientific establishment,

rather that the spurious factual claims delivered by some lay opponents.

Despite London's fluoridation stalemate, in June 1963 the Ministry for Health issued unequivocal approval for all local health authorities to start introducing the measure as soon as possible.[53] Authorities were to instruct their water undertakers and simply inform the Ministry when, rather than if, fluoridation would be commencing. The Ministry of Health also issued a publication, simply entitled *Fluoridation*. The booklet confronted the core criticisms of 'a small but vocal minority' and its tone was urgent.[54] For instance to the question 'Is fluoride a poison?', the anonymous author retorted: 'It would be necessary to drink at one time two and a half bathfuls of water containing fluoride at a concentration of 1p.p.m. before any harmful effects due to fluoride would be experienced.'[55] Scornful, if slightly comical, statements such as this seemed out of place in an official state publication, perhaps only hinting at what views might have been less-delicately expressed behind the Ministry's closed doors. *Fluoridation* also contested the interpretation of an adjective favoured by the anti-fluoridation lobby: 'pure'.[56] Readers were reminded that raw water contained traces of many chemicals. But the more pervasive question about fluoridation had moved to more ideological territory: 'Are personal liberties infringed?'[57]

Popular concern about environmental toxicity was linked to the health-food zeitgeist. A resident of Stoke Newington, an area associated with alternative culture and politics, wrote to the Board in August 1963: 'Surely the only and best way to combat decay in children is more fresh fruit and vegetables, 100% whole-wheat bread, regular meals and brushing clean after each?'[58] Her view was representative of an international swell of concern about industrialised food production. In America, for instance, the publication of *Silent Spring* by the scientist-cum-environ-mental-activist Rachel Carson in 1962 is credited with inspiring the organic food movement and creating the scientific discipline of 'environmental toxicology'.[59] Public outrage caused by the revelations in Carson's best-selling book about chemicals entering the food chain, and killing wildlife, influenced John F. Kennedy to launch a U.S. Government enquiry into pesticides' impact on the environment.[60] This issue infected British scientific and public discourse, but the response in London was also a product of post-war and Cold War concerns about state interference in the private lives of individuals

By the 1960s, one of the more inflammatory phrases used in anti-fluoridation literature in Britain was 'compulsory mass-medication'.[61] In a document entitled *The Ethical Question is Paramount*, the National Pure Water Association wrote the following: '…it is subversive of personal freedom and medically, socially and politically unethical to use the public water supply as a vehicle for administering to the public any substance which is intended to treat the human body.'[62] Reaction to fluoridation's green light by the Ministry of Health in summer 1963 was met with this and many more arguments.

In August 1963 the Board wrote to the London Anti-Fluoridation Campaign (LAFC) complaining that one of the Board's customers had received a postcard from the Campaign with the following message: 'It is proposed to put a poisonous substance in your water supply.'[63] With barely concealed exasperation, the Board's Clerk wrote that the LAFC was warning people that London's water was about to be treated with fluoride, when it already knew that no such decision had been made; at least not by the Board.[64] The Clerk requested the Campaign to stop issuing the postcards, however, by November some 20,000 of these postcards had fluttered through Londoners' letterboxes. *The Times* reported the story, quoting from the besieged Clerk: 'Dozens of people have written to us saying, "Why are you trying to poison us?" and "Stop it immediately". Many of them are extremely angry.'[65]

This correspondence was the start of many years of heated

communication between the LAFC's Chairman, Patrick Clavell-Blount and the MWB. Having served in the RAF as a catering officer, Clavell-Blount did not believe that the war had been fought for a Welfare State system that was, in his view, corrupt.[66] Several anti-fluoridation activists were serial correspondents to the MWB, however Blount was especially prolific. He produced missives such as *Fluoridation: A Monstrous Violation of Human Rights*. That publication claimed that 'fluoridation was one of the greatest infringements of individual freedom ever to have been attempted in a civilised country'.[67] More understandable was his and others concerns about the long-term health impacts of artificially fluoridated water. The LAFC was somewhat dominated by the voice of Patrick Clavell-Blount, but more powerfully placed anti-fluoridation organisations also bore on the fate of London's water supply and, consequently, its population's dental health. Lord Douglas of Barloch, as the President of the National Pure Water Association, wrote to the Board promptly following the Minister's instructions to health authorities to proceed with instigating fluoridation. The Lord claimed that under existing legislation it would be 'illegal for water undertakers to add fluorides to their supplies'.[68] His warning was bound to make London's water supplier nervous about the solidity of the Ministry of Health's legal protection.

In the records of the Board, the file entitled 'Fluoridation: Supporters' is noticeably slimmer than any of the many 'Fluoridation: Objectors' files. One of the few supporters was Marjery Abraham, who wrote: 'I enclose [a] cheque for my colossal rate. I shall feel it is worthwhile when [you] have made up the fluoride content of the water. You have delayed far too long in my opinion. The propaganda against it is misleading and disgraceful.'[69] A second letter pronounced the anti-fluoridation lobby to be 'ignorami and fanatics'.[70] Unsurprisingly amongst other supporters were the British Dental Association and the Royal Dental Hospital.

Whilst London's water remained 'pure', in 1964 Birmingham took the fluoridation plunge. It was the first city to adopt fluoridation as an outright policy, rather than a demonstration. Birmingham's health authority was convinced that it was a sound preventative health-care investment, in a place where 'three-quarters of the city's children had dental caries by the age of five'.[71] Calculations showed that upwards of £90,000 was likely to be saved by the city's health authority in the move from treatment to prevention.

In November 1965, the Minister of Health, Kenneth Robinson addressed the London Boroughs Committee. His speech applauded the capital's complex democracy but decried that it was resulting in the denial of social justice to young citizens. He pleaded with the councils resisting fluoridation: 'I hope all concerned will recognise in their turn the vital importance of their decision to the children of London...[and] not deny the community they serve.'[72] 'All concerned' were not ratifying national health policy and, despite his pleas, London's fluori-

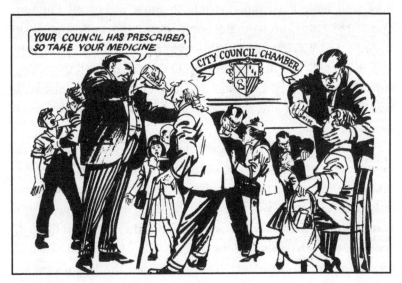

Front cover of London Anti-Fluoridation Campaign pamphlet, 1966
Author unknown. City of London, London Metropolitan Archives.

dation question was still unanswered in 1968.

In the meantime, the Metropolitan Water Board issued numerous stock responses to concerned members of the public stating that health authorities rather than the supplier were ultimately responsible for that fluoridation decision.[73]

Un-Britishness

To clarify the uneasy position of the Board, it wrote to each of the local health authorities to establish which were in favour of fluoridation or not.[74] Responses were tallied in spring 1968. Twenty-four were pro-fluoridation, two had approved it in principle and nine were against the measure.[75] The influential City of London Corporation was an anti-fluoridation island surrounded by boroughs favouring fluoridation such as Southwark and Tower Hamlets. Other opposing borough and county councils were curiously concentrated on the outer edges of the city; Brent in the north and Sutton to the south. Inner city poverty, with resultant poor oral health of many young people may well have been more visible to those in central London. Translated into approximate populations, the opposing areas added up to 918,100 people whilst the pro-fluoridation majority was 6,219,600.[76] Still, the principle remained that the water supply could not be cordoned off to exclude those areas, such was the nature of the technological network and water's very nature as a fluid.

On 26th April 1968 the Board declared an amendment to its own stance on fluoridation: 'That it be recommended to the Board that they take no policy decision with regard to the fluoridation of London's water supply pending the outcome of the Birmingham fluoridation scheme, or the introduction of government legislation on the subject.'[77] In May 1968, a small article in London's *Evening News* publicised the Board's policy decision with the headline 'No Fluoride for Londoners' Teeth'.[78]

As legislation, or a change of mood, in the opposing councils was awaited protest continued into 1969. A statement issued by Patrick Clavell-Blount's London Anti-Fluoridation Campaign was decorated with a list of prominent signatories from the Houses of the Lords and Commons, including the violinist Yehudi Menhuin. '...we do not consider such medication has any place in the British way of life', declared LAFC's supporters.[79]

Even in 2012, fluoride has yet to be artificially added to London's supply. The latest enquiry into the subject, convened by the Greater London Authority, published a report in 2003 and advised against the chemical's introduction. This recommendation was made on the basis of the consent needed from five strategic health authorities in collaboration with four water suppliers.[80] Mass medication was not cited as a reason for the enquiry's conclusion, yet the subject of environmental toxicology is, rightly, remains a current concern.

Public Fountains in Decline

During the span of the anti-fluoridation campaign, a sense of pride and trust in the quality of public water is apparent. That sentiment was perhaps unknowingly reinforced by an international set of *Guidelines for Drinking-Water Quality*, which were first published by the World Health Organisation in 1958. One reason for their establishment was the rise in debate about drinking water safety amongst those enjoying international air travel in the 1950s.[81] Although the United Kingdom was one of the key nations informing the science for these standards, at that point no law for precise drinking water standards had been passed. Faith in tap water did not appear to be affected by absence of legislation in the 1950s and 60s.

Outside the home, drinking water was promoted by modern fountain designs suitable for a variety of potential indoor, public locations. As demonstrated by the drinking fountains in Thomas Crapper's 1954 Puritas range, the modernist bubble jet invented in the 1930s was still in vogue. In gleaming white porcelain and china, the bounty of pure water produced by modern industrial nations could be relished from these hygienic objects.

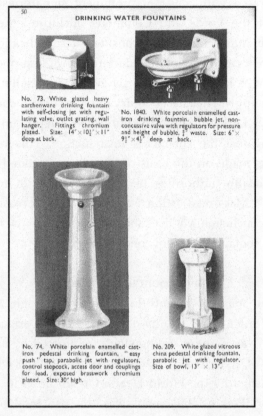

Drinking Water Fountains. Crapper Puritas, Catalogue No. 30, Thomas Crapper and Co. Ltd. 1954, p. 50.

Crapper's catalogue does not tell which organisations purchased and installed the Puritas models, but the range of four designs suggest a demand for drinking fountains as a somewhat utilitarian sanitary ware. Puritas fountains may well have been exported internationally, but it is likely that some of these designs could be found later that decade in schools, hospitals or other public institutions and places of work. Certainly the 1937 *Factories Act* stipulated that a supply of wholesome drinking water had to be supplied by employers.[82] Though the word fountain did not appear in the legislation, a device featuring an 'upward jet' was specified. Thomas Crapper's elegant ceramics would not have survived for very long outdoors, where the public fountain idealism of the post-war years was facing some challenges.

The Metropolitan Drinking Fountain and Cattle Trough Association pointed out the 'menace of vandalism' to supporters in its 1968 annual report: 'It is a regrettable fact that, without close supervision at all times, fountains are only too likely nowadays to be put out of action at the hands of hooligans. Consequently our activities are now largely directed towards the provision of fountains in parks, public gardens, playing fields and children's playgrounds, which can be closed and secured when not in use.'[83] The organisation's retreat from the street had been prefaced by a move from Victoria Street, where it had been based since 1872, to the suburbs in 1960.[84] Though a high profile office location was surrendered that year, a prestigious new pair of drinking fountains were also inaugurated within the walls of London's most iconic public space: Trafalgar Square. The Association's 1960 report noted that its Chairman 'was again invited by the B.B.C. to appear on television in connection with the installation of the fountains'.[85] A public drinking fountain in a striking location was evidently still a newsworthy item.

In an informal survey conducted for this book, many Londoners of the post-war era testified to using drinking fountains habitually. Ron Brooker confirmed that fountains flowed in his south London borough during the '50s: 'At that time Croydon's Park Department ran and maintained the town's parks very well.'[86] One respondent commented on water pressure problems with his local fountain, but still recalled using it. David Khan remembered using the bubble jet 'press-down tap that allowed a flow to bubble upwards, enabling a drinker to partake without any direct contact with the actual outlet'.[87]

Hygiene fears did not seem to preoccupy many respondents, who described how they freely drank from the clunky metal cups, many of which were still firmly affixed to nineteenth-century models. Lesley Ramm remembered of Priory Park, in Hornsey: 'As children we used the old metal cups, attached by chains, to scoop water from basins on hot summers days after playing.'[88] And in Clapham Common, Peter Skuse also used the fountain's metal cups, with this proviso: 'My Dad had told me to dip only my lips into the water in the cup.'[89] At that four-sided fountain, a strict protocol surrounding the cups' use developed: 'As we grew older, we would collectively adopt one cup, and take it in turns, leaving the others free for other children; indeed I recall once at least where we defended a cup against bigger boys, letting smaller girls and boys drink while they had to wait for another to become free. Someone saw us that day, and gave us a bag of Sharps toffees for being public-spirited!' By 1960, he claimed that the fountain was dry, but other areas of London were still in receipt of public hydration. For instance, Virginia Smith recalled of her Hampstead neighbourhood and elsewhere: 'You would always expect to have a fountain in a park, though some were fancier than others.'[90] Bernard Pellegrinetti clearly remembered the 'old fashioned fountain' near Kenwood House, also in Hampstead, where he and his brother regularly refreshed themselves.[91] Lesley Ramm noted a gradual disuse and total disappearance of public fountains: 'I think they were working into the 1970s but when the council withdrew Park Wardens and Gardeners, the park became a no-go area and much was vandalised.' Ron Brooker concurred that 'in later years, one noticed park drinking fountains not working and that was probably due to neglect by the local councils'. The ideals of the welfare state's healthy urban parks were slowly rotting, as the investment in public services from the state dwindled.

One thing that is certain from the 1950s and '60s era of fluoridation and fountains is that Londoners were drinking water, whether it was indoors or outdoors. Valerie Scott, who also responded to the fountain survey, pointed out 'there was no alternative in the days before bottled water'.[92] The anti-fluoridation campaigners were possibly so worried about the proposed additive because they were aware of how intrinsic tap water was to their diets and daily lives. Bottled water's proposition as a more 'natural' product than tap water did not arise in the records of the fluoridation debate that this chapter's research consulted. Possibly this was because fluoride naturally occurs in mineral or spring water sources but, more likely, because bottled water was uncommon and expensive. Mineral waters from Bath or even Schweppes Table Water remained elite, not everyday products. So how did Londoners develop such a penchant for bottled water by the late 1980s?

Chapter Eight

Maggie Thatcher, Jane Fonda and the Water Cooler 1973–2000

Twenty-five years later, it was less what the authorities were
threatening to put into the water that seemed to matter, than the
stuff they were failing to take out.[1]
(*A Journey Through Ruins: The Last Days of London,* Patrick
Wright, 1990)

So wrote Patrick Wright about the state of public drinking water
opinion in London in 1990. His comment reflects the continuum
from fluoridation concerns to the gradual deterioration of tap
water's public image during the 1980s, to the privatisation of the
water industry in Britain in 1989.[2]

This chapter joins the dots between various episodes, and
policies, before and during the 1980s that destabilised both the
perception of tap water and its actual safety record on the world
stage. It builds on the research of four British water books of this
period: *Watershed* by the environmental journalist Fred Pearce
(1982), *The Good Water Guide* co-authored by mineral water gurus
Maureen and Timothy Green (1985), *Troubled Water* by the water
economist David Kinnersley (1988) and *Britain's Poisoned Water*
by Frances and Phil Craig (1989). This chapter shows how the
creation of the bottled water mass market emerged from a matrix
of economic, environmental and political conflicts rather than
from the maxims of artful advertisers alone. Bottled water marketeers were opportunists manipulating a total crisis of faith in
municipal drinking water. However, this thirst for packaged
water — from pristine far-away landscapes — was not a quirky
taste unique to the palates, or pockets, of Londoners. Therefore,
this chapter ventures beyond the M25 (also, incidentally, a child

of the 1980s) into a national frame of drinking water politics and culture.

Authorities and Acts

Although the Metropolitan Water Board had survived the upheavals of the mid-60s during the creation of the Greater London Council, in 1971 its viability was under scrutiny once again. Water management philosophy was changing. Recommendations issued by the Government's Central Advisory Water Committee proposed that the whole river basin's use should integrate plans for water abstraction and wastewater.[3] This holistic view of water management forged the 1973 Water Act. New Regional Water Authorities would oversee all human water needs for drinking, industry and sanitation. The protection of rivers and underground water sources from pollution also fell under the new authorities' remit. Even boating, canoeing and fishing were incorporated under its functions. London's rivers and aquifers became the responsibility of the Thames Water Authority in 1974.[4] However, the Act also dissolved the Metropolitan Water Board.

London's 73-year-old municipal water provider, that had led ground-breaking international research; introduced chlorination; endured the First World War; survived the Blitz and kept afloat during the fluoridation storm was no more. On 28th March 1974 a 'Dinner and Dance to mark the end of the Board's existence', with more than a thousand guests, took place at the London Hilton Hotel on Park Lane.[5] The invite poignantly announced that a toast would be raised to the organisation's 'Glorious Memory' at dinner. Sentimental relief was on offer for the Board's soon to be ex-staff on the dance floors of the Hilton's Grand Ballroom or a 'discotheque' in the hotel's Coronation Room. Elsewhere in the country, boards and statutory water companies weathered the act, but not in London where the whole water and waste water system was rationalised.

Reflecting on this period eight years on, in Fred Pearce's environmental polemic about the state of Britain's rivers, *Watershed*, the journalist labelled the new Water Authorities 'strange hybrid bodies, neither nationalised industry, nor local government'.[6] Despite the authorities' identity crisis perceived by Pearce, the thrust of his critique of these new organisations was directed at their failure to provide much-needed investment for the country's geriatric water infrastructure. In the wake of the economic shockwaves produced by the 1973 international oil crisis, another supranational event changed the course of drinking water more specifically, when the United Kingdom joined the European Community (EC) in 1973.[7]

The 1973 U.K. Water Act repeatedly mentioned the protection of raw supplies for 'wholesomeness', though how this was to be done seemed rather vague. 'Restoration' of the nation's rivers more bluntly hinted that all was not well with the water environment.[8] Strangely, local authorities were to be charged with reporting any failures on the quality front to the new regional water authorities: 'It shall be the duty of every local authority to take such steps from time to time as may be necessary for ascertaining the sufficiency and wholesomeness of water supplies within their area...'[9] This elastic attitude was not consistent with the tone of directives that were being issued from Brussels whose rigour pleased Fred Pearce: 'By the late 1970s almost the only effective kick up the Government's environmental rear came from the EEC. Implementation on the Control of Pollution Act will bring Britain within EEC law on a range of directives.'[10]

Importantly, the 1974 Pollution Act's scope spelled out stringent protection of raw water sources: '...a person shall be guilty of an offence if he causes or knowingly permits a) any poisonous, noxious or polluting matter to enter any stream or controlled waters or any specified underground water...'[11] Precisely what poisonous, noxious or polluting matter the Act referred to (apart from sewage) was not defined, however Pearce was confident that the Act had to implement the directive from Brussels on black list chemicals — mercury, cadmium, aldrin and dieldrin — as well as substances on a secondary 'grey list'. Threats to the health of aquatic life were being tackled, but what about assuring drinking water's wholesomeness for humans? That question was swiftly addressed when the first EC directive on the quality of raw water abstracted for drinking, landed in Westminster in 1975.[13] Member States had to comply within two years.

Dramatic new limits for lead traces in water were proposed in the Directive, halving the World Health Organisation's existing recommendation.[14] Sceptics in Whitehall queried the evidence base for such a drastic reduction. One British participant in the construction of the directive reflected in 2002 on the somewhat arbitrary process that took place inside the European Community, explaining how the value for nitrates was reached: '...we went around the table and various people said it should be 100 ppm [parts per million], 1000 ppm, and finally, the difference was split.'[15]

At the time, in 1976, *The Times* reported a debate about the EC's raft of radical environmental directives, including the drinking water policy, in the House of Lords. According to the Conservative Party's lead sceptic, Lord Sandford: 'The need for the monitoring of lead levels in the atmosphere was not supported by any evidence that there was widespread damage from lead poisoning or any disease attributed to it, and the same applied to the sweeping directive calling for the monitoring of drinking water.'[16] As *The Times'* reporter concluded, the Peers needed some convincing. Some felt that contaminants should be rated in the Directive to be either 'of proven harm to human health' or 'merely undesirable'.[17] Significant funds were required to make these health and quality determinations, which was an unappealing prospect at a time of economic stress.

'Save Water: Bath with a Friend'[18]

An unusual decline in rainfall was recorded in May 1975 and dry conditions persisted throughout the winter across England and Wales. In July 1976 an official state of drought precipitated an emergency Drought Bill.[19] The drought's effect on the capital was not as severe as in the southwest of the country — where stand-pipes replaced domestic supplies for 65,000 households for two weeks — but Londoners were requested to alter their daily water habits. 'Save water, bath with a friend' was one national slogan that was hoped might sustain stressed resources, whilst undoubtedly causing many a raised eyebrow.[20]

Domestic supplies were not lost in London but reserves were low. 'Water Rations on the Way' ran the *Evening News'* front-page headline on 2nd July 1976. The accompanying report indicated a rising level of panic about the prospect of taps being turned off: '...in London it has been a case of July bursting out all over. The Thames Water Authority [has] dealt with 200 burst pipes and water mains in the past month. The capital has plenty of water but the delivery system is threatening to crack under the strain. Public demand has doubled and resulting high pressure is breaking joints in the older pipes, especially in East London. Londoners were warned to turn off their taps or face days without water.' Within a fortnight, the newspaper announced that a Drought Act had been 'rushed through Parliament to fight Britain's worst drought in 250 years'.[21] Ironically, two days later rain broke London's heat wave and the official state of drought. Hydrological effects were still being felt the next month, as this description of the Thames demonstrates: 'In August 1976 it ceased to flow at Teddington (the tidal limit) for the only time in its 128-year record. This was due to a combination of intense drought conditions and the substantial abstractions to meet London's water supply needs...'[22] Fortunately, the Thames did not remain in this state for long but, as some subsequent researchers of this episode summarised: '...for the consumer the drought brought bricks in lavatory cisterns, fewer baths, un-watered gardens, unwashed cars...'[23] Though it is difficult to quantify precisely how many Londoners changed their consumption habits, this experience undermined the illusion of an endless supply of tap water. One British water expert, David Kinnersley — who we will meet properly later in this chapter — reflected that public adaptation to scarcity had been admirable, but cynically added 'this mood is not readily sustained: once the drought broke, normal patterns of consumption soon re-estab-lished themselves.'[24]

When the rains finally did come, accumulated chemicals from agricultural land were washed into adjacent rivers in much higher concentrations that usual. Some mainly rural areas, such as East Anglia, suffered nitrate pollution as a result. Fred Pearce recorded water professionals' worries in 1977 about the potential toxicity of water in the East Anglian region to babies, in the form of the dreaded 'blue baby syndrome', which was fatal. Supplies of bottled water were apparently used in East Anglia, presumably as an alternative to mix powdered milk but perhaps also instead of breast milk if there was real concern that breast-feeding mothers' own water consumption could pass on the contaminants.[25] The details of these personal water fears are not verified in Pearce's account. Clearly the vulnerability of a baby's constitution to toxins, in comparison to an adult, magnified greatly any chemical threat to human health and therefore gave rise to a new level of drinking water awareness and scrutiny amongst the general public.

In subsequent years, intakes of the River Lee for East London's supply were temporarily suspended when nitrate levels were deemed too high for safe human consumption.[26] The necessity of this measure is a reminder of the environmental interconnectedness of rural and urban life, with groundwater and rivers linking and serving both populations. Technically, what is known as the 'water catchment' area describes this holistic relationship. Both pollution and scarcity could now be tangibly associated with public water supplies.

Enter Thatcher

Unemployment in London had grown during the 1970s following the demise of the capital's manufacturing economy in tandem with the impact of the oil crisis. Crime levels were conspicuously rising along with petty vandalism.[27] As the national recession's social impact bit more deeply in the late '70s, the Thames Water Authority's focus shifted from fears of pollution to potential picket lines. Apart from a few unofficial skirmishes, the water industry's manual workforce did not join the public sector strikes during the 'winter of discontent' in 1978–79. During these cold months, public services entered a dirty state of crisis when waste was uncollected and bodies were left unburied in morgues across England.[28] Amidst this state of dysfunction and the highest unemployment rates on record to date, of over three million people, Margaret Thatcher was viewed as a beacon of hope by enough people to be elected as Prime Minister of a new Conservative government on 4th May 1979.[29]

Mrs Thatcher had been a Thames Water Authority ratepayer in her suburban north Finchley constituency, before her salubrious change of address, but was she aware of the rot further down London's municipal and national water pipelines? Under her Government the water industry would have to adapt to the EC's first water quality directive within five years. The Directive challenged the basis of the U.K.'s existing water treatment and testing regime. As an academic water report described the significance of the EC policy's implications: 'First, the shift from relative and negotiated to absolute and regulatory definitions of water quality, based upon maximum permitted concentrations of known pollutants, represents a major change in British practice.'[30] Though the United Kingdom led the world in drinking water treatment at the outset of the century and partic-

ipated in the formation of the World Health Organisation's international drinking water quality guidelines, there was still no
legal basis for these standards, nationally. The EC's new drinking
water quality parameters accompanying the Directive covered
bacteriological, organoleptic (colour, turbidity, odour and taste),
physiochemical (water's naturally variable constituents such as
potassium), undesirable levels of organic and non-organic
chemicals, known toxins such as arsenic and lead, regulations on
artificially-softened water and, finally, microbiological
parameters.[31] Systemically, the troubled water industry had to be
transformed to ensure that the new mechanisms for monitoring
drinking water could be instituted.

Tap water tastes

As the new decade unfurled, at least one company was confident
about the quality of municipal tap water. By transforming it from
banal to beautiful, Soda Stream imagined a whole new
wonderful world of tap water joy. In its 1980 television advert,
broadcast in the U.K., a quirky technicolour-clad cast, aged eight
to eighty, spring collectively from the sofa to mix a smorgasbord
of tap water cocktails. Red water in a wine glass topped with a
cherry, or a plain carbonated draft transformed in an elegant
Martini glass with a slice of lime on its rim.[32] Sipping their
'mocktails', the cast react with a string of contorted, fizzed-up
faces. Coincidentally, as Soda Stream was inspiring people to sex
up their tap water, the first national tap water survey had just
been published.

Drinking Water Consumption in Great Britain was the work of
the government-funded Water Research Centre (an amalgam of
institutions that evolved from its sewage treatment research
remit, originally in the 1890s).[33] 3,564 people from across
England, Scotland and Wales were enlisted to keep a diary of
their drinking water consumption habits over the course of a
week.[34] Although nine geographically and socially diverse areas

of London were included in the survey, these statistics were absorbed generally into the south of England.[35] Any drink that involved turning on one's domestic tap, from plain water to a Soda Stream brew, was included in the survey. Its purpose was to provide evidence about the quantity of drinking water that was coursing through the average British body. The research publication further qualified its objective: 'In recent years a great deal of scientific effort has been expended on the possible relationship between drinking water quality and human health.'[36] In order to establish if positive or negative health factors could be linked to drinking water, daily consumption had to be quantified. Previously, all liquid in-take was merely estimated to be two litres per person per day with no breakdown into different liquids. In 1945, America's Food and Nutrition Board pronounced as a prescription for industrial workers, that 'a suitable allowance of water for adults is 2.5 liters daily in most instances'.[37] Were the British dehydrated in comparison to this standard?

Britain's tap water survey revealed that though the average liquid consumption was circa 1.8 litres per body per day, tap water-based beverages only accounted for 1.1 litres of that total.[38] Tangentially, it also recorded how little bottled water the British were drinking, in comparison to Europeans. France far outstripped any other country's bottled water consumption at 50 litres per-head-per-year, with only Belgium coming anywhere close at 31 litres.[39] In Britain, of the surveyed slice of the population, 70% recorded that they drank no bottled water during the week surveyed and 21% drank one 500ml bottle.[40] Conducted in collaboration with the British Market Research Bureau, any savvy researcher-cum-entrepreneur working on the survey would have done well to note the medical establishment's qualms about the potential relationship between tap water consumption and major health problems, such as patterns of coronary disease, alongside the low national consumption of mineral water. There was clearly a gap in the market that might rapidly widen if tap water was connected with the proliferation of serious diseases.

Arteries, pipes and pollutants

Following the deliberations in the House of Lords about lead in drinking water, in 1977 the Water Research Centre was commissioned to collaborate with London's Royal Free Hospital to carry out a national study. The researchers' task was to determine whether trace elements in drinking water, including lead, and water hardness or softness correlated geographically with heart disease statistics.[41] By the early 80s, water scientists also became concerned about lead: 'Evidence has been presented of the correlation between water lead concentration and blood lead levels ...Lead has also been cited as a causative agent in various disorders including hyperactivity, decreased intelligence, hypertension, mental retardation and renal failure.'[42] These disorders' relationship to lead consumption had been published in high-profile medical journals such as *The Lancet*. However, the water industry was struggling to find a method for the population's exposure to lead from tap water, because of variables in consumer behaviour and plumbing materials. Increased exposure might be caused, for instance, by people who drank the first draught from a tap in the morning rather than those who left their taps to flow for a minute or two, hence flushing out any lingering traces of lead.[43]

1981 was a bumper year for disturbing findings by water researchers. That year marked the opening of a floodgate of evidence about the dangers of organic micro-pollutants, from sewage effluent to trace chemicals found in drinking water, ranging from ingredients of cleaning products to known carcinogens. EC environmental policy was causing closer scrutiny of the contents of its member states water supplies. One research publication exposed concerns about a group of organic chemicals — or compounds containing carbon — called trihalomethanes. Disturbingly, trihalomethanes were produced as a by-product of the reaction of organic materials with chlorine. Fred Pearce commented on the findings: 'It is an unfortunate irony that the chemical pioneered in Britain as the great water-cleanser, chlorine, has become a prime suspect in the organic pollutants controversy.'[44] The prospect of chlorine's safety being de-stabilised was not a good prospect for drinking water treatment professionals (chapter ten returns to this subject).

In 1982, when the Water Research Centre's part in the, now extended, heart disease research programme concluded, accurate methods for determining the population's exposure to lead had been developed. Previous research identified that information about indoor plumbing's 'stagnation curves' and 'household water use patterns' *both* had to be known before lead concentrations could be predicted.[45] The research to date had also concluded that a household's lead exposure was not exacerbated by soft or hard water.[46] Water sitting in lead pipes for extended periods of time, whether it was hard water or soft water, was now conclusively known to present a problem. From the heart disease perspective, medical research continued. The relationship between water's chemical composition and this condition had neither been ruled out, nor proven by the Water Research Council and the Royal Free Hospital's joint study.

Water Workers' Power

Back in the House of Lords, in July 1982, Baroness Birk was concerned. 'Who will deal, for example, with the problem of lead in water?', she wondered.[47] Another heated environmental debate was in progress. This time the subject was the proposed dissolution of the National Water Council. It was the body, born from the 1973 Water Act, which regulated regional water authorities. Apart from the National Water Council's coordinating role strategically, the Baroness also alluded to the Council's more sensitive role in negotiating wage rates for workers. As she spoke, National Health Service employees were the latest public sector workers to dispute their wage packets. Proposals to abolish the Council suggested an ulterior motive: to break up the power base of the water industry's representation of the interests of its manual workforce.

After Parliament's summer recess in 1982, the bill to abolish the Council was presented to the House of Commons in November by Tom King, the Minister for Local Government and Environmental Services. He talked extensively about the evident problems with water and sewerage undertakers' management since the new authorities had been created, however he felt that the National Water Council's role as 'midwife' to the ten newborn authorities had served its purpose: 'Significant costs are involved in the operation of the NWC. We believe that economies can be made.'[48] In the context of high unemployment levels, the Right Honourable Mr Bennett pointed out that the Council's 448 employees would lose their jobs.[49] Despite these concerns, and potential industrial unrest, it was clear that the Bill had momentum. Unions mobilised around the issue by the New Year.

On 18th January *The Times'* Labour Correspondent, David Felton, asked 'Will the water men go over the brink?' Felton explained the situation thus: 'Union leaders see the current negotiations as their last chance of achieving a deal which puts the pay of the 29,000 manual workers firmly into line with the gas and electricity staff...' The same day as this report was published, tension was mounting inside the House of Commons. An M.P. from Birmingham stated in the evening sitting of Parliament: 'Clearly, there is a grave threat of a national water strike for the first time in our history.'[50] That threat had not subsided three days later. An article in the *The Times* on 21st June considered a strike's implications for consumers. 'Waiting for a mineral tidal wave' ran the article's headline. The photograph which illustrated the article, featured the grocery supervisor for

Tesco's Catford branch stacking shelves with a range of bottled water products, including Highland Spring and Perrier.[51] The scene appears to be staged but despite this the products were real and the accompanying article confirms that the sight of such quantities of bottled water in a supermarket trolley was novel at that time.

A peace process set in motion between the water industry's negotiators and the Government broke down two days later. Britain's first national water strike commenced on 24th January 1983, making front-page news in *The Times*. Catford's Tesco branch was in luck because, by the 27th January, south London residents suffered the greatest loss of tap water supplies. Their only alternative to bottled water was temporary street plumbing in the form of standpipes plugged into the mains.[52] No warnings to boil water were issued to Londoners, as was the case for 2.5 million people in Greater Manchester.[53] Unsurprisingly, because of its population density, London had the highest loss of water supplies during that first week of the strike at 2560 households.[54] North of the Thames, the neighbourhood of Finchley also suffered the effects of the strike. Coincidentally, this hit Margaret Thatcher's own constituency, or perhaps it was no accident. In the affected neighbourhoods, nobody knew when they might be able to make tea; brush their teeth; flush their toilets, or use their Soda Streams without having to fetch water from outdoors. For how long could such uncivilised conditions be tolerated?

By the 4th of February, the number of properties in London depending on standpipes had almost doubled from the previous week to 5,061; a sight not seen since the Blitz.[55] Some ten days later Thames Water Authority was blaming consumers for not cutting down their water use.[56] One result of the depleted water workforce was unrepaired mains pipes. Members of 11,417 households were now queuing up for their water on the street.[57] On London's scale, this was a fraction of the resident population (inner London: 2.52 million outer London: circa 4.5 million), however it was the threat of further standpipes springing up across the capital that pressurised the wage negotiators.[58] A potent symbol of the power struggle between the usually invisible hand of water and sewage labourers (such as flushers) versus the state would be blatantly on view.

Not far downstream from Westminster, a Pimlico resident pronounced that he would hire private contractors to repair his area's mains pipe, but the Thames Water Authority warned that such attempts could lead to physical restraint.[59] The risks associated with public hands meddling underground, in the professional sphere of civil engineers, were not to be entertained. Like the smattering of standpipes, this was another glimpse of what risky unofficial arrangements might appear if the industrial dispute lasted for months rather than weeks. On 16th February – some three weeks into the strike – Margaret Thatcher, still defiant, spoke in the House of Commons about efforts to resolve the industrial dispute. '...there is absolutely no point in prolonging strike action, which is causing so much hardship to so many people', she urged.[60]

By 18th February, London remained at the top of the nation's leader board of homes without running water, at 20,022.[61] However, one M.P. declared that 'very little was happening in London' in terms of a loss of water supply, in comparison to his constituents in Cornwall where schools had closed down and ten per cent of people had lost their water during the strike.[62] Such conditions did not deteriorate any further because the strike ended on 22nd February. Water workers had secured their desired wage increase.[63] Thames Water Authority's manual workers went back to work exactly a calendar month after the strike began. David Felton dubbed the episode a 'gentlemanly dispute', arguing that the 29,000 strikers could have unleashed sanitary chaos by not providing emergency cover or 'insisting on strong picketing to block deliveries of chlorine...'[64] He also noted how no major machinery casualties had prevented a catastrophic breakdown in civilisation. For the Government, the greater disaster was the precedent now set by the water workers for other public sector employees. Most notably, the miners' strikes were mounted the next year.

Turning to the Bottle

Another strike victor was the bottled water industry. There is significant evidence that this short episode altered Britain's scale of bottled water production as the temporary panic created an unprecedented demand for the product. Direct as a result of the strike, Highland Spring opened a second source in Scotland and doubled its bottling production.[65] A Dartmoor farmer increased his spring's output from 50 to 1,000 cases and Schweppes confirmed that it had trebled the quantity of Malvern table water in circulation.[66] During the fourth week of the strike, *The Guardian* reported on the bottled water sales phenomenon. Tesco's Finchley branch sold out of a, usually, week-long supply of bottled water in two and a half hours, whilst Buxton's sales trebled.[67] One can imagine bottled water profiteers' disappointment that the strike was so short-lived. Undoubtedly, the strike's demand strengthened the previously weak market charted in the Water Research Centre's survey of British drinking water habits.

Jumping back to 1974, bottled water's position in the marketplace revitalised the market for elite table waters, similarly to the late-nineteenth century. The strap-line for an Appollinaris advertisement bragged that 'Polly is being seen in the best gentlemen's clubs'.[68] The same year, Perrier expanded its small U.K. market with a major advertising campaign.[69] A decade later £3 million had reportedly been spent promoting the brand.[70] As one journalist wrote of the specifically post-strike bottled water boom: 'Ten years ago, scarcely anyone in this country had heard of Perrier. A bottle might be placed on the bedside table of guests in the better country houses, but to the general public Perrier was unknown.'[71]

By the early '80s, a popular new health culture extended the purported benefits of intense hydration to a broader, multi-national market. The popularity of keep-fit classes, including aerobics, was on the rise, particularly for western women in global cities such as London. Pop singer Olivia Newton John's 1981 hit *Physical* was performed in full aerobics kit with choreography. Her 'fitness' moves morphed freely with more sexually suggestive gyrations.[72] The phenomenal success of *Jane Fonda's Workout Book,* and video in 1982, on both sides of the Atlantic, further promoted the looking-good-and-feeling-great merits of personal workouts (along with the joys of wearing very shiny leotards). This fitness fever inhabited a broader, western, global space of popular film culture, magazines and music. Post the feminist movement of the late '60s and '70s, a new generation of women unsettled the male hegemony of the professions, if very slowly in some sectors. Britain's first female Prime Minister was an obvious example of this shift despite the fact that she was no feminist. Underneath the power suits, women's professional bodies could remain lean and mean, yet sexually desirable, through aerobics, fitness regimes and dieting.

The bottled water market also grew up alongside the rise of Young Upwardly Mobile Professionals, or Yuppies. Predominantly male, but also female exponents, of this work and play culture were known for flashing their cash. This 'conspicuous consumption', as London historian Jerry White defines it exemplified the beneficiaries of neo-liberalism's brand of free market capitalism installed by Margaret Thatcher's Government through its economic and social policies.[73] Displays of disposable income, in stark contrast to the general mass of Londoners on average or low incomes, or state benefits, was immortalised by comedian Harry Enfield in his *Loadsamoney* sketches. Money to spare was also met in the City of London by a culture change, noted *The Economist*: '...there is far less booze consumed at lunch than 10 years ago. It is now expected to drink Perrier as an aperitif.'[74] This, apparent, shift in consumption pleased the authors of a new guidebook.

'Drinking Water is fashionable again.'[75]

So said the authors of 1985's *The Good Water Guide*. They cited health consciousness and body image as one of the main drivers for the British bottled water renaissance: 'Mineral water is the health drink discovered by the age that had turned to health foods. It has acquired a sporting image - almost like internal aerobics. ...Women are constantly advised to drink more, to avoid problems like cystitis, and here is a calorie-free way to do so.'[76]

A slim, hardback volume with a glossy jacket *The Good Water Guide* was easily slipped into a handbag or the breast pocket of a suit. Inside its svelte cover, one expects to find lists of fine wines, rather than fine waters. The husband and wife author duo, Maureen and Timothy Green, act as guides for a tour of the elite drinking water world, designed for the British novice. Coincidentally, the Guide hit bookshops just as Britain's legislation came into line with the EC's mineral water regulations.[77] Bottled water producers must have adored the handy little volume.

According to the Greens, it was tap water consumers in London who were the most likely consumers to benefit from the bottled alternative: 'The knowledge in London that the local tap water, while safe, has already been recycled seven times, hardly encourages citizens to quaff great draughts.'[78] It was notable that the Greens were no doubt legally bound to write that London's drinking water was technically 'safe' for human health. However, they implied that though the municipal source was technically healthy, it was not desirable.

A striking feature of *The Good Water Guide* was its transparent exposure of corporate marketing strategies. For instance, the authors revealed quite plainly that Highland Spring leased one of its water sources solely for the use of Sainsbury's. Rebranded Sainsbury's Scottish Spring, the promotion of this pure water from the Highlands had a specific focus, as the Guide explained: 'Advertising from Sainsbury's began to remind the public, and especially Londoners, that, if they wanted to drink a glass of water for the first time, they had better buy it in a bottle.'[79] Second-hand water does not have positive associations, however the hydrological fact that all water is re-used was carefully unmentioned in the *Guide*. It preferred a rather ahistorical relationship to London's civil engineering and public health heritage. Once the sewer and the tap are linked in the imagination, it is not an easy association to banish. Juxtaposing the water siphoned from a pristine Scottish landscape with the industrialised environs of the Thames was a powerful way to influence consumer behaviour - conveniently ignoring the fact that London's drinking water was not abstracted downstream of its own sewers and had not been for well over a hundred years. Granted, abstraction did occur downstream of other urban centres such as Oxford and Reading but miles from where the treated effluent from these towns was discharged and with appropriate timing. Despite these technicalities, municipal drinking water was simply not in vogue, according to the Greens and bottled waters' advertisers.

In the mid-to-late '80s, the advertising for French mineral waters in Britain leant heavily on associations with non-urban locations. *Cosmopolitan* magazine was one medium through which working urban women could pick up tips for feeling and looking good, whilst achieving optimum career and sexual performance. Though it cannot be claimed that *Cosmopolitan's* readership was exclusively London-based, suggestions of how readers might spend their weekends, for instance, were invariably focused on the capital. The first mineral water advertisement of the eighties to appear in an issue of the magazine — in a 1986 health and fitness supplement — was for Volvic (owned by Perrier).[80] A full-page advertisement was split into two halves. The top half featured an arresting illustration of the Auvergne volcanic mountain range in France. Below it, the water's source in the wilderness was embellished with this caption: 'The 25,000 year old volcano that could help you zip up last year's jeans.'[81] The second half of the page contained text devoted to two themes. One focused on the purity of the water and the second on how dieters could benefit from drinking it.

As the '80s progressed, bottled water advertising in *Cosmopolitan* was dominated by Perrier's Volvic. Advertisements sat amongst others for cigarettes, perfume, fitness regimes and the magazine's famously candid articles about sex. Perrier's marketing executives were clearly tailoring their pitches for a sexually liberated readership. In a 1988 campaign, Volvic's origin was represented by 'prehistoric fire' painted directly onto the body of a model whose headless torso was clad only in red paint representing flames, presumably of a volcano, licking up her stomach and breasts.[82] By 1989, only one other bottled water brand competed for *Cosmopolitan* readers' attention. Marketers of Malvern opted for tranquil rather than explosive imagery, matching its 'Original English Water' strap-line with a delicate watercolour of a water lily. The last issue of the magazine that decade also had a feature entitled 'How Will the Eighties Be Remembered?'[83] Bidding good riddance to aerobics and to 'female newsreaders being regarded as freaks', the article was illustrated with an image of a domestic tap in mid flow. Categorised in things 'Loved and Lost', the photograph was captioned 'water we're happy to drink'. The image's specific reference is unclear but its overall message was not: tap water was out. In fact, the photograph was likely a reference to a recent and disastrous incident.

'Poison on Tap'[84]

A major municipal water contamination error had occurred in the southwest of England the previous year, in Camelford. On 7th August 1988, *The Observer* reported that the source of Cornwall's poisoned water had been identified a month after the contamination accident.[85] Residents' symptoms of nausea, diarrhoea and mouth burns had previously been inexplicable. 20 tonnes of aluminium sulphate, usually used as a coagulant in water purification, had been delivered into the wrong tank at a water treatment works and been supplied at an unmeasured concentration to 20,000 households. The South-West Water Authority defended the negligence found by a subsequent government enquiry, claiming that the incident had occurred because of spending cuts forced by preparations for the industry's privatisation.[86] Camelford continued to attract high profile news coverage because of an ongoing campaign to prove the likely long-term health impacts on those who consumed aluminium sulphate-laced tap water. The local residents' campaign succeeded in securing a criminal investigation of the water authority in January 1989.[87] Days after this victory, the Environment Secretary Nicholas Ridley announced that £1.5 billion was to be invested in improving water quality standards before privatisation.[88] Though this figure sounds impressive, it was a third of what the water expert Dr Judith Rees had calculated to be required, in her research on behalf of Friends of the Earth.[89]

Mr Ridley's promised investment did not achieve immediate results. In spring 1989, with the water industry's privatisation looming, the Government received an order from the European Community to conform to the Water Quality Directive's terms, or face prosecution at the European Court.[90] Legislation was yet to be passed on national water quality standards despite the Directive's stipulation that EU member states should have complied by 1985. This embarrassment for the Government was not missed by the authors of a book that would imminently be published: 'As we go to press, the whole privatization scheme appears to be threatened by Britain's failure to meet EEC standards for drinking — and bathing — water cleanliness.'[91] The book was entitled *Britain's Poisoned Water*.

Like the Good Water Guide, *Britain's Poisoned Water* was co-authored by a wife-and-husband team, but this time by the environmental campaigning journalists Frances and Phil Craig. As its polemical title suggests, the book's thesis posited that significant doubt and negative evidence marred the safety of Britain's tap water. And as a work of investigative journalism, it was unsparing in its scathing critique of the state of the water industry and the state of Britain's drinking water. Several inter-views with anonymous or former water industry insiders added to the credibility of the expose's information sources. It was clearly designed to shock and politically mobilise consumers: '...almost half of readers with young families may well be slowly poising their children every time they give them a drink. The poison is lead, and it comes out of the kitchen tap.'[92] On this issue, Frances and Phil Craig noted that a 1983 Royal Commission investigation into the lead problem had advised an action plan, but decried the fact that little had been done about Britain's poisonous plumbing since then.

The concise Penguin pocketbook volume saliently covered the drinking water-related health concerns that were hanging over the tap: Alzheimer's disease (aluminium), children's brain devel-opment (lead) and a host of cancers (nitrates and pesticides). In the case of the latter, the authors admitted that evidence was thin on the ground. Apart from casting blame on the water industry's failings as a result of disinvestment and some of its questionable practices, the book laid out broader concerns about environ-mental pollution. For instance, from a groundwater perspective, the authors exposed that: 'Already 10 per cent of Britain's under-ground aquifers are no longer used for drinking water because of heavy contamination with dangerous chemicals thought to have leaked, in part, from waste dumps.'[93] Man-made chemicals from post-war industrial farming fertilisers and weed-killers, used on a motorways-and-railway-tracks scale, were other water polluting culprits that *Britain's Poisoned Water* pointed out to its general readership. For readers (possibly of an environmentalist bent) who were not already aware, Frances and Phil Craig reminded them: 'In December 1986 Friends of the Earth formally reported the United Kingdom government to the EEC for refusing to obey European drinking water law.'[94] In fact, there was still no coherent law, though there should have been, about drinking water quality relating to the European standards in the United Kingdom, and this failing was potentially jeopardising the terms the U.K.'s membership of the EEC. The anti-tap-water environmental zeitgeist continued to shadow the road to water privatisation. For instance, the Friends of the Earth publication authored by Dr Judith Rees also pointed out 'the monitoring void' for drinking water that was on the cards with a privatised water industry, with only the economic regulator OFWAT checking its economic practices.[95]

Since Friends of the Earth 1986 accusation, the organisation had been compiling a picture of water company failures to meet 'Maximum Admissible Concentrations' (MACS), of five substances with known, or suspected, public health implications (in the absence of a law): lead, aluminium, nitrate, pesticides and trihalomethanes. Evidence was amassed through dialogue with the active participation of the water authorities and statutory water companies. In collaboration with the *Observer* newspaper, the results were splashed across nine pages of the newspaper's Magazine, on Sunday 6th August 1989, in an article entitled *Poison on Tap*.[96]

The feature's second page was dominated by a blonde boy, aged about four or five, clothed only in a pair of red shorts. Down his vulnerable torso, a series of lines connected a water contaminant with the part of his anatomy it was either suspected or known to affect. First, aluminium and lead pointed to the boy's head, for Alzheimer's disease and brain damage respectively. Targeting his heart and lungs jointly were 'pesticides', as suspected carcinogens. Last, the nitrate line linked to the child's stomach represented the question mark over nitrates and abdominal cancers. The feature's remaining pages displayed the survey results with a map for each substance. London's breaches for lead and aluminium were shown to be nil, whilst the southwest, Wales and the north of England all had widespread results contravening the EC's Water Quality Directive. When it came to pesticides, tap water in 25 London boroughs was found to have exceeded the Maximum Admissible Concentration of 0.1 micrograms per litre for individual pesticides and 0.5 micrograms for the total potential cocktail of pesticide-related traces. The European view on the pesticide issue was a sticking point for the Government, which contested the need for such stringent concentration levels to be observed. Fred Pearce — unsurprisingly employed to interpret the results — countered the Conservative's view. He warned readers about drinking water quality apathy in the British political establishment: '...the World Health Organisation is less sanguine. Its study of the dangers of drinking water, published in 1987, says that many pesticides are recent formulations about which we know little.'

Nitrates — residues of nitrogen fertilisers being slowly absorbed from farmland into groundwater sources – were also detected in Greater London, but specifically in eleven of the outer suburban boroughs, including Newham, Croydon and Waltham Forest. Above the nitrate map, a small photograph of the little golden-haired boy hovered, in which he sipped nonchalantly from a glass of water. The final map, showing trihalomethane breaches, with the organic chemicals' potential, though unproven, connections with bladder, colon and rectal cancers showed a relatively small cluster of Greater London outer boroughs had failed the MAC (Broxbourne, Enfield, Epping Forest and Haringey). On the whole, the findings certainly unsettled the argument that rural water was better quality than urban water, at least when it came to these identified substances mostly associated with industrialised farming practices. Proof of pesticide presence in the environment certainly endorsed the motivations of the organic farming movement. *Poison on Tap* did not conclude by suggesting that people inhabiting the cerise-coloured danger zones marked on the maps should rush out and buy a lifetime's supply of bottled water, but could the revelations warrant a wholesale rejection of tap water?

A *Guardian* journalist reported on reactions to the exposé, the following Thursday. Startled by the knee-jerk surge in bottled water sales, Jane Ellison exclaimed: 'Does anyone still drink tap water?'[97] She was not convinced that its contents were laced with poison. The journalist's alarm was sparked when her local wine warehouse erected a sign announcing that it had run dry, of bottled water. Ellison was bewildered that the British public suddenly believed that other EC member states had miraculously acquired supplies of trustworthy potable water, when Britons usually sipped from the safety of water bottles whilst on holiday in those countries. Her voice was a rare left-leaning echo of Water Minister Michael Howard's pleas that tap water was trustworthy. Amidst the pollution furore, Ellison wryly observed that 'new water purifying machines' had made a timely appearance. Like the strike episode, those who stood to benefit commercially from any chink of doubts about tap water safety moved in swiftly to the uncertain consumer's rescue. Those products were not confined to bottled water or the domestic sphere.

Companies that Care

During the mid-to-late '80s, so-called 'sick office building syndrome' was the subject of much discussion in the architectural press.[98] There was a desire to make offices more pleasant to work in and, ultimately, more productive. For instance, a high-profile outbreak of Legionnaire's disease in London demonstrated the unhealthy consequences of failures in modern air-conditioning systems.[99]

By mid-decade, office vending machines serving up well-known instant brands of coffee, such as Nescafé, were all the rage but if one wanted a plain glass of water, it was most likely to have come from the plain tap.[100] In the 1985 edition of the *Yellow Pages* business directory for Central London, the listing for 'water

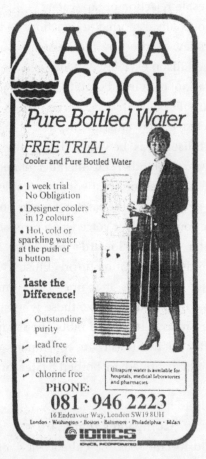

Aqua Cool water cooler advertisement, 1990. Ionics Incorporated: GE Power and Water purchased Ionics in 2005. Copyright General Electric Company; used with permission.

cooler' redirects the reader to 'refrigeration equipment'.[101] Two years later, the *Yellow Pages'* water cooler re-direction instructions is entitled 'vending machines', where Oasis appears as the only company with an entry for a water cooler amongst its plethora of vending wares.[102] However, in the 1988 edition, three suppliers are listed directly under the water cooler heading: Aqua Cool, Holywell Spring and Oasis.[103] In 1989's *Yellow Pages*, the companies touting water coolers had risen to five.[104] 1990 saw that figure doubled.[105] Aqua Cool even had its own illustrated advertisement in the directory.

Aqua Cool's claims of 'outstanding purity', as well as being chlorine, lead and nitrate free seemed to be custom-designed for the U.K. market. Despite these assurances, the advertisement does not explain the source of the water as spring or mineral. It is simply labelled 'pure bottled water'. The advertisement's small print revealed that in addition to London, Aqua Cool operated in Baltimore, Boston, Philadelphia and Washington.

In 1989, the renowned office architect Francis Duffy wrote this snapshot of the city: 'London, as an office centre, is changing rapidly in response to international pressures. Being such an open city — the Hong Kong of the European Community — it is easy to see in every street and skyline the architectural consequences of the globalisation of financial services and all related trades and professions.'[106] At the time, projects such as the construction of Canary Wharf were well underway. The water cooler was a minor response to the market produced by developments in London's global working culture. This was a product that appeared to offer superior quality water to the tap, wherever one was working in the world. The utilitarian tap did not fit the aesthetics of highly designed, materially luxurious office environments. Instead, they could be embellished with a Holywell Springwater Cooler; perfect 'for companies that care about their personnel' or a Buxton Spring Watercooler, with water drawn from a source reassuringly distant from urban pollution.[107] Some twenty different brands appeared in the 1993 edition of the *Yellow Pages*.[108]

The water cooler was also symbolic. It was as much a child of the neo-liberal vision of the free market's entrepreneurial spirit as the drive to privatise the water industry as another 'utility'. Both fitted into the new frame of water as an economic resource.

Pricing Britain's Water

In 1988, a book written by the eminent water industry expert and water economist David Kinnersley unpacked the complex issues surrounding debates over freshwater's value, and therefore the future management and ownership of the water and sewerage industry as it 'stumbled', in his words, towards privatisation.[109] Kinnersley points out in *Troubled Water* how measuring water's value in Britain's economy shifted noticeably with the 1963 Water Resources Act, when protecting river and groundwater quality became bound up with recognising water's value as a raw material for industry.[110] From then, abstraction for commercial use was highly regulated through licences. For Kinnersley, the equation of abstraction from rivers had failed to be balanced with the price of toxic discharges going into rivers. He notes the lag of British Water Authorities in adopting the 'Polluter Pays' principle of other European nations: '...the authorities hung back from serious attention to improving charges for trade effluent disposal to sewers, or promoting in Britain the concept of charges for discharges direct to rivers.'[111] The economist was well placed to be critical of the shortcomings of the water authorities created as a result of the 1973 Water Act. He had been the Chief Executive of one of them.[112]

In the lead up to privatisation, Kinnersley was working in Whitehall as a consultant to the Secretary of State for the Environment. As part of the privatisation policy he is widely credited with masterminding the creation of the National Rivers Authority (NRA); a body that would be independent of the new private water and sewerage companies.[113] The NRA would be responsible for 'administering river basins including deciding and enforcing constraints on all sorts of companies taking water from rivers and putting effluents in them'.[114] He successfully translated his critique of the water industry into this new institution, which would be dedicated to monitoring river abstractions and discharges.

Under privatisation, water's environmental protection looked promising. Another limit on the 'extreme monopolies', as Kinnersley termed the proposed private water companies, included plans to create the Office of Water (OFWAT) to keep an economic check on these water companies i.e. their charges to customers. The efficacy of these structures would only be seen once the switch to privatisation had been flicked. There is no doubt that his 1988 viewpoint demonstrates a fundamental belief that water was a commodity, even on the domestic front.

Kinnersley's argument was based on cultural changes in water's consumption for myriad, arguably unessential uses. For him the change in the function of clean and wastewater services from a public good to a private good was an inevitable outcome of changing standards of living. Though he accepted that the state's role in ensuring safe water and sewers had been needed in an earlier era to protect public health, in his mind that mandate ended in the 1950s, when water consumption became increasingly tied to the use of convenient, water intensive products: dishwashers, washing machines and even multiple bathrooms. As he summarised: 'In short, the water supply and sanitation services have become far more geared to individual ways of life, with the risk of water-borne infection very close to nil, as the service is well-managed. We can say that, in broad terms, this is far more the supply of private goods than of public ones.'[115] On that basis David Kinnersley believed that metering water would best reflect its status as a private good in Britain's modern society. Strangely, he failed to isolate water's use for drinking as distinct from optional water uses in his economic philosophy, though he owned that consumers had little choice over their tap water quality in comparison to bottled water. Surely his theory should have acknowledged that the value of water for drinking and cooking could not be compared ethically to washing one's car or mixing baby food. As a person involved with the foundation of the international development charity WaterAid, in 1981, Kinnersley must have been considering the issue of water justice of some level.

For privatisation's opponents, the argument that water had transposed from a public to a private good was not appreciated. As one 1989 *Evening Standard* article reported when debates about water metering were raging: 'In the general public, of whom 75 per cent are currently against privatisation, there is an emotional feeling about water which did not apply to gas or British Telecom - a feeling that water is not only a natural resource but a vital public health service which is unsuited to being bought and sold for profit.'[116] Regardless of these emotions, privatisation was enacted that year. Other national industries, natural resources and utility-providers already stripped of their 'British' prefix in the hands of Thatcher's Conservative Government, or were in a process of transition to the private sector, included aerospace, airports, electricity, gas, oil, petroleum, steel, telecommunications.[117] In the case of water, like gas and electricity, its status as a 'utility' encompasses amongst other definitions in the Oxford English Dictionary, something that is 'essential to the community'.[118] The notion of essential or non-essential also relates to the dictates of a specific economic system, in this case capitalism, in which the drive towards progress depends on the control and commodification of natural resources. Whilst water for the production of foodstuffs such as rice might be deemed essential in many contexts, it could be argued that a limit to water being channelled into cement-mixing might check the terms of what progress is really needed and for the benefit of whom.

Peter Oborne, then a journalist for the *Evening Standard*, was in the City of London on December 6th 1989, when the Thames Water Authority was rebranded Thames Water PLC. His report described a very public scene, with thousands of would-be water investors queuing at the door of National Westminster Bank for the 10am investment deadline: apparently an outpouring not yet seen for the shift of national assets to the private sector. Oborne captured a very excited reaction from the Minister who seemed giddy by the endorsement of '"popular capitalism"'.[119] Not long after this rush of excitement, Michael Howard soberly announced another limit from the state on the private enterprises' freedom, in the formation of a Drinking Water Inspectorate. This secondary state check on the freshly privatised water industry, alongside OFWAT, was clearly a structure designed to disperse the remaining cloud of doubt over whether the public should trust their tap water or not. From 1990, the Inspectorate was to 'provide independent reassurance that water supplies in England and Wales are safe and drinking water quality is acceptable to customers'.[120] Friends of the Earth reportedly remained sceptical about the new organisation, on the grounds that it was an auditor rather than an independent testing centre.[121] Still, it certainly meant that Thames Water PLC's department of water treatment and examination was under external scrutiny in tandem with its mandate to comply with European water quality standards, now inscribed in the law.

Pollution Prosecution

In spite of the enthusiastic scenes in the City of London endorsing tap water's transfer to the corporate sector, bottled water's marketeers continued to kindle memories of municipal water controversies and failures. *Cosmopolitan's* 1990 summer issue included a feature advertisement for Highland Spring.[122]

The advertisement's opening line was frank about the company's mission to plunder profits from tap water drifters: 'Ever since the growing concern about British tap water, mineral water sales are booming, and one of the most popular in Britain today is Highland Spring.' Readers were invited to send away for a free device for monitoring tap water problems in their area. Once the Drinking Water Inspectorate's work was underway, in 1990, it was probably to the organisation's great relief that drinking water fears that year switched focus temporarily to bottled water. When traces of benzene were found in Perrier, all of its British stocks were recalled.[123] However, filters were also flooding the market by then. Brita was one prominent brand in the U.K.'s filter market. The product for 'optimising tap water' had been invented by a German entrepreneur in 1966, and named after his daughter.[124] In 1990, Brita's 'two-litre deluxe' jugs were on sale in Selfridges department store for £9.99. Plumbed-in filtering machines were also on sale at this store; fresh from American space programme models, for an eye-watering £240.[125] There was certainly a solution to absorb every budget.

To counter tap water's poor image, Thames Water PLC mounted a sustained public relations campaign in the early '90s to reassure consumers about its product. A *Drinking Water Quality* booklet the company published confronted the elephant in the room: 'Water quality has been very much in the news lately. It's good that people are becoming more aware of the importance of water quality, but the messages are confusing.'[126] One reassurance it offered customers was that legal action had also been taken against other EU countries, such as neighbouring Ireland and France. Two leaflets the company issued in the early 1990s acknowledged that many customers feared the safety of their tap water. On the subject of filters, the company emphatically stated: 'We do not consider that water filters are necessary on health grounds and do not endorse particular types or brands.'[127] Customers who worried about nitrates were advised that 'only special resins' could play any role in their removal. Bottled water's share of the market was tackled in a *Water Quality Fact Sheet*. This leaflet argued that bottled water was not healthier than tap water on the grounds that the regulations governing its quality were not as stringent as for piped supplies, particularly on a bacteriological basis. Generously, the corporation issued some guidelines for those whose opinion could not be swayed against using bottled water, including the warning that it should never be used 'as an alternative to boiling tap water for making up baby foods'.[128] Thames Water's marketing department proved that the game of casting doubt on drinking water safety could be as easily played in its own favour. One public relations tactic the corporation employed was the exposure of the shrouded sphere of the water examination laboratory, notably highlighting female staff. Had the communications department decided that highlighting women as the guardians of public water was a positive corporate image? Either that, or it was a true reflection of the laboratory of the 1990s.

Some of the tap water fears Thames Water was responding to may have been rekindled in 1991 when the former South-West Water Authority was fined the relatively minor sum of £10,000 for its liability in the Camelford aluminium pollution incident.[129] Lead contamination also came back under scrutiny that year in the water industry when the Water Research Council was commissioned by the Government to carry out a feasibility study for the replacement of the entire nation's lead-based plumbing, then recognised as the main cause of lead leaching into drinking water. This measure was taken on the grounds that a further European directive was likely to lower the permitted standard.[130] Lead pipes were most likely to be service pipes, transmitting water from the mains to individual houses or indoor plumbing. Responsibility for the former lay with the water companies and for the latter with homeowners or landlords, including of course local authorities. Building constructed after the late 1970s were unlikely to have any lead pipes. In 1992, the report concluded that both companies in England and Wales were faced with a £2,836 million bill for their liabilities whilst homeowners potentially faced a £3,101 million re-fit costs.[131] It was another drinking water problem without an instant solution. Londoners could at least be smugly relieved that their homes were known to be less toxically plumbed than those in the north of England.

The deadliest blow yet to tap water's public image came in 1992 when the long dispute over the United Kingdom's alleged failures on adapting to the Drinking Water Directive, by 1985, came to a conclusion. The European Court of Justice ruled that drinking water standards had been breached because of excess nitrate levels prior to 1989 and that this problem had leached into the early 1990s.[132] Thames Water was exempt from recent failures, but the Three Valleys Water Company serving part of London's outer northern and north-western boroughs was included in the guilty companies list. Records of which specific areas of the Three Valleys supply were affected are extremely elusive in the published archival documents of the Drinking Water Inspectorate. Although the same map of nitrates breaches was reproduced in two newspapers, the detail of the affected areas in London was not spelled out. Whatever exposure London's perimeter had experienced, it was minor in comparison to rural north Anglia.[133] In this climate consumers faced a decision about whether to trust plain tap water, to invest in maintaining a filtered version of it, or to buy water in a safely sealed package from some rural paradise or another country. For the latter, the *Good Water Guide* folks happily obliged by updating their handy little volume in 1994. Readers could now be assured of a far greater choice of superior drinking waters, or so its authors believed, much closer to home.

Sticking with the Bottle

In the Guide's introduction to the U.K.'s own brands, a paparazzi shot of Lady Diana shows her clutching a litre of bottled water along with her tennis racket. Stunning claims were made about the market's growth since the last edition: 'In 1993, people in the U.K. drank 570 million litres…three times as much as they swallowed five years ago and 10 times more than they downed in 1983.'[134] According to the authors' market research guru, this was due to public distrust of tap water's safety and Perrier's successful advertising campaigns. The brand's benzene episode, however, had created a gap for new British brands to fill and sixty homegrown ones were now available. The Guide chose thirty-three of the finest to profile, noting that still water in the nineties had displaced the '80s love of bubbles.[135] Abbey Well was lauded in the top ten British mineral waters, with sales of 14 million litres per annum and described as a 'clean tasting water', 'low in sodium, calcium, nitrate and other minerals'.[136] Northumbrian in origin, it was apparently 'especially popular in London and the south east of England'. Most significantly, the Guide commented on the ubiquity of bottled water's presence in all retail sectors, the largest being supermarkets.[137] Bottled water had become a mass-marketed convenience food.

The shift in public mood away from importing exotic European water was manipulated by Highland Spring, with a hefty dash of irony. A 1996 publicity campaign featured a French model, posing against the shabby chic façade of the Bistrot de Peintre in Paris: 'The Scots can keep their haggis and shortbread. I'll have their Highland Spring.'[138] In a remarkably short space of time, Britain had upended the 1980 Water Research Centre's profile of the nation's drinking water habits which reported that 'the majority of people do not consume mineral water'.[139] Trying to keep pace with the drinking water zeitgeist, a 1995 update of that first survey found that bottled water consumption had risen dramatically and the diversity of brands was particularly noted. For those already in the habit of drinking bottled water, their consumption had risen by a third and the survey also found that these drinkers were 'most likely to be female, aged between 16 and 45, from the Midlands, Wales or the South, and part of a household in which the main wage earner is in a professional/managerial (AB), clerical (C1) or skilled manual (C2) social group'.[140]

Individual servings of drinking water were apt symbols of the growth of a global free market economy. Many of the failings that precipitated the demand in Britain for this highly profitable product are connected to Thatcher's Government's desire to wash its hands of the complex problems faced by Britain's publicly owned water industry in the mid-'80s. In his critical history of neo-liberalism, the Marxist geographer David Harvey interprets, more generally, Thatcher's privatisation policy as a move to 'rid the government of burdensome future obligations'.[141] It is an unfortunate irony that Friends of the Earth also played a critical role in stoking the demand for bottled water and disposable filters during this period. There is no doubt that the third factor in the bottled water market's steady growth was the success of its promotion through prolific advertising campaigns as a fashionable health accessory for stressful twentieth century lives, or even as a less healthy hydration accessory in the ecstasy-fuelled rave culture of the 1990s. Whoever chose to buy it, the stability of the bottled water fad was also tied to one function of the product: its portability. The bottle was a personal, mobile drinking fountain.

Perversely, or perhaps logically, mobile hydration took off just as the desiccation of public drinking fountains was complete. A rather plaintiff entry in the Drinking Fountain Association's annual report of 1985 announced that a poster competition for young people was to be launched the following year with the primary aim of encouraging appreciation of public fountain heritage and a secondary hope that such an appreciation might combat acts of vandalism.[142] As that decade progressed, the Association retreated indoors. It provided primary schools with utilitarian fountains, which was a worrying shortcoming of provision for young people's hydration that the charitable sector was stepping in to fill.[143] Persistent references to 'vandalism' over a period of twenty years hints at the deeper waves of social unrest that was finding expression on London's streets. For instance, 1981's riots in Brixton unleashed the tension between young people and the police over one bloody and fiery spring weekend, and by that summer street violence spread to Dalston in the east, Southall in the west and Wood Green in the north.[144] Slower burning scenes of public protest could also be seen on the civil service picket lines from March to July 1981.[145] The decline of civic services that employed such workers was further helped along by Margaret Thatcher's Government's abolition of the Greater London Council in 1986. With the loss of a strategic Government for the capital, coherent plans for nascent urban services such as waste recycling were negatively affected. In 1988 the problem of street litter was pronounced to be a citywide disgrace.[146]

Disposed water bottles were one the mass-produced disposable products increasingly adding to the volume of consumables in London's daily waste stream throughout the 1990s. By the Millennium, bottled water's transition from novelty to normality was complete.

Chapter Nine

Wasteland and Council Pop: tracking the anti-bottled water zeitgeist 2010–11

When did we get the idea that without constant hydration we'll shrivel up and die?
(*Suckers for bottled water*, Tim Hayward, The Observer, 9th April 2010)

Tim Hayward's exclamation was written in response to a tantrum he witnessed in a London museum, when a teenager howled at her mother for failing to buy her a bottled of water (amongst other crimes). The girl's threat to swoon from dehydration prompted a blog from the food writer. In the teenager's defence, maybe she was aware that her irritability was exacerbated by thirst. The odd drinking fountain has sprung up in London's museums, but a free drinking water source is by no means guaranteed in any public building, except schools (as mentioned in the introduction, not compulsory) or in prisons.

In the Noughties, or 2000s, sightings of Londoners swigging bottled water on the Tube, at office desks or in local parks were commonplace, even banal. Some of the trendiest brands carried by teenagers as accessories masquerade as freshly bought bottles when they are in fact tap water refills. Re-using bought bottles is certainly not a practice confined to young people, but obviously someone has to purchase them in the first place. Finding bottled water is not a problem, anywhere. Corner shop fridges glisten with rows of them, usually with two to three brands to choose from. London's cafés, from the most upmarket to greasy spoons are stocked to the gills with chilled water choices, whilst super-markets invariably dedicate half an aisle, or even more, to bottled water options. Given that the latter comes unrefrigerated, those bottles are most likely to be bound for use at home, or possibly by more frugal bottled water consumers (who presumably plan their extra-domestic drinking water needs). Those who stockpile their water might be relieved to read that the bottles' contents will remain fresh for more than a year. Fresh? The Natural Hydration Council helps by reminding consumers to 'drink plenty' of (bottled) water on behalf of its member brands: Highland Spring, Spa, Vittel and Volvic amongst other corporations.[1] Cooperation between these competing brands must be deemed a worthwhile exercise within the U.K.'s lucrative hydration market.

Between 1993 and 2003, the bottled water market swelled from 570 million litres per annum to a staggering figure of over two billion litres.[2] Consumption did not dip below the two billion mark during the twenty-first century's first decade. That figure does not specify London's gulp of that market but a combination of factors, such as climate, pollution, population and tourism, suggest that even 400 million litres would be a conservative estimate. This chapter investigates the impact of the resulting flow of plastic waste from discarded water bottles and the efforts of environmental campaigners to combat it by reducing demand.

In the belly of the MRF

For each bottle of water consumed, a container is disposed. In the 1990s and early 2000s, London's recycling infrastructure was not as sophisticated as today's material recovery industry but, recycled or not, those discarded bottles usually become someone else's problem. For Jarno Stet, Westminster Council's Waste Services Manager, the seasonal rise in plastic bottle waste from all cold beverages, including water, is a given. The stylish Dutchman, just 30 despite his prominent role in the world of waste, knows that water makes up a significant proportion of that plastic mountain. However, the figures are not precise because the plastic water bottles that do make it into the recycling stream are processed with other clear plastic soft drink containers. One quantity of waste that Stet can be more specific about is the London Marathon, naturally a large-scale water-guzzling affair. He candidly states of the Marathon's five-tonne bottled water footprint: 'They come in and trash the place and we clear it up; that's the unfortunate thing about it.'[3] Hosting the first London Marathon was a coup for Westminster in 1980, well before Stet's time. No doubt the runners and spectators left litter, but certainly not on today's scale. As we learned in the previous chapter, bottled water is highly unlikely to have been available then as an affordable product.

In the 21st century, Stet and his colleagues' swift operation ensures that litter from such major events is invisible. Fortunately, advance planning for inevitable waste production ensures that these plastics do make it into the recycling stream. They are processed in one of two 'materials recovery facilities' that Westminster City Council contracts to deal with its recycling. Like water, the waste management industry has been transformed by European Union environmental policies. High landfill taxes now make recycling an economic imperative for local authorities.

Annually, 6,000 tonnes of potential recyclables from Westminster are sent to a materials recovery facility in Wandsworth, in the suburbs of southwest London.[4] These recycling centres are known in the business as MRFs (pronounced 'murph'). This facility is one of ten across the capital that local authorities can use for large-scale recycling. A further 9,000 tonnes of waste is dispatched annually to a MRF in Greenwich.[5] The Wandsworth MRF, in the industrial suburbs of southwest London, is run by Cory Environmental Services. Intriguingly on Smuggler's Way, its Thames-side location facilitated the transportation of waste by river. Previously, as Stet explains, it was a 'transfer station' built by the Greater London

Council. When landfill dominated, waste used to be loaded directly onto barges bound for Mucking Marshes near Tilbury in Essex. Nowadays, recovered materials are more likely to leave the depot in lorries. A common cargo departing from Wandsworth is a bale of plastic.

Inside the building, a soundproof door separates the reception area from the percussive din of the MRF's enormous waste recovery machinery. On entry, an anteroom provides a gentle start for the uninitiated, though the scale of what lies ahead can be sensed through the sonic bleed into that space. A large conveyor belt runs through it at waist height and a few staff are positioned there to watch out for items to remove from the recyclables stream. Microwaves, for instance, are not uncommon in the flow of disposables. Around the corner, the cathedral-scale machinery is on display, where high-speed belts run at diagonal and horizontal angles. At the mouth of the machinery, a vast concrete pit receives cargo from recycling lorries of circa ten tonnes a load, creating a visual cacophony of waste. Its scale appears to reduce the recycling trucks to toys. Hovering above the pit, a crane arm lowers sporadically to grab two-tonne loads and transfers them to the first conveyor belt. How can the relatively delicate dimensions of a plastic bottle be discerned from this massive sea of waste?

Moving further into aisles of industrial machinery on metal walkways and staircases, the maze of sorting devices starts to reveal some order. 2D and 3D are separated by what look like rows of metal 'teeth'. Cardboard is whipped off high into the air on one conveyor belt whilst another shoots drink bottles along to their next phase of sorting. That stage separates the mass of all bottles into different plastic categories with the aid of a machine programmed to read the mass of the objects, resulting in opaque milk containers being divided from Poly Ethylene Teraphthalate, or PET, soft drink bottles. Using an illuminated heat-reading sensor, on detecting a bottle's mass, that bottle hops via a puff of air onto a separate chute. Bottle after bottle is picked out and 'puffed' away, as a variety of other objects run off the end of the belt and are discarded. But this is not all. As a green bottle approaches the end of the belt, another noise can be heard which signals the need to create a stronger air response: the green bottle is sent to a separate chute from the translucent bottles. The machine's intelligence is not flawless. An operative monitoring its performance calmly pulls out a couple of odd slippers that made it into the clear plastic bottle stream.

All translucent drink bottles, including water, should theoretically make their way into a dedicated chute. The aim is to keep the PET stream uncontaminated so that a bale of clear, coloured or opaque plastic is produced. Depending on the season, the Wandsworth facility recovers between 14 and 28 bales of plastic per day. Weighing in at three tonnes, a PET bale can fetch up to £2000 on the open market. Less transparent is who pays these prices for recycled plastic, or where the bales are destined for after Wandsworth. Westminster's recyclables become the property of Cory Environmental Services once they enter its facility and that private company is not bound to reveal its list of PET clients.

A 2008 research report published by the government-funded Waste and Resources Action Programme (WRAP), instigated to measure the CO_2 impact of exporting recycled paper and plastic bottles abroad, stressed the recent growth of the market: 'In 2007...half a million tonnes of recovered plastics were exported. The principal destination for these exports was China.'[6] The Government agency WRAP concluded that the practice of shipping containers of plastic bales to China was environmentally sustainable on the basis of the CO_2 emissions that it calculated at that time, however the system of cost and profits from plastic recycling between the public and private sectors seems ethically dubious.[7] More positively, a local client for PET bales that Jarno Stet highlights is Dagenham's Closed Loop Recycling centre on the periphery of East London. At that centre, another phase of recycling produces re-usable plastic for either new drink bottles or other forms of food packaging. The centre proudly claims on its website to be the U.K.'s first 'food-grade plastics recycler'.[8]

These glimpses of the world of waste management — often out of our sight in industrial estates on the city's fringes — reveal well-oiled businesses; ones that are part of a sector valued at over £11 billion in the United Kingdom (2011).[9] Certainly, many jobs are created by the waste industry but the notion that the polluter pays, in the case of products such as bottled water, is far from established. Most plastic water bottles do not make it into the recycling stream at all. Stet demonstrated this fact by an experimental survey of plastic bottle waste in a selection of Westminster's bins on a hot July day.

Donning a pair of a member of his team's gloves, he sorted through Piccadilly Circus's bins after a single morning of waste disposal. As a passionate advocate of recycling, for him it was a sobering confrontation with the items that will never make it into the recycling stream. This is 'contaminated' waste, in which plastic bottles mix with the dregs from disposable coffee cups and half-eaten sandwiches, for instance. Such waste, at least in Westminster, is no longer bound for landfill. Stet puts this waste policy in a nutshell: 'Throwing it into a hole in the ground is just silly because it sits there and doesn't do anything.' He is a subscriber to the philosophy of waste-as-resource. Instead of land-filling, all of Westminster's contaminated waste is burnt in a high-tech 'Energy from Waste' facility. The excess power produced is sold to the National Grid.

Even so, the human labour involved in clearing up and trans-porting these materials, and the carbon footprint generated in the process, is significant. Westminster City Council subcontracts the recruitment and management of its waste collection and recycling to the multinational company Veolia. 500 people are employed in Westminster's waste and recycling operation alone. Two of these operatives, who usually start work at 4.30am, assist Stet with his experiment in their Chinatown depot. They pile the would-be recyclables into neat mounds of plastic, paper and cardboard. Apart from his gloves, Stet looks incongruous performing this whiffy task in neatly pressed suit trousers and a crisp, stripy shirt. He appears dismayed by the results. Not one bag is devoid of plastic water bottles. In fact, they dominate the other soft drinks type by three to one. From six bags, more than thirty water bottles are extracted and that is only one morning of consumption, in one small patch of the capital. Multiply this average of four-to-six bottles per bin by the 2,000 waste receptacles on Westminster's streets (give or take a few), and the figure for a morning's contaminated water bottle waste is upwards of 8,000 bottles. Given the climbing temperatures on the hot July morning of the experiment, the figure is bound to be higher than on a drizzly February morning, but it remains alarming. Strikingly, a plethora of water brands were represented in the extracted bottles, testifying to the fact that for those who passed through Piccadilly Circus, on that morning at least, there was no favoured water tipple. Brand choice seemed arbitrary and therefore it suggests that drinkers are more concerned with the bottles' contents rather than the claims printed on the plastic strip glued around their middles. Some of the bottles reveal that only a few swigs were taken before they were discarded. Schweppes Abbey Well is one brand that was recovered from the general waste stream. This was London's 'official water' for the 2012 Olympic Games, an event purported to be a bastion of sustainable innovation.

The Cause

Post-Millennium, as climate change became a mainstream topic of debate, bottled water arose as a campaign focus in the agendas of some London-based environmental campaigners. Sustain was one of the first organisations to target bottled water consumption as an environmental problem from its 'better food and farming' perspective.[10] The charity has an umbrella membership working nationally but is London-based. As a food product, bottled water fell under its remit. Sustain published a report in 2006 entitled *Have You Bottled It? How drinking tap water can help save you and the planet.* The publication's author undermined a notion that was central to mineral and spring water consumers from Queen Elizabeth I to 1980s Yuppies: that bottled water was a health product. By querying the virtues of twenty-first century plastic packaging, in terms of the chemicals involved in its production and the uncertainty over whether those could leach into the water, or even absorb external toxins, the rows of bottled water illustrating the report take on a more sinister hue. Chemical leaching from plastic is a common health concern on many American websites that question the merits of bottled water, but little conclusive evidence exists to prove that the substance in question — 'bisphenol a' — is a health risk.[11] Sustain's anti-bottled water stance, however, is more firmly planted in the concept of water miles: 'The concept of food miles, and the environmental damage they cause is now well-established but bottled water can also travel all around the world before we drink it.'[12] This voyage certainly does not promote the notion of bottled water's freshness in comparison to tap water. Most importantly for the report's authors, choosing to drink tap over bottled water fulfils the ultimate goal of the internationally accepted priority of the 'waste hierarchy', ideally to *reduce* rather than recycle or reuse.

In 2007, after Sustain's report was published, an entrepreneur contacted Waste Watch's Maria Andrews about his Hydrachill product, a tap water vending machine.[13] Waste Watch was situated in Shoreditch just down the hill from Sustain's Islington offices. As a plastics expert, Nick Davies might have seemed an unlikely ally to Waste Watch, however he had designed a bottle specifically with tap-water-refilling in mind. His bottle tackled a flaw in the mouthpieces of other refillable bottle designs which were a choking hazard for some user groups. However, it was not the bottle but how it could be refilled that caused Nick Davies to contact Waste Watch. He had recently convinced Water UK to have a prototype of his 'Hydrachill' vending machine installed at its headquarters. The Hydrachill mirrors the design aesthetic and proportions of a common soft drinks vending unit, yet it plugs into a mains water supply to 'vend' filtered drinking water. When Maria Andrews heard about the tap water vending machine, she was hooked: 'You can talk about recycling, you can talk about re-use but the word *reduce* is really hard [to show].' As 2007 progressed, Waste Watch collaborated with Hydrachill, Water UK and Thames Water to promote the installation of ten trial vending machines in public spaces, funded by the latter. The project managers besieged London's local authorities with presentations about how Hydrachills could reduce waste. One organisation was pinpointed strategically as the most attractive, high profile partner for hosting the trial units: London Underground. Given the annual posters that appear in Tube stations during hot summers advising the public to carry bottled water, the proposal seemed to match a gap in Transport for London's service. Curiously, the organisation was not cooperative. Maria Andrews explained in March 2010 that, in her experience, 'if you try and talk to Transport for London which we've done on a number of different occasions, they asked us to do a feasibility study on where their water mains are — they were saying it would cost us 50k to go and find where the water access is'. Rather than see the proposal as an opportunity, Andrews felt that Hydrachill was treated as any other commercial marketing proposal or sales venture: 'If I was a franchise, say I was Burger King, I would have Transport for London running around after me.' What further frustrated Andrews was that the Greater London Authority's collaboration with Thames Water for the

London on Tap promotion campaign should surely have compelled its transport department to engage with a prominent Mayoral strategy: Ken Livingstone's, at that time. The Hydrachill sales team managed to secure two sites in Hammersmith Bus Station, with some sign of a willing Transport for London outpost, and the Museum of London. However, the planned October 2009 launch was stalled when the Chief Executive Officer at Thames Water changed. Hydrachill was not infecting everyone with the same enthusiasm as its promoters.

Aspects of Hydrachill might not persuade ardent environmentalists, let alone Transport for London officials, whose job description does not stretch to facilitating tap water promotion projects. Visually, the vending machine unit is not elegant. The advertising hoarding façades may attract users through scale and strident colours, however the unit's dimensions seem to exceed its main functions of cooling and serving piped water. A third function of dispensing branded refill bottles is one defence of a larger bulk for storage, but it is the aesthetic of vending as a design concept that seems an uneasy counterpoint to the commodification of drinking water. There is another reason for the vending likeness: Hydrachill's promoters proposed that a charge of 20 pence per refill would fund the project's continuation. For Sustain employee Christine Haigh, this sent out a confused message about the pro-tap water zeitgeist amongst environmentalists, about which she was blunt: 'Either it is free, or it is not.'[14]

Ideologically similar voluntary organisations can rapidly dissociate themselves from each other on the question of how best to achieve their goals. By design, Hydrachill importantly addressed the public space provision issue, albeit with the need for shelter and electricity. Sustain raised the spatial aspect of bottled water demand in its 2008 publication, *The Taps Are Turning*: 'Streets, parks, bus and train stations, museums and galleries, for example are woefully poorly served with public drinking fountains. Given how difficult it is to get access to the public water supply in public places, it is small wonder that people have opted to carry bottles of water with them.'[15]

The report's seemingly innocuous list of spaces in reality throws open a breadth of categories and reveals the complexities inherent in proposing where or by what means public water might flow freely. Another issue that the report raised also plays an important role in the tap versus bottled water equation in public life: political will. Sustain's report patted Ken Livingstone on the back for his administration's discouragement of bottled water provision at meetings. In 2008, his tap water commitment became patently high profile when the Greater London Authority collaborated with Thames Water. *London on Tap* was born. It was a campaign, the like of which had not been mounted since the post-privatisation years to market the capital's tap water.

Tarting up the Tap

London on Tap was launched in February 2008, with a specific remit 'to promote tap water in London's restaurants, cafés and pubs'.[16] The campaign's first press release was timed to coincide with the BBC's broadcast of a Panorama programme provocatively entitled, *Bottled Water: Who Needs It?* Journalist Tim Heap's investigative piece on the global bottled water industry presented stark images of environmental devastation, such as the carcass of a bird on a Dorset beach whose stomach showed that it had ingested 'nurdles'. These minute particles of plastic waste represented the environmental pollution caused by plastics generally, including disposable water, and other drink, bottles. The film, coupled with the *London on Tap* campaign, signalled that the anti-bottled water zeitgeist was not confined to environmental activists on the fringe, but that it was an issue endorsed by the water industry itself, the BBC and the Mayor of London. Anti-bottled-water activism had gone mainstream.

From the outset, *London on Tap* was openly anti-bottled-water, with supporters such as the Green Party in Livingstone's cohort at City Hall. The campaign focused on the message of de-stigmatising requests for tap water in London's restaurants. As Livingstone was quoted: 'My message is very simple: don't be embarrassed to ask for tap water when you eat out. You will save money and help save the planet.'[18] Thames Water adopted the quality assurance stance, when the company's then Chief Executive, David Owens, stated: 'Luckily in London we have probably the best drinking water in the world...in a recent independent taste test rated higher than 20, more expensive, bottled brands.'[19] He may well have been referring to Waste Watch's 'Tap Water Challenge', from which Maria Andrews reported that 90% of tasters could not distinguish between bottled and tap water (apparently the secret was to chill the water).

Designer bottled water emperor's-new-clothes effect was alluded to in *London on Tap's* competition for an 'iconic carafe' to turn diners on to tap water. The competition was judged by a high profile panel, including the Crafts Council's director Rosy Greenlees, architect Zaha Hadid and the environmentalist Tony Juniper. By the time the competition's winning design was announced, in December 2008, Boris Johnson had been elected Mayor of London. Despite party political differences, Johnson picked up where Livingstone had left off. In fact, his enthusiasm for tap water soon became as renowned as his love of the bicycle. Announcing the winning carafe design, the Mayor commented: 'Many congratulations to Neil Barron, who has created Tap Top, a top-notch water carafe for London. I am sure it will be snapped up by businesses and organisations across the capital in order to make tap water an easier choice. At a time when we are all tightening our belts, choosing tap water over bottled water makes more sense than ever, whilst also helping people to cut their carbon footprint.'[20] Visually, the industrial designer's winning carafe mimicked the familiar contours of a standard kitchen tap, but with dimensions stretched to the scale of a wine bottle. Like the top of the tap that one habitually turns, the carafe's neck has four ridges to grip, suggesting this familiar 'tap top' aesthetic whilst performing the more functional role of trapping ice in the carafe. With a choice of clear, bottle green or topaz-like blue, the carafe's elegant design might have enticed even the finest of the capital's restaurants to buy into the *London on Tap* campaign.

However, the plan for the carafe to become as common a sight on restaurant tables as the tap in one's kitchen has not transpired. Resources lavished on the initial campaign were perhaps not sustained for the project management of the ambitious scheme's next phase. Media partner to the campaign, the *Evening Standard* only covered the launch and the winner's announcement despite the fact that its editorial position is now firmly in the anti-bottled water camp. Perhaps there was no more news to relay about the 10,000 carafes that were released to infect restauranteurs' enthusiasm. The only eatery *London on Tap* parades its association with in press releases is the celebrity chef Aldo Zilli's chain (Zilli also happened to be one of the judges). One reason for the reluctant uptake could be that restaurants which encourage tap water consumption already have their own jugs, so they are consequently not willing to pay £120 for a box of designer carafes.[21]

Given the economic climate at the end of the Noughties first decade, restaurant owners would have to be pretty ardent environmentalists to both invest in the carafes and actively dissuade customers from buying bottled water. The product is by no means a benign profit issue. It is true that many of London's trendiest eateries do earnestly advocate tap water as a more ethical and sustainable food culture has taken root in recent times. For instance, Emma Reynolds, the dynamic young manager of a successful trio of sushi restaurants prides herself on the company's commitment to source fish from only avowedly sustainable sources. The same sensibility led to her trialling the second branch of Tsuru, when it first opened, as a bottled-water-free eatery. Many customers did not take to the lack of drinking water choice. Consequently, Reynolds now ensures that chilled tap water is always available to customers, but only as an alternative to the ubiquitous fridge stocked with bottled water. Some figures she quotes reveal why many businesses might not be so keen to push the tap over the bottle: 'We pay 30p for a 500ml bottle of water, charge £1 and pay 20% V.A.T. on the sale, so we make 50p per bottle.'[22] It is a persuasive profit margin for businesses weighing up environmental sustainability commitments, green kudos and consumer desires.

Twenty-first century philanthropy

The environmental zeitgeist in the restaurant industry that *London on Tap* hoped to connect with bubbled up elsewhere in 2009: outdoors, in Hyde Park's grade-one-listed environs. A local jogger noticed the world famous park's lack of hydration facilities. That jogger also happened to be a property developer involved in the largest regeneration project in central London in the late Noughties: King's Cross. Michael Freeman was also a trustee of the charitable foundation associated with the Royal Parks. When he proposed bestowing a gift for his neighbourhood park, the idea of a drinking fountain arose. Sara Lom, the Royal Parks Foundation's Chief Executive, recalls how she was cautious about matching the gift with the needs of Hyde Park's users and managers. Following consultation with the park's management, the project was welcomed as a public service and as a means of tackling the vast volume of plastic waste from water bottles discarded in the park. Ensuring the gift's actual benefit to park users and managers was dependent on an appropriate location. The chosen spot near Cumberland Gate, at the Marble Arch end of the park was identified as a place where the paths of riders, runners and walkers intersected. A small plaque not far from where the new fountain would be installed marked the spot where an ostentatious nineteenth-century drinking fountain — sponsored by the Maharajah of Vizianagram — once stood.[24] Like the Maharajah's offering to the Royal Park, this object would also be a unique artwork, though with a more muted aesthetic sensibility.

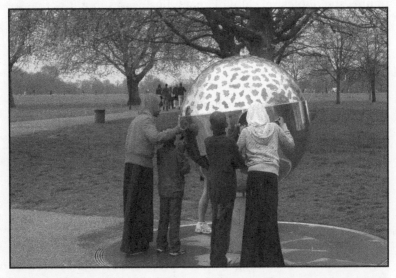

Freeman Family Fountain, Hyde Park, 2010. Author's own photograph.

Sculptor David Harber translated Michael Freeman's £30,000 donation into a globe of mirror-polished, marine-grade stainless steel.[25] At 1.2 metres in diameter, the shiny plinth-mounted object is visible from a distance to approaching joggers.[26] If one stands close by, a runner's laboured breathing can be heard as she or he runs on the spot whilst sipping from the fountain, even steaming up its mirrored surfaces on wintry days. At close quarters, Harber's nod to the hydrological cycle can be appreciated in the subtle shades of the fountain's bluey-green petals. During the sculpture's creation, the Royal Parks Foundation's consultation also involved working with young people from nearby St Vincent's Primary School who, as Sara Lom enthusiastically recounts worked on 'a project about why plastic bottles were bad and what they would want to see in a fountain'. Their ideas were fed back to David Harber, so it is no coincidence that young users of the fountain today can be observed benefitting from the design's three drinking spouts positioned at various heights. A fourth bottle-refilling spout is a notably twenty-first century design feature. The fountain's unveiling in September 2009 signalled the start of a London fountain renaissance, at least an outdoor one, when it was heralded as the first new drinking fountain to grace the Royal Parks in thirty years.

Whilst the finishing touches were being put to the Hyde Park fountain, Sustain began a project to translate its tap versus bottled water polemic into activism. Coincidentally, the initiative was focused on parks and fountains. Off a side street, near the bustle of Angel Tube in central London, the two women behind the Children's Food Campaign (CFC), at the charity Sustain, operate from an office densely packed with environmentalists. Their core campaign is to counteract the damaging effects of junk food mass-marketing targeted at young people and to secure better 'real food education in every school'. Jackie Schneider's and Christine Haigh's part-time posts are funded by the British Heart Foundation (at the time of the interview, in 2010). Their time is tight and the task is mammoth. Sustain's research on bottled water and the public space connection resonated with Schneider, also a primary school teacher. Fountains are a familiar topic amongst her pupils: 'Most schools aren't equipped for the whole class to have drinking water at once. Children get quite stroppy about that if they've forgotten their water bottle or drunk it all at playtime and they can't refill it. They are actually quite keen to drink water when they're thirsty.' All schools have fountains (often donated), however Schneider explains that the problem is the quantity. A lack of sufficient fountains is a common complaint voiced by student councils nationally. From a health perspective, the case for promoting drinking water as an alternative to sugary drinks was an obvious link for the CFC but Jackie Schneider underlines how it is also a crucial issue in the battle against childhood obesity: 'Young people can be confused that their body is telling them they are thirsty and they mistake it for hunger.' Water UK agree that obesity, diabetes, and some cancers, such as urinary tract, could be avoided later in life by children having better access to hydration and education about why it is important.[28]

When the bottled water issue became a prominent focus for Sustain, the CFC managers saw an opportunity to connect the public-space-water-access-deficit with children's play spaces (outside the context of schools). In summer 2009, they mounted a national census of park fountains. As predicted by the activists, the results were poor. One hundred and fifty responses were tallied, but only fifteen parks with drinking fountains were recorded and some of those had more than one fountain.[29] Desiccated civic fountains are a common trope of British parks, usually designed in the late nineteenth or early twentieth centuries. Out of the fifteen parks in the survey results, thirteen working drinking fountains were recorded. Though the research was conducted across the U.K. (fountains stretching from Ashford to Wolverhampton were tallied), ten of the fifteen parks with fountains identified were in London. A mere nine were reported to be functional.

Sustain's *Thirsty Play* report acknowledged that the results represented approximately a three per cent sample of the nation. An on-line message board associated with the campaign was overwhelmingly supportive, however concerns about vandalism and 'dog poo' contamination did surface. With limited personnel and time, they hoped the project would add to the momentum of other environmental groups tackling the bottled water problem and *London on Tap*. Christine Haigh further explained their philosophy: 'We could go down to the level of a national campaign and try to get a law that says every park must have a fountain but frankly we don't think that's the road to go down.' These campaigners prefer a democratic, bottom-up approach to the issue.

Find-A-Fountain

Parallel to Sustain's foray into park landscapes, a fresh-faced drinking fountain enthusiast was on his bike mapping London's drinking fountains. Like the CFC's results, he found that most of them were in a state of dereliction. Guy Jeremiah was a successful environmental consultant; that is until he became an anti-bottled-water zealot (easily done). As he recalls in summer 2011, a couple of years previously he was about to board a train in London to his hometown of Sheffield, when he realised that the only drinking water he could access was from a shop — in an expensive, environmentally unfriendly package. Mentioning this experience to his mother, she retorted '"Why don't you do what your dad does!"' It turned out that Dad simply refilled a used bottle from the home tap on his excursions. Jeremiah was not satisfied with this solution. One hung-over day in May 2008 he was lolling with friends on London's Primrose Hill and the thought of the tap water refilling came back to him (dehydration can induce such drinking water fantasies). After sketching the 'squashy thing' he was imagining, one friend was immediately impressed with his mock up. That friend is still a shareholder in what became a new product and a company: Aquatina (now rebranded 'ohyo'). Jeremiah's inner designer was on the loose.

Aquatina is a collapsible plastic bottle, intended to be as portable as keys or a mobile phone. The accordion-like bottles come in an array of bold pink, blue and green shades but the product took a long time to translate from his foggy-headed sketch to a mass-produced object that can be purchased in a couple of clicks online. Jeremiah brought his sketch to a product design firm in Sheffield, where it was translated into a 3D version that fulfils his collapsible vision whilst materially withstanding any possibility of chemical leaching. Moulded from 'category four' plastic, the Aquatina can claim to be free of any trace of the chemical Bisphenol A (BPA) potentially associated with negative health effects from long-term plastic

213

degradation. This environmental professional was not content with 'marketing Tupperware', as he puts it. He also wanted to tackle the public space facet of where such a vessel could be refilled with water, for free.

Jeremiah explains how he set about the fountain search with his colleague: 'Paul in a crazy fashion did a Freedom of Information request to every council in the country, pestered them all and some came back really enthusiastically and gave us all these rough locations of fountains. Most bizarrely did, so we mapped them all.' This spatial plotting, on the ground in London, was done with the aid of Google Maps and the same software was used to put together a crude website. Find-A-Fountain was born. Jeremiah is aware that his fountain promotion might seem too green to be true: 'Cynically people can look at this and think Find-A-Fountain is just a PR campaign. I hope it does raise PR but at the same time with the amount of effort we put into Find-A-Fountain. If I was a hard-nosed businessman it would be, forget that: put all the money into marketing Tupperware.' At sales of over 60,000 Aquatina bottles (as of September 2011) and purchases from major retailers, such as Robert Dyas, the marketing end of things is going well though Jeremiah is adamant that many more need to be sold for the operation to stay afloat. The refill market is getting crowded. One competitor particularly irks Jeremiah. The Water Bobble pipped the Aquatina to the post for supplying London's Science Museum shop. Apart from a loss of sales, and the product's American origin, Jeremiah disapproves of its unique-selling-point: a built-in filter: 'What are they filtering?' In his mind, those in the business of advocating tap water refilling should not be raising doubts about quality, because 'they're giving the impression to those who go into the Science Museum that for London's water to be safe, you have to filter it'. Jeremiah might be comforted to learn that the only bottle presently on sale in the Museum's shop is not the Water Bobble but a designer glass refill model that is starkly devoid of any brand name or filtering apparatus.[31]

Jeremiah does not mention the embodied energy in the production of his plastic product but Aquatina's website does state: 'Refill your Aquatina just three times and it's carbon neutral compared to buying bottles.' For those consumers in the habit of buying disposable bottles and not reusing them for fear of leaching, the product is a better option. Jeremiah is evidently passionate about improving access to free tap water in London and beyond. Aquatina's presence at the Prince of Wales 'Start' sustainable living garden party attracted the interest of the Garfield Foundation and Charles himself is said to have declared the design to be '"genius"'.

Find-A-Fountain now has a sophisticated website on which an interactive map of all the working, and dry, fountains Jeremiah and his colleagues located appear. Anyone can send in details of a fountain they find; whether outdoor, indoor or defunct. No map of London's drinking fountains has been published since the Metropolitan Drinking Fountain and Cattle Trough Association issued maps attached to its annual reports in the 1870s, but they were soon suspended as an extravagance when funds were running low. It is apt, therefore, that the same organisation in its contemporary guise — The Drinking Fountain Association — is working in partnership with Aquatina's founder on this contemporary mapping project that takes full advantage of the digital age and locative media.

"Refill on Tap"[33]

A new fountain, which appeared on Find-A-Fountain's radar in 2010, became the darling of the tap water refill market. This would be no bombastic Victorian-style restoration but a suitably twenty-first century civic amenity. Victor Callister, the Street Scene Manager for The City of London Corporation, was keen for sustainability policies to be transposed from the comfort of digital files to the messier realities on the ground. The edges of

Callister's Mancunian accent may have been softened during twenty years down south, but he is hard on the waste issue: 'We don't have many litterbins in the City [an anti-terrorism measure]. There's a lot of street waste...so in the general cleansing there are high volumes of bottle waste. It seems unnecessary that people are buying bottled water and not refilling their bottles.'[34] He issues this statement within an elegant glass-fronted boardroom, which forms a contemporary façade to the medieval Guildhall complex. Nestled in one of the world's most historically resonant spaces of global finance, his anti-bottled water stance comes as a surprise. Despite his distaste for plastic litter, Callister explains that the new fountain design will embrace the use of bottles, as long as they are re-usable: 'We think it's more about topping up bottles rather than drinking from the jet fountain.' Despite the project's small material scale, the human resources being poured into its production are evident from the account of its production that Callister shares.

With highly qualified urban designers and architects in situ, the Corporation's planners are usually in a luxurious position (the economic climate have already changed that). Part of the planner's job is to observe and respond to changes in the use of urban space. Victor Callister explains the significance of the chosen site for the pilot fountain: 'When I started to work in the City, it was a business city. It closed down in the evening, it closed down at the weekend and it was really only people coming in to do maintenance work on buildings. There was no retail because there was no business then. That's fundamentally shifted. You come around St Paul's at the weekend and it's one of the busiest places in central London.' These new residential and transient tourist populations form new publics. They consume and they make waste. One location where the City's diverse groups of workers, residents and visitors intersect is in the outdoor space of Carter Lane Gardens.

From a bird's eye view of St Paul's Cathedral, Carter Lane

Gardens is a slice of pedestrianised breathing space sandwiched between the road running along the south of the church and the Thames. The semi-circular little plaza-cum-garden has planted beds and benches dotted around it. Tourists, office workers, construction labourers and local school children alike all take breathers from their exertions there. Standing in the garden's centre and tilting one's head up to the right, the full height of the Cathedral looms, whilst to the left the Millennium Bridge's dramatic walkway shoots across the Thames to the feet of the Tate Modern. Pedestrians moving from the mammoth contemporary art gallery to one of London's première heritage tourism draws can pause in the tranquil space of the landscaped garden before entering the City proper. Here, the minor architectural wonder of the new drinking fountain lies.

Just before eleven on the scorching morning of 21st May 2010, a modest group of circa thirty people gather to launch Refill on Tap. Standing at just over a metre high, the polished cast iron rectangular slab of the fountain forms a sleek, elegant casing for the single water pipe out of which a sturdy, gleaming brass spout protrudes. Its Spanish designers, Santa and Cole, state that their concept for *Atlántida* – an off-the-shelf landscape architecture accessory – was to break 'with the classic design of an ornamental fountain'.[35] The only other feature is a grate in the ground for an essential function, which is drainage. Drinking directly from the fountain's brass spout would require a feat of acrobatics. It points firmly, almost stubbornly, downwards.

For the launch, a temporary street sign is in place to the side of the fountain, announcing: 'This is London's first fully approved drinking fountain in thirty years.'[36] Given that the Hyde Park fountain was the only other high-profile public fountain project in London at this point, it is hard not to interpret the statement as a slight to that project's integrity (green kudos a much-sought after accolade). The acronym WRAS, standing for Water Regulations Advisory Scheme, is emblazoned on the sign.

This stamp of approval certifies that the plumbing fittings encased in the cast iron slab, and the spout's design, protect both the health of its users and the wider water supply from contamination. Approval also encompasses the design's prevention of water waste. Santa and Cole's *Atlántida* had to be adapted for The City of London Corporation to meet these precise regulations. Callister is very clear that the fountain being shut down as a public health hazard would not look good and the fountain project officer, Henry Smith, looks harassed by remembering the lengthy process of securing the WRAS stamp of approval.

At the launch, Smith and his colleagues appear to be letting off steam. Ties are loosened and the team enthusiastically doles out custom-designed refill bottles to passersby, some of whom linger momentarily to see why such a fuss is being made about a visually underwhelming object. A compass is even embossed in the necks of the refill bottles (for lost tourists?).

The launch's atmosphere is convivially filled with animated chatter, until the hubbub is broken by the crackle of an amplified voice. That voice belongs to Bob Duffield, the charismatic Chairman (2010) of the City of London's Port Health and Environmental Service Committee. He issues the necessary acknowledgements to the regulatory bodies involved before launching into a passionate, political speech about the environmental cost of bottled water. Everyone seems hooked as he momentarily transforms Carter's Lane gardens into his own Speaker's Corner. Those lolling on benches languidly with their bottles of Evian perhaps had not banked on a late-morning snack of polemic. Firstly, Duffield outs himself as a hydrophile but the real meat comes as he states: 'There is no contest when it comes to cost. Tap water at two-tenths of a pence per litre is a hundred and forty-one times cheaper than the best-selling mineral water, which is Evian, and which, even if you buy it in a supermarket, costs over thirty pence a litre. Civil society begins and ends with effective plumbing and we should remember clean water on tap represented a quantum leap in human history and it is a tragedy that so many people in the world are remaining without clean running water.'[37] Duffield is an anthropologist by training, which goes some way to explaining his humanitarian stance on the subject. He makes it apparent why he believes the modest installation is, in fact, a seriously political move. Evidently not a shareholder in Evian, he reminds those gathered that a cargo of this brand, on a truck from Lake Geneva to Edinburgh uses '15.77 gallons of diesel and emits 350 pounds of carbon dioxide'. As buses and cars pass in a steady stream on Carter Lane and the air is thick with heat, the taste of carbon emissions is tangible.

Moments after Bob Duffield's speech concludes, runners from the City of London's marathon team canter over to hydrate and a queue forms at the fountain. Its slight proportions are overshadowed by the bustling milieu of planning department and environmental health officers who enthusiastically chat about their role in providing this alternative to bottled water in the City.

This fountain does pose an alternative to the notion that the surrounding shops, cafes and supermarkets should be profiting from the commodification of drinking water. As the launch crowd dissipates, a Water Delivery Company vehicle turns down an adjacent street and pulls up beside an office block. The company's cargo contains 'Spring Water and Water Coolers for your Office or Home'; a timely reminder of the powerful water culture the City planners are up against.[38] Presumably the modern office building has plenty of taps inside its premises, but this vehicle suggests that plain old London tap water does not meet workers' hydration tastes. This is somewhat ironic, given that many water cooler suppliers merely re-package tap water. Across the park from my own home in East London, tucked behind a corrugated fence under a railway arch, one such bottling plant busily fills up water cooler products with a filtered version of tap water. A peek behind the fence reveals the operation's convoluted apparatus, presumably for the removal of lime from London's naturally hard water (understandable), but no underground spring or mineral water source is being tapped under this semi-industrial cavern. I doubt this semi-industrial location is the provenance imagined by the people who drink from their office water coolers. The lucrative market for office water, some twenty years from when it was established, suggests it is now a cultural norm for offices to provide chilled water despite the environmental or financial cost and the availability of tap water from kitchens. In some settings, consciousness about the dubious merits of water coolers ensures the success of 'ethical' brands, such as AquAid. A portion of its profit is donated to countries with poor water infrastructure. AquAid, in partnership with Christian Aid, even strives to encourage existing clients who purchase coolers filled with spring water to consider moving to their more environmentally sound mains-fed systems.[39] As morally enticing as this company's agenda may sound, it still boasts a range of six different water cooler products, which is not exactly environmentally kind.[40] Combining corporate water profits with environmental and social ethics is a dicey public relations business.

Olympic Hydration

Tensions between contemporary urban sustainability agendas, modern consumer desires and the role of corporate sponsorship were blatantly displayed in London's plans for the Olympic Games. London Mayor Boris Johnson proclaimed his enthusiasm for public fountains back in 2010 when the Freeman Family Fountain was launched: 'I applaud the arrival of a super stylish new public drinking fountain in Hyde Park. ...I am a massive fan of drinking fountains and we are currently considering other ways of encouraging better access to tap water including drinking fountains.'[41] As the Greater London Authority was one of the main public agency drivers of the Olympic Delivery

Authority, one imagines that the high sustainability claims for the Games encompassed a free drinking water vision.

Published in 2009, the London 2012 Sustainability Plan *Towards A One Planet 2012* mentioned only one drinking water goal: 'To reduce the amount of drinking water used in the Olympic Village homes by 35 per cent.'[42] The publication also stated that 'games-time water management policies will be developed by LOCOG as part of the venue operational management plans'.[43] Initial discussion about water in the sustainability agenda was entirely couched in the rhetoric of water stress. Therefore, the fact that the London Organising Committee for the Olympic Games (LOCOG) was in receipt of major sponsorship from Coca-Cola could remain comfortably off the sustainability agenda until the event's operational phase began. A minor reference in the 2009 policy document briefly raised the issue of food packaging waste, including drink bottles as a recycling concern.[44] In the 103-page document, the word plastic appeared only twice, and that was in relation to construction materials. These omissions are rather disingenuous from a sustainability perspective, given that Coca-Cola Great Britain launched its new branding for the 2012 Olympics in March 2009.[45] As we saw from the brief forage through Westminster's bins, that very brand, Schweppes Abbey Well, is already in circulation. Coca-Cola's stake in the Games had not escaped the attention of Jenny Jones, Assembly Member of the Greater London Authority for the Green Party.

In a 2009 London Assembly session where LOCOG presented an update about its planning, Jenny Jones was first off the starting blocks: 'What are the requirements of Coca-Cola and McDonalds in relation to the catering arrangements at Games' venues?'[46] LOCOG's Chief Executive Officer, Paul Deighton, responded: '[Coca-Cola's] right is to be the exclusive supplier of non-alcoholic beverages in the Park....Coca-Cola, of course, has a wide range of products...also juices and water. The second thing I will just say to you is we have already committed to providing free drinking water in each of the venues as well.'[47] Jones pressed Deighton further, 'So can people bring in their own water, for example?' His rejoinder: 'Yes. Absolutely.' Perhaps it was planned by London 2012, but drinking water's first prominent mention in its published documents appeared in a press release about catering plans, coincidentally a couple of months after this very meeting: 'LOCOG has confirmed that free drinking water will be made available at all Games venues.'[48] Whilst LOCOG's commitment to a free drinking water offer, as the event delivery arm of London 2012, could be seen as commendable, this provision is stipulated as important for all public events by the U.K.'s Health and Safety Executive (HSE).[49] It is not really a choice in an event of the Olympics' profile. For every 3,000 people, one water outlet is advised by the HSE. Such licensing guidelines are well known by one of the designers of the Olympic Stadium.

Architect Megan Ashfield, of the architectural practice Populous, is softly spoken, but the strength of her passion about designing sports stadia is clear. She a strong advocate for embedding sustainable principles in the design of stadia but yet she is more than aware of the challenges this building typology presents. As one of the designers for the Sydney Green Games' ANZ Stadium, Populous experimented with alternative water systems: 'We actually used the roof as a water gathering and water harvesting device.'[50] Sydney's grey-water harvest was employed for both sanitation (flushing toilets) and pitch irrigation. For London 2012, she is a chief architect for the main stadium, or 'the world's biggest stage', as she calls the building. Thus far, the sustainability focus for its construction had been on ensuring that the embodied energy in the production and transportation of materials for the Stadium was kept to a minimum. Existing gas pipes, for instance, were used as structural components rather than freshly manufactured custom elements. With a circumference of almost a kilometre, the 'giant bicycle wheel on its side', as Ashfield describes the design, must reflect the project motto conceived by the architects, 'embrace the temporary'. London's challenge of scaling capacity up for the Olympics to 80,000 and back down to a minimum of 25,000 afterwards made the Meccano set concept for the building appropriate, as a skeleton that could be fleshed out as required. Some design elements in this skeleton were essential to its final use, such as toilets, however the architect explains that 'drinking water is one of those factors which can go either way'.

It is evident that Ashfield is ambivalent about the merits of drinking fountains, in sport stadia anyway. One reason is the intermittent use of the stadium as a building typology. She explains that 'unlike any other building type, they only open for a certain number of days per year. The average is about 26 days per year'. This fact makes Ashfield concerned about water stagnating in pipe-work when the building is not in use. Another concern is the queues fountains might cause, in a building designed for fast circulation of people between sporting events. She worries that a quick gulp from a fountain spout might not satisfy thirst over long periods of spectatorship. Despite her reticence on the fountain front, Megan Ashfield owns of drinking water: 'It's a given that you must ensure that people have access to that need.' She explains how an 'event continuation supply' must also be available in an emergency, but that is a larger plumbing issue. With respect to the general free drinking water commitment that LOCOG announced in its press release, Ashfield says there are two likely options, which are either mains-fed tankers or bottled water. And in her opinion, the bottle is the best choice: 'In terms of flexibility of supply, bottled water is actually the most efficient just because you can order one palette, or you can order 100.' Coca-Cola's distributors are likely to nod furiously in agreement. Whatever the architect might have advised at meetings, the final decisions about this were not hers. Bizarrely, these negotiations involved another team at her architectural practice. LOCOG contracted a team at Populous to provide the 'overlay' — the term for the temporary infrastructure that would flesh out the venues — but for reasons of client confidentiality, the two teams were not at liberty to discuss their projects beyond meetings convened by London 2012. Because of the design process, the drinking water solution was added on, rather than integrated to the venues' final uses.

For James Bulley, LOCOG's Head of Infrastructure, drinking water was only one issue in his daunting mission to prepare each venue for the Olympic and Paralympic Games. Given his hectic schedule, he agreed to a telephone interview with ten months to go until Games time, late in 2011. Bulley had been involved with London's preparations since the bid stage. His first response on the free drinking water question is candid, given that his paycheque was part-financed by Coca-Cola: 'One of the commitments we've made is that, for spectators at our competition venues, we will supply a source of drinking water...irrespective of what the legislation may require us to do...'[51] As previously mentioned, this is really a question of best practice rather than a sustainability choice. However, the method and prominence of the free drinking water offer can be widely interpreted. Drinking water provision first came onto Bulley's radar early in 2010 when spectator experience and security were discussed. When those customers entered the private, golden-ticketed realm of the Olympic village or other venues, they were not allowed to bring any drink bottles in with them; at least full ones. He describes the security protocol as 'airport style'. His colleague Paul Deighton's promise back in 2009 that people can bring in their own water clearly preceded this security protocol.

Airport-style security rules means that if LOCOG did not provide free drinking water facilities, their customers would be forced to buy bottled water. Given the profile of the positive environmental claims of this Olympics, that issue is unlikely to have slipped under the radar of LOCOG's Sustainability Team members who, as Bulley exclaims 'have a bearing on everything' (this is comforting to hear). He confirms that the sustainability advisors influenced the decision about free tap water provision, however it also involved input from members of the London 2012 Food Advisory Group. Sustain has been a member of this group throughout its planning but despite the organisation's groundwork on bottled water issues, its representative, and Sustain's Policy Director, Kath Dalmeny, had this comment on the drinking water discussions: 'On tap water, I wouldn't feel comfortable claiming a strong or pivotal influence. We were certainly one of several voices asking for this, but if memory serves me correct[ly] this included the Mayor himself, lots of people in the media...organisations on the Food Advisory Group, and just generally a kind of cultural sense of this would be the right thing to do.'[52] Some further research reveals that the drinking water element of the food policy (not sustainability as previously mentioned) was in print as early as December 2009, when many of the venues could still have had drinking fountains plumbed in: 'London 2012 will not only provide free drinking water at the Games, but will also work with venue owners to urge them to make sure it continues to be available in the Olympic and Paralympic venues beyond the Games.'[53] With such strong words, one wonders why this was not written into briefs for the world-class architects tendering to design the venues. More attention to detail at that stage might have resulted in some fountains being integrated into the buildings from the outset. Architects may protest that this level of detail does not appear so early in the design process, but, if it does not, such details will inevitably get left out.

Early in 2012, LOCOG's Head of Venue Development, Paul May, sheds more light on the free drinking water plan. For him, the permanent infrastructure built under the Olympic Delivery Authority contract simply cannot meet the drinking water commitment.[54] When asked about pre-existing drinking fountains in the venues; he can only confirm that the temporary basketball arena building (the one with the elbowed-out skin) was kitted out. It is evident from the conversation that drinking fountains are, unsurprisingly, not a must-have feature of the Olympic venues. May struggles to remember which venues, if any, have them. This poses a problem for the overlay team.

May reveals that the free drinking water offer for spectators will be a convoluted injection of temporary plumbing installations throughout the venues. Strangely, this contract is not with London 2012's official 'provider' for water and sewerage services locally — Thames Water — but with a Dutch company MTD. May qualifies: 'They're actually the world leader in this sort of infrastructure. They've done previous Games before and major events so we have quite an experienced supplier.' Where possible, MTD plugged into Thames Water's mains pipes, but for venues where this is practically difficult, such as Hyde Park, water was to be transported via a bowser (water tanker). MTD was also tasked with installing the 'drinking water outlets', or temporary drinking fountains. May promises that these facilities will be well signposted, though what they will look like was unknown when we spoke. A quick browse on the company's website shows, under the heading 'accessories', an image of utilitarian stainless steel trough-like sinks.[55] Design-wise they certainly do not overwhelm or excite me, but modernists may well applaud these plainly functional forms. For London 2012 staff, May was also confident that they would have water on tap in their dining quarters via 'bubblers' provided by the caterers (mains fed water coolers), to which MTD were to distribute mains water. From a spectator and staff perspective, therefore, the possibility of choosing the tap over the bottle seems plausible.

The people with less choice, from the plans described, were the athletes and the media. Both Bulley and May stress the need for portable water. May explains: 'Welfare of athletes has to come first, so they'll be very mobile, they'll need a bottle water solution so they can carry it around.' What did Olympic athletes do in the 1950s, I muse? For the international sports' media representatives, free bottled water is an entitlement that comes along with their Olympic press accreditation.

Even if no London 2012 spectator or employee chose to buy a bottle of Schweppes Abbey Well — the only unflavoured, still water option that was available inside Olympic venues — 10,500 athletes and 20,000 media personnel to be kept hydrated.[56] Bottles of Schweppes Abbey Well have to be transported by some means from Morpeth in Northumberland, where 'every last drop has been naturally filtered through water bearing white

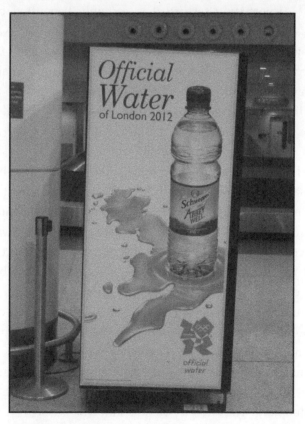

Vending machine, Heathrow Airport, 2012 . Author's own photograph.

sandstone for at least 3,000 years', as Coca-Cola's website states.[57] Morpeth is 298 miles from London, with an estimated journey time of five hours and thirteen minutes from the Olympic Park in Stratford. Comparatively, Thames Water's Coppermills Water Treatment Works, in Walthamstow, practically neighbours the Olympic site. Moreover, pipes rather than vehicles transport the latter's product.

Dedicated Schweppes Abbey Well vending machines across London stoked with 'the Official Water of the London 2012 Olympic Games' signalled that the unsustainable face of Olympic hydration will be spilled far beyond the confines of the official venues to the global city's most profitable tranches of public retail space.[58] Airport-style security has certainly benefitted bottled water sales. The seemingly unstoppable flow of bottled water to locations, such as airports, where demand for hydration is high and access to tap water access is limited, or unavailable, is something that incenses the founder of tapwater.org, who would 'really like to see Coca-Cola's sales plummet'.[59]

Council Pop

Michael Green calls tapwater.org a movement rather than an organisation, despite its title: 'When all's said and done its H_2O; there's no difference between what's in a plastic bottle and what comes out of your tap. They can call it what they want. It hydrates your body.' His no-nonsense view of the subject stems from a Yorkshire childhood, as he explains: 'Me and my brother would come in from playing football all sweaty and go to the fridge and there'd be nothing. Me mother used to say "well get some Council Pop"' i.e. tap water. His mother's witty tap water 're-branding' stayed with Green. When his London-based environmental movement was incubating, he decided that tapwater.org was probably a more sensible title than councilpop.org. The latter's potential ambivalence was an association that might dilute Green's polemical stance on promoting tap water. So tapwater.org was born, with a mission to make piped water access outside the home or workplace easier, and tastier.

The movement's founder is an unlikely environmentalist and anti-capitalist campaigner as a former property developer; and a successful one. Foreseeing the 2008 economic crash, he sold his property stock and headed for Sri Lanka. There, he put his carpentry skills to use on a post-tsunami rebuilding project. He recalls how this interlude, which morphed from four weeks into four months, allowed his long-standing antipathy towards bottled water float into the foreground, quite literally. One episode was on New Year's Eve, when he saw a Sri Lankan beach awash with plastic drink bottles. Having been a WaterAid volunteer at five Glastonbury festivals, Green was versed in the global injustices surrounding water and sanitation. He wanted to do something to address the production of plastic pollution, but he realised that his battleground lay where the choice between tap and bottled water presented equally safe products.

When he returned to live in London, Green was spurred further on his mission when he read a newspaper article about Neil Barron's carafe design for *London on Tap*: 'I rang him up and asked him if he would be interested in designing a bottle for me. And he is mad passionate about the hatred of plastic: just the same as me.' The refillable bottle that Barron and Green conceived is stainless steel, with vacuum insulation to keep its tap water contents well chilled, for up to twenty hours, as the website claims.[60] For Green the pièce de resistance was the design for the bottle's cap, which is now patented. The cap hides a secret storage compartment where tapwater.org's brand of flavoured tablets can be stashed. Dissolve these tablets and Thames water is swiftly transformed by orange, strawberry, or peach flavours, or with 'more exotic red tea and sea buckthorn flavours' (one 5 pence tablet apparently enlivens 500ml of water).

Barron's 'lifebottle' is an object with high design values that took some two years to develop and perfect. Lifebottles can be purchased from tapwater.org's online shop, which was launched in 2011, and seems to operate as slickly as any retailer (clearly, Green's commercial acumen comes in handy). The bottles sell in a strident matt orange colour; an opaque white coat, or in a raw, utilitarian (and hygienic) stainless steel. At £12 for a 350ml bottle and £15 for a one-litre bottle, the income their sale could generate might not be unsubstantial. Even so, Green is adamant that his project is not profit-driven: 'The fact that we sell bottles is irrelevant to the scheme. You do not have to have our bottle. It's open to everybody.'

Like Aquatina's inventor, Michael Green's cohort is equally interested in where the refilling takes place, however, there is a critical difference as Green explains: 'I don't think that drinking water fountains in the twenty-first century are a viable working option personally. They're strong words them. I'd love to think in the great, glossy romantic world they'd be fabulous but what you have to understand is that the councils won't adopt them, they won't clean them because they don't have the finances to do that;' (or possibly the will?). Green's alternative strategy is to gain access to pre-existing taps by convincing businesses to join the refill movement. Those locations then join the tapwater.org map, which can be used as a downloadable phone application. Cafés across London have signed up as free drinking water sites and the 1,000 mark was surpassed during the week of this interview, in August 2011. Michael Green summarises the philosophy thus: 'We thought, everybody has a tap so here you've got the perfect possibility to advertise, to promote small businesses. We're never going to get Costa on board. We're never going to get Starbucks. That's great for me.' Volunteers have signed up to help Green recruit these businesses and, then, it was London-centric. Green recounts how one volunteer, Ursula, 'completely blitzed her area. There's more [business on the map] in Chiswick than anywhere else'. A paid employee keeps the tap-water blogs flowing, with posts that reflect a distinctly internationalist feel for the issue. Green's other colleagues are freelance, but, when we spoke, he was bankrolling the whole operation himself.

Tapwater.org promotes its work at university green days, hoping to prevent the next generation from bottled water apathy and mobilise tap water enthusiasts. Green explains that this strand of work was initially driven by the organisation, but that university sustainability officers started requesting tapwater.org's participation in 'green' events. Consequently, it audited the drinking water offer in one London university and found that it had 135 bottled water machines. Not only was this quantity disturbing but, as Green utters incredulously: 'Guess what they're buying? Tap water!' He would not name the institution in question. With students, Green finds the most successful anti-bottled water argument is economics. Top of the list on the Frequently Asked Questions page of the organisation's website is a calculation for what the average person apparently spends on bottled water and other soft drinks in a lifetime: £25,000.[61]

Given that Michael Green's anti-bottled water polemic is so focused on the huge profit margins made by bottled water purveyors, another of the entrepreneur's ideas seems incongruous. He wanted to see refilling stations outside tube stations. Similarly to the Water UK, Waste Watch and Thames Water project, he also suggests that users should pay, for refills, '10p for a still water and 20p for a fizzy water'. Green argues that the charge can be justified because a service is being offered: 'You're getting water, you're filtering it and you're adding CO_2, so then they're not buying tap water.' Like Wastewatch, the organisation is no doubt thinking of ways to keep its operations afloat in the long-term, however such debates drive a fissure through the principle of free tap water as an alternative to expensive, unsustainable bottled water. The notion of an organisation other than a water company charging for tap water is potentially a dubious practice, one that would undoubtedly need to be scrutinised by OFWAT, as the water industry's economic regulator.

A single issue that London's pro-tap-water lobby does concur on the quality of the product that they are in effect promoting. Twenty years ago, faith in tap water quality is something that environmental campaigners, such as Friends of the Earth (FOE), were unlikely to have been as gung-ho about. FOE recently urged its supporters not to consume bottled water: 'Drink water from the tap instead — our water is much cleaner than it was 15 years ago thanks to EU laws, and is perfectly safe to drink.'[62] This wholesale endorsement of tap water is mirrored by tapwater.org and Sustain, however their rhetoric is supported by sparse information about how tap water quality is actually delivered and assured. They applaud the product but do not explain in any detail why, suggesting that the facts might bore readers. For example, the language used on tapwater.org's website to tout piped water is rather bland: 'Independent tests show UK tap water is among the safest in the world.'[63]

How is such a vociferously agreed quality stamp achieved, particularly in the case of London's, mythically, oft-recycled tap water? Should we implicitly trust the product endorsement delivered by the water industry, its inspectors, the Greater London Authority and environmentalists?

Chapter Ten

21st Century Tap Water: 2011–2012

It's not a product like biscuits on a shelf. You can't do product withdrawal: it's online all the time.
(The Chief Inspector of Drinking Water in England and Wales, Professor Jeni Colbourne)[1]

Public concern about London's tap water surfaces sporadically. Hangovers from the water quality issues of the 1980s are materially displayed in the staple stock of water filtration products on supermarket shelves and their aisles dedicated to bottled water. Those bottles are also ubiquitous in pretty much any retail outlet with space for a fridge, where they can be highly profitable sidelines: gyms are a good example. Clearly convenience plays a role in the non-domestic-use bottled water market, but the presence of the product as a staple in supermarkets does point to home consumption either as a health-based preference to sugary drinks, or as an alternative because of, some, genuine fears about tap water's long-term damage to health.

One accidental interviewee for this book was a successful painter who I met working part-time at a hair salon. She was performing pre-cut hair washes to help pay her bills. Originally from the modestly populated city of Belfast, the painter instinctively felt mistrustful and even physically repelled by the idea of drinking London's tap water when she moved here. Despite her financial struggles, the artist continued to buy Evian.

This instinct to reject London's drinking water could be attributed to two facts that do separate piped water from the product in a plastic or glass package. First, tap water is derived from *both* ground and surface water sources and, second, surface water requires more treatment than ground water. In the case of spring or mineral bottled water, this substance is siphoned from aquifers or springs rather than rivers and therefore consists solely of groundwater. The latter product is also sealed in a way that tap water cannot be; perhaps a characteristic that some consumers find reassuring as a guarantor of purity. Just like tap water, under EU regulations, all mineral and spring water must be tested to ensure that it is bacteriologically, chemically and radioactively safe for human consumption. However, a unique selling point is that bottled water remains chemically untreated, or, more correctly, unsterilized. The only treatments permitted under current legislation for mineral water include 'an authorised ozone-enriched air oxidation technique'[2], filtering to remove 'unstable elements'[3] (for example iron and sulphur compounds) and either the introduction or elimination of carbon dioxide. Spring water is also permitted to have either of the latter procedures or ozone treatment.

English law states that that the 'treatment of natural mineral waters and spring waters with ozone-enriched air shall only be carried out if it is for the purpose of separating compounds of iron, manganese, sulphur and arsenic from water in which they occur naturally at source.'[4] For many consumers, the notion of non-sterilised and therefore chemically untreated water is appealing. As the above list of naturally occurring substances shows, nature can also be toxic. Still, it is understandable that we might perceive rivers to be more volatile and susceptible to pollution, particularly from illegal sources, than enclosed groundwater. Could it follow that those who remain doubtful about drinking from the tap relate its outflow to the quality of London's river water?

This chapter enters the expert realm of contemporary drinking water production and inspection to find out if there is any basis to mistrust the safety of London's tap water.

Police and Producers

Thames Water's media team did not initially welcome the opportunity to facilitate a conversation between this little known drinking water enthusiast and the drinking water experts inside the industry's private gates, or entertain a site visit.[5] In the context of England and Wales, this barrier is also a reminder that tap water is produced by a corporation rather than by the public sector. Thames Water, or any other private water and wastewater service provider in England and Wales, has no duty to furnish me with access onto its private land to observe how drinking water, or sewage, is treated. One can appreciate Thames Water's reluctance to grant a visit to me on the grounds of the state of high alert for potential acts of bio-terrorism in London, though I would have happily been screened on that basis. My communication with Thames Water's press officers leaves me with the feeling that they prefer to keep enquiries for more information, beyond the scope of the company's website, at bay. This is a shame given that no other popular book dedicated to the subject of London's drinking water has been written prior to this one (certainly by November 2012). I am grateful that Thames Water has deposited the records of its predecessors at London Metropolitan Archives (City of London) where the general public can access the rich industrial and social heritage of this city's water supply. For any lay person to gain a more contemporary appreciation of the engineering, environmental and scientific issues facing today's water industry, only one London water company actively encourages schools to visit its facilities at the time of writing (Sutton and East Water PLC).[6]

Working with a sociotechnical approach to human water consumption, the Australian academic Zoe Safoulis is critical of the water industry's voice of authority because it often excludes the possibility of cultural and social dialogue about the interdependence of consumer behaviour and technology.[7] Safoulis dubs this authoritative stance by water industry professionals over the perspective of the user as 'Big Water'. Grand water engineering conquests such as dams and desalination plants display the industry's expertise, as well as its economic power and technological control over access to natural resources.[8] End users cower under the monumental scale of these grand feats, with little possibility of critiquing their conception or continuation as best models of practice. Such big technologies obscure our view of what goes on inside the water industry and whether we have any agency to shape its operations as consumers.

Highly mediated public relations strategies limit our gaze into the water industry. On Thames Water's website, one can read all about the amazing Ring Main, via which 1,300 million litres of water can be circulated, in a tunnel twenty metres below the depth of the Tube. It can serve Londoners up a freshwater cocktail with a dash of groundwater (from the New River for instance), mixed with a good measure of Lee or Thames surface water, or both. Virtually, one can snatch glimpses of the inner sancta of the water industry, but these corporate videos do not let the viewer linger over the messier process of abstracting raw water and its eventual refinement at the water treatment works. On the website, simplified pedagogical graphics simulating the water treatment process are useful on one level, but they cannot replace a more visceral, complex experience of the technological realm of the twenty-first century water treatment plant and an insight into the views of the people who are responsible for the production of up to two billion litres of water daily. Fortunately, a follow-up letter to the Chief Executive Officer of Thames Water prompted my enquiry to be revisited. Steve White, Drinking Water Strategy Manager for Thames Water, offered a telephone interview, explaining that physical access to a drinking water treatment works was not possible because of internal logistics coupled with my stated deadline (naturally, this was some months after my initial contact). Fortunately, White was generous with his time on the telephone.

At the Drinking Water Inspectorate (DWI) my request for an interview with a senior member this organisation was met with a degree of surprise, perhaps about the need for science professionals to engage with my lay approach to their fields of expertise.

Fortunately, the Chief Inspector of Drinking Water at the DWI, Dr Jeni Colbourne, did agree to meet in person to discuss her extensive knowledge of London's drinking water. Her organisation, formed post-privatisation in 1990 as chapter eight explained, is tasked 'to check that the water companies in England and Wales supply safe drinking water that is acceptable to consumers and meets the standards set down in law'.[9] On the DWI's website, common consumer concerns about tap water in England and Wales are reflected in the main subject headings of the DWI's choice of downloadable advice leaflets. Fluoride; Lead; Nitrate; Pesticides and Pharmaceuticals are a few of the titles one can peruse.[10] Most of the leaflets are designed to dispel all concerns. Lead is one substance that still lingers in the pipes of some homes that were built before the late 1970s (make sure to check that the pipes connecting your home with the mains supply have been converted to non lead-based materials).

Despite the organisation's title, the DWI does not carry out primary tests. It audits the tests that the water companies perform themselves and also the laboratories where they take place. A 2009 review of the organisation's practices pointed out that 'since 2007 [the] DWI has fundamentally shifted its regulatory approach to one which is focused on risks to water quality and safety', suggesting that testing is rather run-of-the-mill.[11] In Jeni Colbourne's *Drinking Water 2011* report (published after my interview with the Inspector) Thames Water was documented for some quality concern 'events', yet overall the company achieved a 99.98% rating for its product in that year.[12] One event categorised as 'significant' happened when a procedure failed at the Hampton water treatment works for a period of one hour.[13] Part of the chlorination process seems to have been the issue from the published notes, but details are minimal. It is clear that even such a one-off error, even for such a short time could potentially have extremely serious consequences.

Before Jeni Colbourne became the Chief Inspector of Drinking Water for England and Wales she explains that she 'was responsible, in various ways for the testing and the safety of London's drinking water supply from 1974 to 2003'.[14] Her responsibilities started at Thames Water Authority in 1974 and continued post-privatisation at Thames Water PLC. Despite the fact, as she puts it, 'that the badge changed on the door several times' during this period, Colbourne believes that her job has always been public health protection. She seems proud that her first post in the industry was as a scientist in the 'world's leading laboratory for microbiology' (the first designated Drinking Water Quality Centre of Excellence). She worked in the purpose-built water examination laboratory, constructed for the Metropolitan Water Board (MWB) in the late 1930s on Rosebury Avenue in Islington. A place, she comments, that is now 'posh flats'.

Our conversation takes place at the Inspectorate's Thames-side offices, just a few hundred metres from the Houses of Parliament within the Department for the Environment, Farming and Rural Affairs (DEFRA). Inside the open-plan office, the only hints of the industrial water environment are some yellow hard hats peppered about on coat stands. Refreshment is offered: a glass of water, naturally.

The grey-haired, yet youthfully exuberant, Professor pinpoints the factors that make London's water heritage so precious locally and on the global drinking water research stage. For instance, the MWB was the first organisation to publish drinking water examination data: 'The unique thing about London was that it was transparent. You've got 110 years of records.' Colbourne continues to inhabit the examination and research sphere that Dr Houston created, but now she is removed from the production of drinking water. Steve White, on the other hand, is on the front line of supplying 6.6 million people with drinking quality water, daily, on behalf of Thames Water.[15] Unsurprisingly, he moves in the same professional circles as Jeni Colbourne. Despite her public sector status as an inspector of his private sector sphere, they collaborate strategically amongst a highly specialised pool of experts. As a drinking water strategist, White's role 'involves understanding the quality of our drinking water and making sure we are doing, and planning to do, what is necessary to make it safe to drink'.[16] Colbourne emphasises, 'testing the water doesn't make it safe' but its method of supply and treatment should.

From Wholesome to GAC Sandwiches

Safety is a constituent of the legal term used to define water that is fit for human consumption: wholesome. The term is loaded for water industry professionals. Spelled 'holsome' in the sixteenth century[17], its basic meaning — that water should be a good element of one's diet — has endured, but our understanding of water's role in health, and food hygiene, has utterly transformed. In England and Wales' current drinking water quality legislation, wholesomeness refers to water supplied 'for such purposes as consist in or include, cooking, drinking, food preparation or washing'.[18] On the basis of this consumption and use it must not contain 'any micro-organism…or parasite…or any substance at a concentration or value which could constitute a potential danger to human health'.[19] The list of twenty-six chemicals in the legislation somewhat dwarfs the microbiological tally of four potential pathogens, however all water experts working at Colbourne's and White's level must have a proficiency in biology, chemistry and understand engineering processes and technologies.

By telephone, Steve White relays in a pondering voice the

stages via which London's water should arrive at the wholesome benchmark. He seems to pause at the well-stocked shelves of his mental water library, before swooping in on the precise word or phrase he is searching for. When he finds them, his enthusiasm for his job is evident. Abstraction, White explains, is actually the first stage of drinking water treatment; particularly in relation to surface water. Groundwater is less treated than surface water. Selecting raw surface water can be critical to the treatment it needs: 'You imagine, there's a plume of pollution coming down the river - the first thing you do is shut your intake so you can avoid that plume.' Abstraction also involves the physical screening of water through structures such as metal grilles, which, as White says, 'keep the canoeists and the dead sheep out!' Smaller screening devices also sift out natural debris such as leaves and twigs.

The supply's next treatment stage is storage, utilising the precious time factor that Dr Houston advocated so vociferously a century ago. Principles governing storage in water treatment have little altered since Dr Houston's days, according to Colbourne: 'It's a completely natural process and it uses sunlight and temperature and about ninety per cent of all purification of water supply happens just standing it in those reservoirs.' This is certainly a revelation. Steve White adds sagely that 'storage is about providing time'. Whilst potentially pathogenic bacteria are starved of sustenance, particles of organic and inorganic solids also drift to the bottom of the reservoir. Most of them, obligingly, stay there. Storage's power of bactericide also explains why groundwater requires less treatment, given its natural incubation period (groundwater can also become more intensely polluted because of the difficulty of diluting it).

Because Thames Water inherited most of Greater London's storage infrastructure accrued during the nineteenth and twentieth centuries with privatisation, the natural water treatment benefits of this method can be employed on a London scale. Though reservoir capacity is critical to water quality, it is equally critical to managing the quantity of water that London consumes. Professor Colbourne believes that the land purchased by private water companies during the industry's expansion in the late eighteenth and early nineteenth centuries has played a vital role in preventing London from a water crisis: 'They actually bought sufficient land in the area where most of the abstraction takes place from the upper Thames, you know around Hampton, Heathrow Airport and also to some extent up on the River Lee. They bought enough land to be able to build works with, what some people might say in this modern day was over capacity, as a result of which...London has survived.' Some of the land that used to house water treatment infrastructure has become redundant, as technologies have been streamlined. This provides a lucrative bonus for Thames Water shareholders in residential property development (such as the New River Village). But the vast reservoirs remain in situ. For instance, Queen Mary reservoir in west London has a capacity of 30,360 million litres. It seems extraordinary to consider the waste of any of this water, post-purification, being flushed down the toilet.

A cycle around the exterior of one of Thames Water's main water treatment works, in East London, helps to visualise the scale of a reservoir. Water held in the Walthamstow Reservoirs (which looks more like a lake) awaits transfer to Coppermills Advanced Water Treatment Works. The reservoirs are something of a suburban wildlife paradise. Anglers and birdwatchers can revel in these bio-diverse sanctuaries for an affordable daily or annual fee: impressive fishing catches from the reservoirs can be seen on angling websites.[20] On the road bisecting the reservoirs from the treatment works entrance, one side borders a wilderness-like scene behind a high metal fence. Birds set off on flights from an island in the centre of the reservoir and water gently lapping against its edge provides a soothing counterpoint to ambient urban noises. Across the road, behind another high

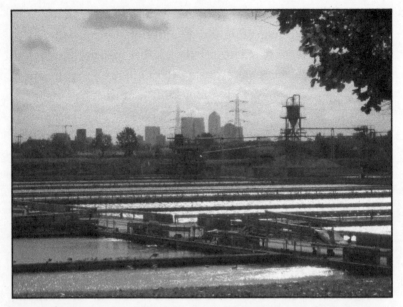

Coppermills Advanced Water Treatment Works, Walthamstow,
London, 2012. Author's own photograph.

fence, a more rational industrial scene unfolds.

The Coppermills Advanced Water Treatment Works is not the kind of place you would stumble across, though some residents on Coppermill Lane have good views over the slow-sand filter beds with Canary Wharf's skyscrapers looming in the background. In a recent book entitled *Edgelands*, its authors are preoccupied with the significance of the land morphed between the city and the countryside, where places such as sewage treatments works are located: '...they toil anonymously in the edgelands, never to be looked at, hidden away from business and residential areas, unvisited.'[21] Certainly, sewage works have good reason to be more distant, from an olfactory perspective at least, than drinking water treatment works, but there is no denying that Coppermills is obscured from the daily views of most East Londoners who rely on its product to survive.

A slightly unnerving statutory health and safety sign posted on the fence warns locals what to do in the event of a major chemical accident involving chlorine, sulphur dioxide, ammonia, liquid oxygen or fuel oil: 'Go indoors, stay indoors and seal all external ventilation until emergency services announcements are relayed on the radio.'[22] This gives more of an idea why the water industry might want to keep a low profile.

Behind the sign, the next stage of water's journey towards wholesome is on display. Vast field-like rectangular filter beds are filled with 'crops' of water. The development of slow-sand filtration during the nineteenth-century radically improved the quality of drinking water, however those innovators were not aware of the full extent of the microbiological good they were performing in the process (until the Franklands research proved it, as we learned in chapter four). During slow-sand filtration, water percolates through a layer of fine sand, which is supported by a layer of gravel. Sand filtration is highly effective for ridding water of any unwanted fragments of iron, rust or manganese; however, as a biologist by training, Steve White is also enthused by the removal of organic material such as algae, bacteria and parasites. As he puts it, the slow-sand filter 'reduces substances that are amenable to biological degradation'. Not so amenable, are some synthetic chemicals.

Chemical Challenges

When Steve White started working at the newborn Thames Water in 1989, the toxic chemical controversy was at its height. The problem had to be tackled by the corporation in order to comply with the law that adopted the European Drinking Water Directive as part of the terms of the industry's privatisation. In terms of nitrates, the distance of London's abstraction of river water from farmland relieved its levels of fertiliser by-products (in comparison to East Anglia for instance), but the slower process of nitrate seepage into groundwater sources was a slower-burning problem. Local to London, the large-scale spraying of the chemicals Atrazine and Simazine to suppress weeds on the edges of roads and railway lines in and around the city introduced a toxic substance into the aquatic environment. Addressing these chemical presences caused slow-sand filtration technology to be 'tweaked around', to use Steve White's modest description of what was, in reality, many years of engineering and scientific research in the early-to-mid 1990s. The case is a reminder of how there is no quick fix to complex water pollution problems, which is why pollution needs to be prevented by industry and the Environment Agency and why the 'polluter pays' maxim should be strictly enforced.

During those years what is now known in the industry as 'advanced water treatment' evolved. This involves a modular system of processes and technologies that can be targeted at specific water pollution culprits. For instance, if required, ozone dosing can take place before water enters the slow-sand filters. Steve White explains how this 'highly reactive form of oxygen gas breaks organic molecules down into material that's more readily digestible by microorganisms' and therefore builds up a 'biological community that adds to the natural cleaning process' within the filter. Filtration's other change is more materially solid. It employs a substance known as granular activated carbon (GAC), lodged between sand and gravel. Steve White describes it as 'a slow-sand, or a GAC, sandwich' and he clearly enjoys sharing the industry slang. GAC's principle function is the removal of pesticides but the treatment process is also capable of conquering other chemicals. 'It's a good thing for water treatment', White emphatically states about GAC. Londoners have benefitted from advanced water treatment since trials were completed in the late 90s. This technological evolution shows how polluters and pollutants have demanded costly new technologies and research programmes to be mounted in order to meet European drinking water standards, now U.K. law. Steve White was also personally active in the campaign that successfully banned the herbicides, or weed-killers, Atrazine and Simazine.

Chemical Concerns

Negotiating strategies for the prevention of toxins entering water catchments is still a facet of Steve White's work, in partnership with the Environment Agency (the rebranded National Rivers Agency) in its capacity as an environmental police force. He claims that he is 'less reactionary' than he was earlier in his career, meaning that he now considers the perspective of farmers more sympathetically in the agrichemicals-versus-water-pollution equation. It is important to note here that there is a distinction between synthetic and natural chemicals in pesticides. Choosing the latter is one of the bedrocks of the modern organic farming movement, but some scientists argue that any chemical, naturally occurring or not, can be toxic in high concentrations and that synthetic pesticides in safe quantities are no more carcinogenic than their naturally occurring counterparts.[23] No doubt that debate about synthetic chemicals and an evidence base will continue to grow throughout the twenty-first century.

Under current legislation, the permitted concentration of an individual pesticide in a sample of tap water is 0.1 microgrammes per litre, or one part in ten billion.[24] Some people would understandably have concerns about any trace of *any* pesticide entering their bodies, on the basis of fears that the cumulative effects of gradually absorbing multiple toxins in our environment can eventually cause cancers to develop (known as 'environmental toxicology' in academia). Proving this is, of course, very difficult given our exposure to so many substances involuntarily and as lifestyle choices, not to mention the lottery of genetic predisposition and the rise of epigenetics. The World Health Organisation's 2001 *Guidelines for Drinking-Water Quality* confronts this valid public health concern. In fact, the topic appears prominently on page one of the current 564-page edition of the publication, suggesting the perceived importance of this issue: 'Safe drinking water, as defined by the Guidelines, does not represent any significant risk to health over a lifetime of consumption, including different sensitivities that may occur between life stages.'[25] Its authors' certainty is reassuring. The same definition of safety is enshrined in the 1998 EU Drinking Water Directive on which the U.K.'s current drinking water quality law is based. It states that the combined total of pesticide residues in a sample of water must not exceed 0.50 microgrammes per litre, but this measurement only applies from 25th December 2013.[26] Reassuringly, Thames Water's website states that this is already the Maximum Admissible Concentration (MAC) of combined pesticide concentration that it observes.[27] Of course, a substance can only be ruled out if it is on the industry's search radar in the first instance. Pesticide compounds should all be detectable as their use in the European Union has to be licensed but there are measures in place to search for known illegal, or unknown, chemicals too.

In 2007 Steve White thought his days of worrying about pesticides were over. Another water company detected traces of a chemical compound called Metaldehyde.[28] The ingredient contained in some slug pellets was previously not thought to be capable of entering water sources. Metaldehyde's 'discovery' precipitated the creation of a national Metaldehyde Stewardship Group.[29] This group set up a 'Get Pelletwise!' information website to encourage and educate farmers about protecting water when using the product.[30] Thames Water recorded eight failures for the pesticide in 2009, out of more than forty thousand tests.[31] These breaches were minor and of no immediate concern for human health, but they had to be resolved because they transgressed the permitted MAC for a single pesticide. Thames Water recorded no Metaldehyde failures, from water produced in its own works, in 2010 or in 2011. The current emphasis on tackling the latest pesticide challenge is preventative, as the synthetic chemical compound stubbornly eludes all treatment processes apart from reverse osmosis.

Since 2001, the Voluntary Initiative — a national coalition of agricultural organisations — has been working to encourage pesticide education and offers technical advice on how to reduce the negative impact from pesticides on the environment, as an alternative to the introduction of a pesticide tax. The Voluntary Initiative's foci are protecting biodiversity and water, whilst continuing to permit agricultural professionals to use approved pesticide products. Its metaldehyde leaflet offers guidelines on the quantity of metaldehyde to use per hectare of land, along with instructions not to apply the substance within '6 metres of a watercourse' or when 'heavy rain is forecast'.[32] For the environmentally-conscious farmers this might work well, but what about when they are under pressure to protect their crops from a slug invasion? It would be extremely difficult, if not impossible, for metaldehyde detected in a water catchment to be traced to a specific farm or farm worker. The Royal Society for the Protection of Birds, which is represented on the Voluntary Initiative's steering group, and its supporters advocate education for pesticide users but argue that regulations to enforce the reduction of the most harmful pesticides are still needed.[33]

Sue Pennison, an agrichemicals expert at the DWI, is aggrieved that the word pesticide immediately raises alarm bells for many people: 'All pesticides have to be assessed for their effect on vertebrates, invertebrates, all of the food chain...'[34] Her defence of the potential toxicity of some products is reassuring on one level, but to meet the minimum legal standards for the concentration of such substances in the public water supply, great expense is clearly involved. In this respect, the polluter is certainly not paying anything. Our Rivers, an environmental campaigning coalition, including the World Wildlife Fund (UK) and the Royal Society for the Protection of Birds, argues that the cost of this 'diffuse pollution' (pollution from a range of unknown, multiple sources) is a clean-up cost that is met by the water companies and therefore ultimately water consumers.[35] The same group also questions the Environment Agency's efficacy in preventing diffuse pollution of rivers. Criminal charges can be brought against perpetrators under Environmental Permitting regulations, with fines of up to £50,000 if convicted.[36] Viable alternatives to synthetic pesticides do exist. Organic pesticide use is advocated by the Soil Association, which has published a comprehensive list of products that registered organic farmers must use.[37] There are plenty of slug-killing options that the Association recommends, proving that substances such as metaldehyde are not essential, even to farms not registered as strictly organic.

Whilst pesticide politics continue, the 1980's concern about the organic chemicals (trihalomethanes) produced during chlorine treatment has abated. Steve White believes the furore that trihalomethanes caused in the water research community was an over-reaction to the early evidence of their toxicity: 'We've now got a more rounded view, so the [current] WHO guidelines for trihalomethanes are more relaxed than they were back in the mid-eighties.' Therefore, the use of chlorine in water treatment has survived into the twenty-first century, but, interestingly, not primarily as a disinfectant. Colbourne gets excited about this point, exclaiming: 'There's no law in this country that says you must add chlorine to the water; there never has been.' The Inspector adds: 'What is a legal requirement, is to disinfect the water but that doesn't mean using chlorine and in fact many water companies don't use chlorine as the primary treatment these days.' (Remember, Houston only introduced chlorination in 1916 when ordinary water treatment processes were threatened by potential coal, and therefore power, shortages for filtration and pumping.) The Netherlands has controversially pioneered the production of chlorine-free public water supplies. Disinfection can now be assured with new technologies and processes such as fine membranes, ozone or ultraviolet treatments. Chlorine's role in London is apparently a matter of 'hygiene' rather than disinfection per se. By this, Colbourne means that low levels of 'residual chlorine' are added to the treated water at the very last stage of the treatment process to protect it, particularly in London, on the long distribution network from the treatment plant to the tap (some Londoners have valid concerns about the hygiene of the pipes between treatment plants and their homes, which is a topic that Thames Water would do well to discuss publicly). It is the accepted use of such chemical processes that we should reasonably question as water consumers, to understand why they are necessary in perpetuity, if they indeed are. Why do water industry professionals believe their use should not be a health concern? Such questions need to be publicly, transparently debated so that scientists can unpack the expertise informing these treatment choices. But first, let us return to the production line.

During chlorination, either by gas or liquid, the water moves through maze-like structures called baffles, so that no water escapes treatment. Ammonia is also used to prevent any adverse reaction between the chlorinated water and iron pipes, which could potentially cause a more discernible flavour of the chemical's residue.

Acceptability

In Steve White's department of Thames Water, a revolving team test the final drinking water product for taste and odour at least five days a week. He relays how tasters only make the grade if they pass a vital stage of sampling stock solutions. These 'organoleptic' tests also involve using smell and sight to evaluate the water sample. If a taster fails to identify its contents correctly, she or he is instantly dismissed from the water-tasting elite as not 'fit for the task'. Fortunately, it seems that Thames Water has enough staff with sufficient olfactory, visual and taste-bud talents to make the grade. This rather more subjective aspect of the drinking water world is tied to another critical concept to the legal requirements of the water companies: acceptability. Regardless of what scientists might say about the quality of the drinking water that has been supplied to a household, if the Drinking Water Inspectorate can prove that a reasonable consumer does finds the appearance, odour or taste of their water to be unacceptable, the water company has failed to supply wholesome drinking water. Coincidentally, I made a 'phone call to Thames Water with such a legitimate complaint about my water flavour, coincidentally during this research, and the person in the company's call centre had no idea what I was talking about when I said that my drinking water was 'unacceptable'. Nobody called me back to arrange an inspection and, after a couple of days, my tap water tasted normal and I let the matter drop.

The importance of 'acceptability' as a value has been enshrined in the World Health Organisation's drinking water guidelines since they were established in the 1950s. In less industrialised and democratic global locations, this can be a critical protection for communities where the assurance of safe water supplies can be a lottery. As Colbourne qualifies: 'If water's not acceptable, it still could be safe...but if they [members of a community] reject the water because it looks dirty, that's an unsafe thing because they will go off and find another water source that may appear clear but could have harmful things in it.' Acceptability is legally sheltered under the umbrella of wholesome and it is a concept that Colbourne notes 'most lay people don't understand'. This is a shame because it is a critical consumer right. The term certainly does not pop up with an easy explanation in a search of the DWI, Consumer Council for Water or Thames Water websites.[38] It is another example of insider knowledge confined to the realm of experts and industry jargon, rather than being deliberately withheld from the larger public.

Recycled Tap Water

One sure way to arouse a sense that water might be unacceptable is the often-posed argument that the average glass of London tap water has passed through several other bodies and kidneys before it reaches the kitchen tap. What does this claim actually mean? Surely the very basis of the hydrological cycle is the constant re-use of water?

Both the unfounded fears and the realities of water pollutants are tied to the persistent myth that London's supplies have been ingested and excreted by several bodies because of the population size, i.e. that the capital's drinking water is somehow *more* recycled than other towns or cities' drinking water.

On this subject, Steve White offers what sounds like a stock response to people who query the reality of this myth: 'All water's recycled. It's been through whales kidneys!' To separate what is mythical about London's drinking water from fact, it is essential to define what recycled water is imagined to be. When White uses the image of the whale, he is quite simply referring to the hydrological cycle in which water flows from rivers to the sea, evaporating into clouds, then becomes rain and so on. Water by its physical nature is impossible to trace precisely because of its natural mutability. As a chemical compound however, a strong characteristic of water is its efficiency as a solvent. So when we think about recycled water, we are conscious of what used to be dissolved and carried along with those molecules of H_2O and therefore what traces of those other substances might still remain concentrated in our water supply.

For instance, an issue that gained prominence in the mid-90s was that London's drinking water contained higher concentrations of substances derived from the birth control pill than elsewhere in Britain. Concern that this was causing oestrogenic effects was aroused when *The Lancet* medical journal published the results of a study into male sperm count in the Thames Water region.[39] If the fertility of male Londoners was under siege from tap water, it would actually have been as a result of pill consumption upstream, in Oxford or Reading, rather than within the capital itself. The mainstream press picked up on the research. An article in *The Independent* fanned the popular scientific speculation by failing to mention that other environmental factors had not been ruled out in the study.[40] Further flurries of publicity erupted and subsequent levels of public concern led to Europe-wide research into the plausibility of residual substances from the birth control pill being present in public drinking water supplies.[41] Scientists arrived at two conclusions. First, the chemical's presence at points of abstraction was rarely detected and could therefore be ruled out as a public threat on that basis. Second, where it was identified as a minor chemical constituent of abstracted raw water, conventional water treatment was found to eradicate all traces of these synthetic chemicals.[42] As the Drinking Water Inspectorate's information leaflet on endocrine disruptors states: 'The perception that London's drinking water is particularly at risk is also a myth...'[43] Testing for other pharmaceuticals follows a similar research protocol devised for the contraceptive pill, to detect any instances where abstracted water requires treatment for 'nanogram levels' of any substance (1 part in 1 million times 1 million).[44] Chemicals can be eliminated as a threat using this methodology. Colbourne explains that 'you don't go testing for substances that you've done the tests for, to show that they can't possibly get into water'. Caffeine is routinely used as a barometer for concentrations of what might be entering the water, at the sewage effluent stage, because it is so widely excreted after tea and coffee consumption. If caffeine is present, that suggests that other human waste products might also be.

Another more psychologically unsettling association with tap water's production is how we imagine wastewater evolving into drinking water. This perception forms a staple criticism of London's tap water as a densely populated place. Treated sewage does flow into the Lee and Thames upstream of where London's drinking water is eventually abstracted, but that effluent is not from London but places upstream of the capital. 95% of London's permitted sewage effluent discharges enter the Thames in its tidal part, with the closest point of discharge to the capital being Beckton. A 2004 Environment Agency report stated: 'There are large consented discharges of treated sewage effluent directly or near-directly into the River Thames as Cirencester, Oxford, Abingdon, Reading, Little Marlow, Windsor and Kingston-Upon-Thames.'[45] Jeni Colbourne rather nonchalantly explains how 'at the top of the Thames on the route to where London's water supply is abstracted out into the big reservoirs, there are some towns' effluents that go in, at a volume that overall helps to add to the mass balance but at a quality that supports the life in that river and encourages nature's processes of purification all the way down the river'. Her logic is clear, but visualising the effluent itself is less so.

These 'point source' effluent discharges from sewage treatment works are considered by experts to be of far less concern than untreated, and often unknown, agricultural effluent. Demystifying wastewater's contents and quality might reassure those 'recycled water' sceptics, however finding such details is rather a smoke and mirrors affair. On the Environment Agency's website, which polices the permitted quality of these discharges, no easy definition of sewage effluent pops up in a search. Any relevant, jargon-laden, documents are targeted at water industry professionals, or representatives from businesses who need to comply with discharge regulations, and these seem to assume that the reader is already well versed in effluent speak. Fortunately, the European Union's website has a handy 'urban waste water' glossary for the novice. Two helpful explanations reveal that effluent can be discharged after either primary or secondary treatment, depending on how the receiving water is categorised in terms of sensitivity i.e. industrial wastewater or domestic sewage.[47] In terms of future abstractions for drinking water the need for secondary treatment is evaluated by levels of remaining nitrate concentration. Other secondary treatment issues relate to wildlife protection in the areas local to the point of discharges. Effluent quality is determined by the amount of dissolved oxygen in the water, which indicates if there is a micro-biological population and therefore the presence of sewage, or not; a standard known as BOD5.[48] A clear explanation of sewage effluent does not surface in multiple searches on the DWI or Thames Water websites, nor how the substance's discharge relates to rivers and subsequent drinking water abstraction. What we do know is that all harmful bacteria and viruses are removed from sewage through the combined processes of wastewater treatment, natural river purification and drinking water treatment. However, clearer information about sewage treatment and effluent quality would be a helpful demystification of the high-technological realm of effluent production and management. If this information was available, tales of recycled water could at least be more factually grounded and some Londoners might obsess a little less about water purity.

Many non-water professionals might not be aware of the Water Framework Directive's significance. This ambitious piece of European environmental policy was integrated into English and Welsh law in 2003. Implementation of the plans to achieve 'good status' for all ground and surface waters by 2015 is now in motion. An Environment Agency document summarises that 'DrWPAs will be designated as safeguard zones that will have investigations and measures applied'.[49] These designated zones could be compared to the land owned by bottled water companies which they closely protect to ensure their products' purity and therefore ongoing profitability. Back in 1989, the authors of *Britain's Poisoned Water* mentioned that trials of such 'water-protection zones' had been effective in West Germany, Italy and Switzerland. The time lag between then and current policy implementation is frustratingly long. Drinking Water

Protection Areas success as a project remains to be seen but for it to succeed illegal diffuse water pollution will have to cease, permanently.

Successful adaptation to the standards of the Water Framework Directive does not mean that the quality of the final water we drink will be any better, at least if the drinking water quality standards remain as they are now. Its real significance as an environmental policy is that the energy expended in treating water should be dramatically reduced and less chemicals should be used in the process. Whether in the current treatment regime or a more resource-efficient system in the future, the notion that such precious potable water should be flushed down toilets seems absurd.

Steve White is not convinced about the notion of separating water supplies into potable and grey water categories, and not just because of the complicated engineering that policy might unleash. He says that some people in his industry believe that grey water use is a backward step and he concurs: 'How dirty would you allow your water going into your toilet to be? You want to maintain a clean toilet. You don't want brown water going into your nice white sanitary-ware because then you've got a major cleaning job. It looks like you're not being clean yourself.' Other forces might be shaping the forward-looking technological vision of his employer, as well as this preference for stain-free ceramics.

Thames Water took a significant technological leap forward when it invested in the construction of the U.K.'s first desalination plant amidst the large-scale regeneration of East London. The Thames Gateway Water Treatment Works started operating in 2011. In the short film on Thames Water's website publicising the merits of the desalination plant — *Keeping London on Tap* — the only use of water that is specifically mentioned, or visualised, is for drinking.[50] Only a plain glass of water represents the corporate product. People are not shown wallowing in baths, washing their cars, luxuriating in showers or flushing their toilets. None of water's many industrial applications in the city, such as cement mixing or beer brewing are shown. When we consider such omissions, the glass of drinking water is a rather benign, even misleading, representation of London's plethora of domestic and industrial water needs and desires.

The frontier of high-tech water engineering fits with the ambitions of Kemble Water Limited, which 'acquired' Thames Water in 2006 for £8 billion.[51] It is complicated. Kemble Water Limited is actually owned by Kemble Water Holdings, which is itself buoyed up by a consortium of investors. More than fifty per cent of the Kemble Water Holdings consortium includes various factions of the global finance company, the Macquarie Group.[52] Part of this group, Macquarie Infrastructure and Real Assets, is the largest manager of civil infrastructure assets in the world. As Macquarie's UK arm of the corporation announced in 2011, '9.9 per cent of Kemble Water Holdings Limited (Kemble), the ultimate holding company of Thames Water' was sold to Infinity Investments, according to Macquarie's website, 'a wholly owned subsidiary of the Abu Dhabi Investment Authority, for an undisclosed sum'.[53]

Of course, Thames Water's investment in desalination fulfils its licensed, regulatory commitment to keep London's taps flowing but ultimately the investment must also please shareholders. Desalination is clearly at the cutting edge of modern water management and treatment amidst global freshwater and climate change politics. Turning salty water into drinking water is quite simply technological alchemy in a century where water wars have already taken place and future conflicts over freshwater are sadly predicted. The grand technology of the Thames Gateway Water Treatment Works has many critics. Steve White admits that desalination is a 'horrendously expensive' water treatment process. External critics are more concerned about the wisdom of simply meeting ever more demand, rather than managing demand, when London has been classed as 'seriously water stressed' along with the rest of southeast England, since 2007.[54] Desalination, in the context of London, rather than its usual application only in extremely arid regions of southern Spain and the Middle East, does seem to be a rather extreme move. In 2011, both London's former Mayor Ken Livingstone and the Green Party's Darren Johnson argued that Thames Water should be conserving existing water supplies by preventing well-documented leakage.[55] The company's defence, reiterated in its promotional film for the plant was that leakage repairs were exceeding targets but that consequent savings would not meet water demand during a drought — particularly with anticipated population expansion in the intensely regenerated Thames Gateway region.[56] Theoretically, desalination should have been in operation during the 2012 drought, so swathes of East Londoners might have been unaware that they were swallowing their first draughts of desalinated water.

A search for further details about the desalination plant leads to the DWI's copy of a public relations strategy for the project, produced by Thames Water. The campaign's aim, evidently shared with such stakeholders was to 'move customers from uninformed', to 'informed', to 'reassured' then, finally, to 'acceptance'.[57] The need to shoe-horn sceptics into this narrative might relate to a drinking water practice that had been unorthodox since the Metropolis Water Act was first enforced in 1855: abstracting water from *below* Teddington Lock. We must remind ourselves that the river has 16 nautical miles (29 kilometres) to dilute any effluent from the Mogden Sewage Treatment Works near Isleworth in west London. We might also take comfort from the fact that, Beckton's unique 'four-stage' reverse osmosis technology apparently strips the water so bare in its purification process that it has to be re-mineralised before going into distribution. Quality assurance is needed whilst plans for a Thames Tideway Tunnel, popularly dubbed the 'super sewer', necessitate revealing how much untreated sewage regularly enters the river during periods of high rainfall, due to overflows from London's combined sewage and rainwater pipes (CSOs). Serious pollution incidents have hit the headlines, for instance in June 2011 when thousands of tonnes of sewage decimated thousands of fish, as reported by BBC News. Less porous ground and more hard surfaces, as the built environment ever grows, contribute to a quantity of rainwater that Bazalgette's drainage system was not designed to absorb. This situation makes the desalination plant's location *downstream* of the CSO pipes less appealing. Hopefully, because the desalination plant powers into action only in dry times (according to Thames Water's public relations literature), its intake is less likely to suck in untreated sewage. After reverse osmosis, the water will still be wholesome, but the desalination works location certainly explains why Thames Water had to craft a tight public relations campaign to convince stakeholders, even within the industry, of the system's merits. Having heard Steve White and Jeni Colbourne heap praise on the natural processes of water purification, the desalination works seems strangely out of kilter with their philosophy. But desalination is all about quantity, not a modest glass of drinking water.

From large water to little water

Although Thames Water is adept at producing and managing such grand infrastructure, when the company was approached about the relatively minor infrastructural issue of a proposed drinking fountain for the City of London, in 2010, it was flummoxed. The question of public fountains only surfaced recently in Thames Water's short lifespan. When the project manager for the City's pilot fountain project contacted Steve White's colleagues to ensure that all was above the regulatory parapet, White recalls, with some embarrassment, that the fountain project manager was 'bounced around different departments'. No public water department existed to catch the query.

Decades of dried up fountains had left Thames Water without an up-to-date policy. Consequently, these objects were considered to be a low priority risk on its radar of external contaminants that could tamper with the integrity of the company's supply. In fact, it was the City's query that pushed Thames Water into drafting a new policy on the subject.

Steve White enthuses about producing *Policy and Procedure for Drinking Fountains in Public Areas* between 2010–11.[58] 'On principle, it's great. Having water available for people when they're outside. Fantastic. An impediment to use is one of maintenance and how do you make sure that the water we deliver to that fountain actually stays as clean as we want it to? A lot will depend on what the last person has done with the fountain' but some of that behaviour, according to White and the City of London's urban design team 'beggars belief'. Though he did not supply graphic details, White gave the impression some unsanitary uses were involved. The City's urban design officers had meticulously done their homework on the design and installation of the fountain with respect to the plumbing and water supply, but maintenance issues are riskier. In order for a new public fountain to meet the regulations, two other parties must sign it off. In a water company's supply area, it needs to approve the fittings and maintenance to assure the risk of mains pollution is minimal in terms of design, installation and maintenance. This process follows the letter of the law, outlined in the Water Regulations Advisory Scheme (WRAS). The relevant local authority's environmental health department must also be on board the approval chain to perform its duty in safeguarding public health for fountains on its land and also for any 'onward distribution system' on land outside the local authority's direct control, but on its territory. The Royal Parks is a good example of a case where it must take responsibility as the landowner, yet the local authority also has a duty of care to the public who might consume from a fountain, in Regent's Park for instance.

If readers are confused by this convoluted regulatory maze so, it seems, were employees of Thames Water. The Chief Inspector of Drinking Water throws some clear light on a water company's duty as operators: 'If somebody connects a gizmo, they can do something that gets back and contaminates the wider supply.' Any fountain that is attached to Thames Water's mains supply immediately becomes a node in its highly regulated drinking water network. Thames Water could be liable if that supply became infected.

Colbourne is more than aware of the company's dormant public drinking fountain policy because she was involved in writing one when she worked there herself. The potential for contamination that she highlights falls under specific water fittings regulations.[59] In 1999 a new law supplanted the Byelaw Inspections, under which the fountains of the post-war period sprang up and subsequently faded. Responsibility lies with the water company supplying a fountain to inspect a device and ensure that the installation conforms to the fittings standard. Though the owners of all private buildings have to meet plumbing standards for protecting drinking quality water, when that premises is a public place (the definition embraces indoor and outdoor), the water issues become murkier. For instance, the DWI must ensure that environmental health teams in local authorities are abreast of any new installations available for public use.

Another point in Thames Water's drinking fountain policy has significant implications: '...all water used by the drinking fountain must be metered.'[60] Every non-domestic supply the company feeds is metered, therefore whether it is a general private supply including a fountain as one outlet, or a separately-metered supply created for just one fountain, the object's categorisation as a private water supply is not just a case of property ownership: it is a case of water ownership too. When The City of London Corporation publicised its new drinking fountain in May 2010, any mention of Thames Water was conspicuously absent. As Victor Callister clarified about the relationship between the object and its contents: 'We're buying the water off Thames Water so we're not necessarily promoting their involvement because we're just buying a service off them.'[61]

This is a point on which the success of a free water project, incubated in London's current Mayoral administration, since September 2010, depends. As Boris Johnson bombastically declared: 'If this place is generally getting hotter and people are going off buying bottled water I think we should have a new era of public fountains.'[62] When Jeni Colbourne was asked if she was aware of the Mayor's ambitions, this was her response: 'He's been wanting to bring back water fountains and all sorts of things, bless him. I don't have any problem with it at all as long as it's done in the right way. There's a right way and a wrong way and as long as it's done in the right way, great. If they do it in the wrong way, we'll do something about it to make sure they do it in the right way!' What, then, would Colbourne view as the wrong way?

So is the free public drinking water revival likely to ensure more free drinking water oases for Londoners? It certainly seems that neither London's drinking water quality or quantity present any barriers, but who is committed to jumping through the considerable regulatory hoops, footing the bill and ensuring that resources are perpetually maintained? And even if this is achieved, is it possible that Londoners might give up bottled water for good? Do outdoors fountains get used? Are indoor fountains more suitable for London's needs and climate? How should the drinking fountains of the future be designed?

Conclusions and Questions

The Mayor's vision is to encourage people to keep hydrated and reduce the demand for bottled water by ensuring free and easily accessible drinking water is made available across London.
(Greater London Authority, October 2010)[1]

High quality tap water is embedded in the network of technologies that serve the twenty-first century city. Understandably, our most common experience of accessing that resource is within our homes via our kitchen taps at a fixed price for an unlimited supply (for unmetered customers). The question of that water entering non-domestic spaces, whether private or public, indoors or outdoors, remains a fraught one. As we have seen, the free water access issue has arisen with green activism and politics in the first decade of this century. Even a modest public drinking fountain can therefore represent loaded social attitudes and values in tandem with its mere functional presence.

'Free access to drinking water across London', from which the above quote is extracted, is a Mayoral initiative that was launched in 2010 but has had little publicity to date (at least not at the time of writing in October 2012). As we have seen, public water provision is certainly not a new idea. It is worth briefly rewinding through some nodes of the narrative covered in this book's earlier chapters to establish how distinctions between public and private water evolved.

In the medieval City of London, the Corporation's involvement in the provision of outdoor water facilities was delivered in a marriage of private finance and public sector management. Conduits depended on the labour of human water carriers to transfer the liquid from public sources to homes and businesses, if it was not consumed outdoors (for instance in the thriving street market on Cheapside). The development of water

262

pumping technologies in the sixteenth century saw the birth of London's piped water supply corporations, whose founders invested in the creation of the city's first network technology (as Mark Jenner pointed out). Though it was a long journey for this distribution system to democratically connect all citizens with even basic provision for domestic and sanitary water uses, piped corporate water *indoors* permanently transformed the basis for why public water sources *outdoors* might also be needed and used in London.

The seventeenth-century parish pump clearly represented the continuation of a free public water resource for consumption at street level, or for transportation into homes. As the private water network grew during the eighteenth century, bottled mineral water became an elite health commodity for the wealthy, or for desperate hypochondriacs. The commodity was dispensed by coffee houses or sold in exclusive shopping districts. This product was not an alternative to ordinary drinking water, even though it is difficult to ascertain how much domestic tap water was used purely for drinking. We do know that the eruption of public concern about London's piped water quality did not occur until the late 1820s. At that point, groundwater pumps were still a part of daily life for many Londoners.

Then and until the mid-1850s, the parish pump brand of drinking water was considered by many consumers as superior to piped water, both in flavour and temperature. Post-cholera, the Metropolis Water Act of 1852 gave more of a guarantee that piped water did not contain London's wastewater, when it could only be drawn from above Teddington Lock and also 'effectually' filtered. We have also learned that it is somewhat of an urban history myth that alcohol was widely considered to be safer than water by Victorian Londoners, though some may have held that view post-1854's cholera epidemic and, three decades later, post-germ theory's discovery. These were moments or spells of concern, rather than pervasive beliefs held over decades. Certainly, the disrepute that the common street water pump suffered as a result of John Snow's research into cholera's 'mode of communication' was one plank on which the Metropolitan Free Drinking Fountain Association rested its case for a better-managed form of public hydration in 1859. Even though the true motivation for the charity's foundation, and swift progress, was to cure the drunkenness of the poor and working classes, its literature reveals a prevailing belief that corporate water was safer than the parish pump (this view failed to hinder John Snow's evidence about piped water's role in spreading the disease). Clearly, the construction of London's revolutionary sewerage system in the 1860s also immeasurably transformed the likelihood of sewage and drinking water mixing. A sanitary problem that did dog this period in the city's poorest communities was the fact that many people shared communal water butts fed by piped water. Therefore, many different, and some unwashed, hands and vessels potentially mingled to spread disease. 1871 marked a legislative turning point for more equitable domestic water supplies: companies were bound to provide a constant supply (even on Sundays) and landlords had to ensure that plumbing was in place to serve all tenants and all storeys of their buildings.

In the scientific and sanitary revolution that dominated the last fifteen years of the nineteenth century, the ethical debate over water's control, ownership and quality assurance swelled into a full-blown political campaign. This eventually resulted in piped water's transition from a corporate good to a rateable public service in 1902. Much of the ethical water question was focused on quality for public health. Achieving guaranteed tap water safety to all London homes was the task of the Metropolitan Water Board's department of water examination — in the first two decades of the twentieth century — under Dr Alexander Houston. His team's groundbreaking drinking water research made the provision of health-guaranteed piped water inside every Londoner's home an imperative. Sustaining this standard of production was threatened during the economic climate of war, which led to the introduction of chlorination in 1916. London's example influenced water engineers and examiners in other industrialised nations and the age of high-tech chlorination advanced during the 1920s. In these seismic changes focused on the democratisation of domestic water supplies, it not surprising that the issue of public fountains, at least in London, was not at the forefront of public analysts' and sanitarians' minds, or even architects, nor the new discipline of urban planning (in London anyway).

In the 1930s, the bubble jet fountain's arrival did show a flutter of concern for the extra-domestic tap. Its design offered a more streamlined, modernist approach to the common drinking fountain suited to indoor workspaces, such as the 1937 Factories Act demanded. We also saw a revival of enthusiasm for public water provision post the Second World War, when London's parks were revamped and socialist ideas were set into the built environment. The last example is the only government-led public fountain policy that I encountered during my research until that of Boris Johnson's administration. The drinking fountain has therefore somehow managed to connect the political left and right across many decades as a civic idea.

The nascent scheme of Boris Johnson's administration is heavily dependent on the goodwill and finance of charitable people (that is nothing new). Even though the scheme has not been publicised, those in the drinking fountain or anti-bottled-water campaigning realm are well aware of the Mayor's project. Some have even tendered to deliver the vision. There is a catch for them. The Greater London Authority's (GLA) policy document reveals that proposals have been sought from organisations 'to assist in the delivery of the Mayor's vision to provide free and easily accessible drinking water to Londoners on the move at no cost to the GLA or participating stakeholders.'[2]

Recalling my many conversations with fountain enthusiasts and passionate tap water and anti-bottled-water campaigners over the last two years, I wonder how precariously funded voluntary organisations can benefit from a scheme that offers no finance to support projects? Clearly it would be unwise for an organisation to snub such high profile political support. The attractions of Mayoral endorsement for the voluntary sector's existing projects offers input from urban planning professionals and powerful publicity opportunities, yet after my research it is apparent to me that creating a viable alternative to the bottled water market in a large city requires significant investment in people, hardware and, potentially, new legislation. An impressive aspect of the GLA's approach to the issue has been its consultation with various stakeholders, reflecting a respect for the knowledge and experience that already exists and therefore a democratic process, even if the project might well be inherently unsustainable. The niche social sphere of public drinking fountains and free water devotees is not free from its own politics.

John Mills, Chairman of the Drinking Fountain Association since 1982 (the current incarnation of the Victorian fountain charity), sounds a note of caution about the recent interest in public water. 'Yes, suddenly everyone wants drinking fountains; Boris and then the Lord Mayor and all the local authorities. They think they're going to do it for nothing. It comes and goes', he professes knowingly.[3] Mills is well aware that the delivery of any drinking fountain is not cheap in terms of materials, project management, maintenance, or even water supply (at least permanently). As an architect, Mills has designed drinking fountains in his day job. His architecture practice installed many a vandal-proof fountain for its client the Home Office, in Her Majesty's prisons. They are one of the few buildings where drinking fountains must be provided by law. In his voluntary capacity, Mills also works on local fountain builds or restorations (when I meet him, he takes me into a room adjacent to his office where he is tinkering with adjustments to a stainless steel outdoor fountain prototype). He feels that community-led fountain projects often succeed where the public sector fails. 'The local authorities are a bit disinterested [in drinking fountains]', he states candidly. If this assertion is largely true, it does not bode well for Johnson's vision. Both historical and contemporary examples, however, do testify to the influence of personalities on the fate of free water missions. Sustaining these projects until they become a social norm after initial passions have abated is more of a concern, from my evidence.

Before his re-election in 2012, the Mayor of London declined my request for an interview to discuss his drinking water vision. Some context for the scheme is provided in his administration's London Plan (2011) and in the environmental policy, 'Securing London's Water Future'. The latter policy reiterates that if free drinking water does spring up, it will do so 'at no cost to the taxpayer'.[4] As precedents, the policy cites six public fountains that the GLA has recently facilitated to some degree, though not paid for directly.[5] It is a modest number but a move in the right direction. A sudden proliferation of fountains in public realm design projects is unlikely, when the London Plan states that 'social infrastructure', in which drinking fountains are bracketed, should be incorporated into public realm design 'where appropriate'.[6] Appropriate is a rather loose term to interpret.

The GLA's vague note signals the limits of where the organisation can prescribe the detailed design of places it does not govern. Limits on the state's authority over the design and management of the public realm is partly a product of neo-liberal ideology that surrendered so much 'public space' to the market-place. More recently, state agencies are fond of sub-contracting the maintenance of the public realm out various service providers. Civic oases are few and far between, regardless of their managers. Importantly in the 'free' (or affordable) water access debate, thinking of the often-blurred boundaries that morph between public or private and indoor or outdoor is critical. Spatial nuances matter. For instance, in a model where free drinking water access is mapped on a website and navigated on the internet, or with a mobile phone application and promoted via social media, another layer of public space mediates between the actual café or park fountain, whether privately or publicly owned. Like tapwater.org, Find-A-Fountain and similar international schemes, for example Blue W in Canada, private sector sympathy for free tap water access may provide a more pervasive solution than a public sector revival of civic drinking fountains; precisely because businesses occupy such a large percentage of the extra-domestic spaces we use. One can also see the attraction for businesses to brush up against progressive social movements, or even tout their involvement as a corporate social responsibility exercise. It goes without saying that businesses, business owners and employees are no homogenous mass. Their influence on how the city looks, feels and works is enormous. Individuals' politics and influence play an important role in determining alliances. Whilst a water access lottery can create dynamic surprises, it also provides no guarantee that a café which joins a free water map will sustain this arrangement if it proves not to suit the business, or if the management, or even ownership, changes hands. Weighing up the evidence amassed during this book's research, I believe this is a gamble for a public drinking water solution that actually requires legislation to force the hand of *both* corporations and the public sector. Systemic change is needed to alter the built environment, just as campaigners for better public toilet facilities advocate.

Despite the surrender of much 'public' space to commercial ownership, the public sector still retains a great deal of power over the design, use and management of vast swathes of London's public realm (even by sub-contracts). Mayoral control over the daily operation of Transport for London and therefore the London Underground presents one example of a vast public spatial network that is ripe for a free drinking water trial. As we learned in chapter nine, the Hydrachill tap water vending machine promoters did not succeed in their mission. Embedded in the unit's design is the inherent contradiction of charging (even nominally) for tap water access, coupled with a pretty undemocratic approach to tackling the broader question of drinking water access on the London Underground, by mooting only one design possibility. Yet these environmental campaigners raised a pertinent question about a powerful strategic target. Architects, planners, product designers, station managers, Thames Water and Tube users would all need to be involved in a sophisticated consultation process. Reminders for Tube passengers to carry bottles of water during hot weather could be rebranded to promote refill facilities within stations or even on platforms (rather than boost spring or mineral water sales).

If a state or a public-private partnership did come to fruition, it would be the first professionally planned scheme of free drinking water in London.

The GLA's current vision does acknowledge that conventional drinking fountains may not be the sole solution to affordable water access, equally parading the notion of 'refill stations'. What should the fountains of the twenty-first century look like, who should be responsible for funding them and how might they succeed where others have desiccated? Some recent projects have got the ball rolling and deserve to be mentioned.

Ultimate Designs

During my research for this book, the Royal Parks embarked on an international architecture and drinking fountain quest (there has certainly been a strong zeitgeist propelling this history book into the present tense). Once the Freeman Family Fountain project in Hyde Park was in situ, the Chief Executive of the Royal Parks Foundation, Sara Lom, was hooked on the free drinking water topic.[7] About that time, Tiffany & Co. Foundation had set its sights on the Grade One-listed environs of Hyde Park for a project to mark its tenth anniversary. Following a stroll around Hyde Park with the person from Tiffany's, Lom consulted the Park managers about the prospect of splashing this cash on more drinking fountains. Hey presto, in 2010 a competition for an 'ultimate drinking fountain' was launched to find a design suitable for replication throughout the Royal Parks.[8] Under the banner of *Tiffany's Across the Water*, £1,000,000 was donated for the development of a new drinking fountain template, along with the restoration of 43 historic drinking fountains in the Royal Parks and some decorative water features. In collaboration with the Royal Institute of British Architects, the competition attracted over 150 entries from 26 countries. The specialist design and sanitary-ware expert judges could not settle upon an ultimate design: joint winners had to be declared. Announced in 2011, prizes were awarded to the elegant, elongated bronze *Trumpet* by Moxon Architects and the granite human-and-dog-friendly *Watering Holes* of Robin Monotti Architects.[9] In January 2012, the first *Trumpet* was inaugurated with a live fanfare by the Band of Life Guards in Kensington Gardens and a Watering Hole was ready for drinkers to use in Green Park by June. Olympics year was not the reason for these celebrations but it was certainly another motive to get the amenities installed and functioning.

A little trumpeted fact about the Royal Parks is the precedent of an existing drinking fountain restoration in Regent's Park for the Millennium.[10] Originally installed in 1869, the opulent structure of the Readymoney fountain, situated prominently on the main pedestrian thoroughfare of Broad Walk, was bequeathed by a gentleman from India's Parsee community during the philanthropic fountain craze.[11] Back in 2000, anti-bottled water debate was not high on the environmental agenda when climate change was still gaining profile as the issue of the new century. Consequently, this restoration was not heralded for

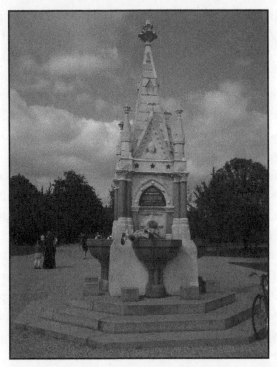

Readymoney drinking fountain, Broad Walk, Regent's Park, 2010.
Author's own photograph.

its green credentials. The restored fountain is not just a heritage showpiece. Readymoney dispenses water constantly, particularly on hot days, to Broad Walk's walkers and bikers. If the Royal Parks does roll out the ultimate fountains across its hectares of land, the popularity of Regent's Park facility bodes well for their use. Waste reduction could be significant if drinking fountains prevent bottled water sales in the Royal Parks because 37 million visitors a year reportedly enjoying these environmental lungs.[12] In order for large-scale behaviour shift to occur people have to be aware of these amenities. No easy alternatives would help, such as retailers selling bottled water within metres of drinking fountains. On my last trip to Hyde Park, in September 2012, I checked the café outlets and found that they were well stocked with Harrogate Spa water at £1.60 for 500ml. Parting with this sum for a convenient bottle of chilled, quality-assured, drinking water has simply become habitual. Beyond Hyde Park, retailers who align themselves with environmental policies of waste reduction, or addressing food provenance, often still stock bottled water but of so-called ethical brands. Even for those who claim to be environmentally responsible consumers, purchasing water in a bottle seems to reassure them. Conversely, many café and restaurant staff now make a point of serving tap water to show they are doing their bit to lubricate culture, and therefore, behaviour change. Bottled water is usually still available alongside their offer.

This study could not stretch to learning more about the reasons that motivate complex consumer choices in London today, but it is clear that, outside of commercial retail spaces, tap water access is problematic. Long-term, for free tap water resources to dent the bottled water demand and supply equation, they have to become a basic expectation in public places. In short, drinking fountains or any tap water refill facilities must be plentiful and located where they are most likely to be heavily used and well advertised. Only then can they make their transition from novel to normal.

Tiffany's and the Royal Parks also hope that its template fountains might crop up in parks and public spaces internationally, as a legacy of their competition. The ultimate drinking fountain quest certainly seems to have breathed fresh inspiration into what twenty-first century drinking fountains might look like, how they function and why they should be supported by public space managers. Enquiries from abroad have started, though Sara Lom is coy about divulging from where. Given Tiffany's involvement with funding the incredible High Line Park, on a disused railway line in New York, these prototypes could spring up in some equally fantastic locations on Tiffany's home turf, America.

Illustrious fountain locations understandably attract benefactors more readily than more banal public environs. Who, for instance, will fund fountains in railway stations? Some are, admittedly, more glamorous than others. In 1949, the Metropolitan Drinking Fountain and Cattle Trough Association announced its triumph of installing fountains in London's mainline train stations. Euston, St Pancras, Victoria, Liverpool Street, Fenchurch Street and King's Cross all received donated fountains.[13] British Rail evidently had more of a penchant for easing this civic provision than its successor, Network Rail. Now, every available square metre of space in railway stations, save platforms and essential thoroughfares, is filled with retail 'opportunities'. In the freshly regenerated St Pancras, the cathedral-like station is awash with drinking water choices, as long as you are happy to pay for your choice of bottled water brand from the saturated shop shelves. Nowhere in that bastion of modern, world-class, public space is even a small drinking fountain to be found. Under the new canopy of its refurbished neighbour, King's Cross, the impressive expanse of a spider's web-like white steel structure is not a shelter for even a minor hydration amenity. Both stations have been re-designed by internationally acclaimed architectural and urban master-planning practices whose work spans other cities of global stature such as Dubai, Moscow and Shanghai.[14] In architectural and engineering projects on these scales, the minor detail of a drinking fountain might simply be overlooked or specifically unwanted by clients. Such omissions pose a deep challenge about how to argue the design of this amenity *into* daily life, like they must appear in prisons or are more commonly found in primary schools (the latter is, incredibly, not a legal requirement despite the obvious case for sufficient hydration easing mental concentration).[15] Contrast King's Cross station with a similarly traffic filled public building, which has embedded the need for hydration into its very skin.

Users

On the Find-A-Fountain website's drinking water map, a blue-grey dot on the Euston Road marks the British Library. The dot represents one of only 28 indoor working fountains logged by volunteer researchers across London (not a lot for a population of millions).[16] Each floor of the Library contains two robust, yet elegant, stainless steel fonts. They are set into the walls of the communal areas where the library's users, known as 'readers', frequently pass by. These amenities are required for a building where water cannot be permitted to enter the reading rooms containing rare books. What is so notable about the British Library's drinking fountains is their integration into the current building, designed by Colin St John Wilson architects. Not clumsily piped in as an afterthought; these fountains are stitched into the fabric of the building. Readers and other visitors can sip perfectly chilled water at the spotless fonts either by using the thin, biodegradable paper cone-shaped cups supplied, or by refilling their own vessels. These fountains are heavily used. Located in close proximity to the building's toilets, they are just far enough from the loo doors to endow them with entirely sanitary associations. Even so, the British Library's restaurant, cafés and vending machines continue to stock bottled water choices (sadly like the Royal and Olympic Parks). Given the regular use of the amenities, with short queues often forming, one wonders what would happen if bottled water was totally withdrawn from the building's shops? A riot?

In the current consumer and retail climate, I wonder if we can ever imagine a shop not selling bottled water? Given that even environmentally progressive retailers opt for 'ethical' water brands such as Belu or One water, for instance, to propose the complete absence of the product seems revolutionary. Notably, that revolution has started in Bundanoon, a town in Australia just a couple of hours north of Sydney where shops agreed to stop stocking bottled water in July 2009.[17] This move might be the only way that customers will be forced to think about why they purchase expensive bottles of water and for stockists to think about how its drinking water profits can be met, if needed, some other way.

Back in central London, just west of the British Library along Euston Road, another dot for an indoor fountain on the Find-A-Fountain website represents University College Hospital. Inside the clinical white and mint-green-hued tower, which opened its doors in 2005, a cathedral-scale atrium with equally vast floor-to-ceiling windows permits natural light to flood in. Tucked in the corner of this state-of-the art medical facility's entrance, an inconspicuous Water Logic mains-fed dispenser cowers. On an early field trip for this book, I find that it is out of cups. When prompted, the receptionist rummaged around in a few cabinets before producing some plastic disposable vessels. While I should commend any free hydration resource — sighting one was extremely rare at the outset of my research in 2010 — it seems remiss of the designers for such a recent building, and its client (the National Health Service), to not have included a purpose-built public water source functionally and symbolically for human health. Also in the University College Hospital atrium, a newsagent is conveniently situated to relieve those thirsty medical professionals, patients or visitors who, unsurprisingly, fail to notice the Water Logic cooler (as I mentioned, it is rather slight in stature). Whilst I was parked on a stainless steel bench observing the mains fed water cooler's use over half an hour on a warm day, not one person approached it. Conversely, people emerged from the atrium's in-house newsagent equipped with their choice of bottled water product. Aqua Pura from Cumbria at £0.90 for 500ml, Volvic at £1.20 per litre, or the charmingly named Very English Spring Water from Kent at £1 for a small bottle were all available. Without conducting an intrusive survey, I cannot be sure if their water purchases were a deliberate choice of bottled over tap water, or potentially for the convenience of a portable container.

Either way, Dame Yves Buckland, Head of the National Consumer Council for Water would lament their choice. In an interview with *The Guardian* back in 2008, she noted that 'it's really hard to get a glass of tap water if you're in a hospital, or if you're in a railway station. You're almost compelled to buy bottled water because there's nothing else available'.[18] She is an advocate of the high quality offer we have on tap. Perhaps at least some NHS Primary Care Trust executives or estate managers tuned into the podcast and were inspired by her words, but without a design commensurate with the grand proportions of spaces such as the grand UCH atrium, the mains fed cooler is practically invisible and therefore unlikely to be used. Good design matters and off-the-shelf solutions do not always fit with the space in question, as functionally adept and low maintenance as they may be.

The Hospital example is even more galling because indoor public buildings are ripe for fountain experimentation. Praise must be bestowed on a neighbour of UCH, the Wellcome Trust medical history centre, which has installed two big, striking stainless steel (chilled) tap water fountains in its library in attractive and, importantly, highly visible units. As a tribute to London's stunning contribution to the sphere of drinking water's role in health internationally, the Trust might also consider providing such a resource in its busy lobby, perhaps through a commission of a fountain artwork, to draw attention to the drinking water issue symbolically as well as functionally.

Indoor fountains – particularly in London's temperate climate – are pragmatic because they provide plumbing, shelter and, hopefully, maintenance staff. If the managers of publicly used buildings, and architects of the future, emulate the principles of the British Library fountain model to any degree, there may be hope that widespread, high quality facilities in public buildings could stimulate a change in the perception of drinking fountains and, consequently, behaviour. On a practical basis, indoor facilities potentially provide a more stable environment and infrastructure to support drinking fountains. Yet that comfort has not stopped some optimists from the challenges of outdoor spaces.

The Great Outdoors

Another researcher has, helpfully, spent some time observing public fountains from the perspective of urban design. Could they, he asked, 'reduce the city's carbon footprint' by reducing the use and consequent waste of bottled water?[19] In June 2011, Roberto Cantu's first case study was on Trafalgar Square. This fountain was bequeathed to the square in 1960 by the Drinking Fountain Association and retrofitted to working order by the Greater London Authority. The amenity is a low-key mural design, only slightly ruffling the smooth lines of Trafalgar Square's eastern wall. The mural fountain is practically camouflaged in comparison to the way this world heritage site's bombastic ornamental fountains flaunt themselves. Visually, there is little to draw thirsty people to the free water source, instead of opting for the plethora of packaged water brands in nearby newsagents. Over three hours, Cantu counted a mere thirty drinkers on a mid-summer's day. One of those drinkers was a local street cleaner.[20] The snapshot in Cantu's report of that fountain user reminds me of Charles Melly's claim about urban labourers before his fountain was installed on Liverpool Docks: 'It was almost impossible for anyone to procure a glass of water without going into a shop and buying something — spending, in fact, what he might otherwise have economised' (1858).[21] Whilst his point is uncannily resonant today, the street cleaner's sup from the fountain is further layered with the irony that Westminster City Council's street cleansing team, some of who we met in chapter nine, are employees of the sub-contractor Veolia Environmental Services, in turn a subsidiary of French-owned multinational Veolia Environnement which is one of the largest water management operators on the planet.[22] Aside from the question of who is controlling and managing the civic provision of 'free' water, those who work outdoors are an important user group to consider in the public drinking fountain equation. At least this street cleaner did know about the resource but others may not have realised it was available. Over time, it is likely that word-of-mouth would play a role in promoting the use of clean, functioning fountains such as this one.

Cantu concluded that one reason for the Trafalgar Square fountain's low level of usage was a lack of signposting to the facility, compounded by its poor visibility. The researcher also noted that the proximity of an open rubbish bin to the fountain was unappealing. However, he rated the device's automatic

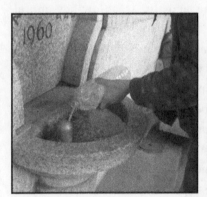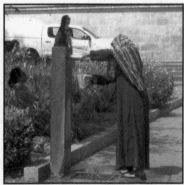

Left: Trafalgar Square drinking fountain, 2011. Photograph by
Right: Carter Lane Gardens drinking fountain, City of London, 2011.
Both photographs by Roberto Cantu, reproduced with kind
permission.

sensor highly on his 'usability' register, encompassing a range of differently enabled users, whilst pointing out that the 1960s design did not account for the needs of wheelchair users in terms of access.[23]

At the designer's next observation post, the bottle-refill fountain on Carter Lane Gardens — which we attended the inauguration of in chapter nine — access standards were better. Cantu chalked up 191 drinkers on his chart. Unsurprisingly, it was the hottest day of 2011.[24] His data affirms that an attractive, functional fountain will be used given the right weather conditions and the visibility of the amenity, as long as the user has a vessel handy to refill. At the City of London Corporation, there is no lack of investment in maintaining the appearance and cleanliness of the public realm of global finance's mise en scène. Many local authorities do not have this wealth. Even so, the money potentially saved by eliminating the cost of clearing up and processing water bottles as waste or recycling is one avenue for arguing the financial sense of installing and maintaining some strategically-located fountains. Routine maintenance, of a high standard, is critical to promoting the use of facilities, if built, and therefore potentially stimulating behaviour to change from bottle to tap water consumption. A conventional promotion campaign could also raise the profile of the modest fountain as a topic for public debate.

Funding-wise, Thames Water's shareholders might be convinced to part with some of their profits for public fountains as part of a corporate social responsibility strategy? In the financial year 2010–11, Thames Water Utilities Limited made a profit of £225.2 million and in 2011–2012 the corporation's Chief Executive Officer, Martin Baggs, earned almost £900,000 in salary and bonuses combined.[25] The cost of a few, or many, drinking fountains is clearly a drop in the ocean of Thames Water's profit margins. It would certainly be an appropriately civic gesture from the company's shareholders to Londoners, not to mention being a positive endorsement of its excellent product. Another incentive for the water industry to engage with drinking fountains is, perhaps counter-intuitively, to promote water conservation.

Just Enough

With good designers, materials and maintenance, drinking fountains should play an important role in rising to the twenty-first century's climate change and freshwater challenges. The fact that we only drink what we need from a fountain makes it sustainable *both* in terms of reducing bottled water waste and freshwater use. A well-designed, well-located, well-maintained drinking fountain gives appropriate access to 'little water', to invert Zoe Safoulis's term for the inhumane scale, and socially detached stance, of 'big water' engineering.[26] The social historian John Burnett reminds us in *Liquid Pleasures* (1999): 'Water remains the principle liquid drunk in Britain, although this takes a very small proportion of total water usage of 135 litres per person per day.' (Large uses are activities such as toilet flushing, bathing or showering).[27] The 1995 survey that Burnett quotes found that average tap water use was 1.14 litres. This figure was not broken down into water used in the home or outdoors but, even so, we know that the quantity of public drinking water that we need to counter bottled water is small fry in the bigger freshwater demand equation. More problematic is the promotion of unnecessary levels of hydration to rationalise the pallet-loads of bottled water that are shifted from juggernaut, to warehouse and newsagent fridges daily.

In a seriously water-stressed place like London, the idea of providing a resource where people can drink just *enough* for their hydration needs fits with forward-looking strategies of organisations such as Waterwise. Bottled water-sized packages are prescribed portions of water, but, when using a well-designed fountain, we can have agency over the quantity water we consume with the simple push of a button. Freshwater resources sucked out of the ground into bottles hundreds of miles away can be saved, as can the energy to transport them to us and for refrigeration. Water is heavy, as so many people around the world well know. Whilst refilling and carting around water is not a problem for some, for others who are already cycling with heavy loads, walking with luggage, or dealing with pushchairs and associated baby paraphernalia, water is an extra burden for the pedestrian and not an inconsiderable one. It is also easy to forget to bring water out, hence many impulse sales of bottled water (these add up over the years). But in order to make these choices, we have to know that drinking water is widely available and accessible, *everywhere* beyond our kitchens.

A hydration lottery will not work, as people will simply revert to bottled water. The bottled water market relies on our instinctive craving for water, often in favour of any other hydration product. For public water resources to change London's consumption and waste habits significantly, and those of other cities or towns in Europe and beyond, fountains are not only needed as amenities in parks, they need to be provided in indoor, or at least sheltered, locations in the city and beyond; such as motorway service stations, shopping centres, supermarkets and train stations to name but a few places. Where is free drinking water to be found in the vast swathes of space owned by Asda, Sainsbury's, Tesco or Westfield? With decent budgets from such wealthy corporations, a whole new fountain, public tap, or refill station lexicon could be unleashed (I have a particular fantasy about rain-water harvesting drinking fountains that, somehow, purify in situ). Through planning legislation, the Community Infrastructure Levy could certainly be another fountain funding stream, which all developers of publicly used buildings must pay towards civic infrastructure (at a fee per square metre). Section 106 fees that property developers must pay to local authorities are also a source of cash for this much-needed 'social infrastructure'.[28] How that need is translated successfully into the built environment for the benefit of users and the managers of buildings and public spaces does need further analysis and research to ensure sustainable solutions. Legislation may well be the only way to force those owners of our most frequently used daily spaces to actively promote the de-commodification of drinking water and make one healthy contribution to a more sustainable city. Similarly to the hospital example in terms of scale, supermarkets or shopping malls would need to install a highly visible fountain in order to distract any consumers from bottled water.

Drinking water ethics

Through whatever combination of fountains, refill stations, or water transported by individuals from their own homes, a permanent public drinking water revolution for London could actually eliminate the need for bottled water. A perpetual flow of piped tap water and bottled water into the city is simply not necessary. Of course, this mirrors the story of many packaged, highly profitable consumables but the difference with water is that we really do need some of it, if not in those quantities or through those modes of production.

A mirror of the overlap between this city's public and private space interests was seen in the planning for the 2012 Olympic Games, particularly because of its public-private funding partnership. Some eco ambitions were thwarted by Coca-Cola's sponsorship which dictated that its product had to be supplied alongside free tap water. Tales from inside the Olympic Park recounted impossibly long queues for the free water sources, with one of my interviewees explaining how her mother had given up the wait and bought a bottle of Schweppes Abbey Well, in order to make it to the next event (tickets were hard fought for).[29] Culturally, there is a certain resignation to parting with £1.60 for a bottle of water, simply because the products are so ubiquitous and it is hard to imagine a time when they were not available, like so many disposable consumables. Positively, ticket holders at London 2012 were permitted to bring empty plastic bottles into the Park. Also, at the temporary hydration stations, no cups were provided to help combat unnecessary waste production. The efforts of the sustainability people working inside the Games can be felt in these important, intelligent choices. My inside observers concurred that demand for the free water well exceeded what was available during busy spells. If bottled water had not been available, more free drinking water sources would have been essential, particularly in the light of the airport-style security preventing ticket holders from bringing their own tap water into the venues. The strain between sustainability rhetoric and the stake of, some, sponsors is evident in the twin drinking water arrangements.

Coca-Cola met potential accusations of hypocrisy head on, in a now-familiar style of corporations acknowledging inherently unsustainable practices. A form of reverse psychology is employed to green-wash what is really un-green-washable. Take this statement in one of London 2012's sustainability reports: 'Millions of drinks will be consumed during the Olympic and Paralympic Games and the company recognises that their product packaging will contribute significantly to the recyclable waste stream. The Coca-Cola Company is therefore working in partnership with LOCOG to develop a compelling campaign to encourage visitors to recycle.'[30] The corporation certainly seemed confident from this statement that the tap water choice would not dent its sales at the Games. This paradigm shows how ludicrously profitable drinking water has become in London, and globally. One persistent defence from bottled water manufacturers is that their product is essential in emergencies, which is unfortunately true for places such as Haiti. There, the 2010 earthquake led to an outbreak of cholera which is reported to have caused more than 7,000 deaths and has been mired in controversy about where responsibility for the cause and cure for the disease should lie. The United Nations itself has been accused of causing the spread of cholera.[31] It is immoral and unacceptable that such a poor nation has to rely on bottled water for an assured supply of safe drinking water. Like many places where water quality cannot be guaranteed, the poorest people are forced to buy bottled water or use the services of water 'vendors', who profit from these endemic infrastructural malaises. Those are political and environmental failures that most developed world nations are extremely fortunate *not* to confront.

Drought is a natural disaster that must be considered in the U.K. and other developed world nations and hence the concept of a national water grid is rightly on the environmental, political and water industry agenda. That is simply not a drinking water issue because of the quantities of consumption in question. As stated at the beginning of the book, hosepipe bans are an inconvenience but not being able to pour a glass of water out of the tap is practically unimaginable and could soon be solved from alternative sources without the need for emergency bottled water, with appropriate planning.

As well as countering the flow of bottled water products, issues of social justice and welfare also need to be factored into the hydration equation even in industrialised nations. If we forget to refill a bottle from the tap to bring outdoors with us, should our only hydration recourse be to pay an unethically high price for drinking water, or to beg an employee in a café to hand over some free water? What if that thirsty person is ill, heavily pregnant, elderly, a toddler, penniless or homeless? Or what if that person is none of those vulnerable categories, but simply a thirsty citizen in need of a modest quantity of water to rehydrate? Water is fundamental to maintaining all of our bodily functions, so how can citizens be effectively denied access to it? How does the United Nations landmark announcement in 2002 that access to safe drinking water is a core human right translate to the context of the developed world globalised city?

Published in 2001, economist Riccardo Petrella's polemic *The Water Manifesto* argues for a World Water Contract to ensure basic and consistent access to water 'for every human being and every human community'.[32] His critique of the transition of water's management in many countries from the public to the private sector and its valuation in market-based terms, rather than as a 'non-substitutable common social asset' remains valid in England and Wales today (notably not in Scotland, where the water and waste-water industry was not privatised in 1989). As a Dubliner originally, I was downcast to read in Petrella's account of water's commodification that an international agreement about re-categorising water as an 'economic asset', convened by the United Nations, was forged in 1992, in my home city.[33] Less than ten years later, this economist was making a different plea to the international community, on the basis that water is not interchangeable with other commodities, particularly water needed for drinking. In Petrella's words: 'Basic access for *every human being* means that he or she can enjoy the minimum quantity of fresh drinking water that society considers necessary and indispensable to a decent life, and that the quality of this water is in accordance with world health norms.'[34] His thesis has been hugely influential. In 2003 the United Nations published its conclusions from a committee interrogating drinking water's place in the International Covenant on Economic, Social and Cultural Rights: 'The Human Right to water is indispensable for leading a life in human dignity'. The Committee further resolved that 'the right to water is also inextricably linked to the right to the highest attainable standard of health'.[35] Even though we might imagine that the need for this right to be addressed by the United Nations was legitimately focused on global injustices, particularly between the northern and southern hemispheres, the committee elaborated that the organisation had been 'confronted continually with the widespread denial of the right to water in developing as well as developed countries' (I emphasise that the health inequities between countries with and without adequate water and sanitations are intolerable and unjust).[36] The United Nation's recommendation about water rights within the covenant does, however, define the limits of that human right to water spatially to the 'household, educational institution and workplace'.[37] If this spatial definition was broadened, then it could legally oblige public and private bodies to provide drinking water in the environs they own and manage. Employers, for instance, have to ensure that sufficient drinking water is available for their staff, as a statutory health and safety requirement.[38] Hence the success of water cooler companies whose workers can be seen unloading their wares from vans in most of London's office districts on a daily basis. Water coolers are children of America.

Fountains Abroad

Across the 'pond', there has been prolific anti-bottled-water activism in the last decade. The town of Concord in Massachusetts followed Bundanoon's example and banned bottled water from its shops in 2010.[39] A particularly vocal critic of the bottled water industry's ethics and the decline of public drinking fountains is the water scientist and environmental campaigner Dr Peter Gleick. He is clearly incensed by the ubiquity of bottled water in his book *Bottled and Sold*: 'Water fountains used to be everywhere, but they have slowly disappeared as public water is increasingly pushed out in favor of private control and profit.'[40] Gleick concludes: 'If public sources of drinking water were more accessible, arguments about the convenience of bottled water would seem silly.'[41] The environmental journalist Elizabeth Royte is equally incensed by the murky ethics of bottled water production. Her book, *Bottlemania* cites aspirational water drinking as one reason for the success of imported products in America when she recalls a time when 'ordering imported water was classy; it improved the tone of a dinner party. Once that idea took hold in America, there was no going back'.[42] Some anti-bottled-water activism in the U.S. has focused on the use of oil in bottle production. For instance, the documentary *Tapped* exposes the horrific health impacts of poor air quality on residents living beside a plastic bottle manufacturer, with evidence of high rates of premature deaths from cancers associated with this industry's production of air pollution.[43]

The Pacific Institute, of which Dr Peter Gleick is President, recently launched a website, in partnership with Google, to map America's public drinking fountains and a downloadable app, called WeTap Map. At the time of writing, the project is in its infancy but it adds to information in the public domain about free water sources and is a stimulus for viral communication.

On WeTap's blog, one enthusiastic contributor has posted a link to a list of Paris's public fountains. Tourist blogs about Paris wax lyrical about the free hydration offer of Les Fontaines Wallace, or the Wallace Fountains. Their benefactor, the Anglo-Frenchman, Sir Richard Wallace donated the fountains to Paris following the destruction caused to the city during the Franco-Prussian War in the 1870s. Sir Richard was politely offered advice from the Metropolitan Drinking Fountain Association but the playful aesthetic of his fountains suggests that he did not pay much heed to the English style of public fountain.[44] His interpretation of the amenity type was rather different from England's sombre granite fountains. Generously, Wallace personally financed over a hundred fountains to be built across Paris and his payback has come with immortalisation in a much-loved social architectural offering. They still serve the city today. Les Fontaines Wallaces' distinctively decorative style in delicately wrought, yet robust, ivy-green cast iron features four Caryatids — female figures employed as structural supports — representing kindness, simplicity, charity and sobriety, who guard the precious public water. These fountains are lauded as a part of Paris' architectural heritage and benefit locals and tourists alike. Their visual flamboyance seems to attract users and suggests that a little novelty factor can work well in some contexts. Also, the water they dispense is evidently trusted. A recent visitor to Paris told me that she and her extended family availed of the Wallace Fountains on their holiday trek around the city over several days and saw others using them constantly. She recalled that they did buy bottled water initially, but then re-used those containers once they had located the fountains (not an uncommon practice and a reason why the refill bottle market jostles with lots of great designs, but, like umbrellas, water containers tend to go missing).

Given that Paris, like London, is awash with bottled water, it seems naïve to imagine that decades of habitual purchases of mineral and spring water will suddenly cease. My recent visit to Athens during the sweltering summer of 2012 showed a city also awash with bottled water but, curiously, there is a rather humane pact between sales outlets that all bottles retail for €0.50. This price is considerably less outlandish than bottled water sells for in most capital cities. In Greece's dismal economic situation, even that price seems immoral when temperatures are 38 degree centigrade plus. I spotted a sole public fountain during a week in Athens (admittedly, that was not the focus of my trip), at an entrance to the national gardens. The amenity was not in great condition but one man, who appeared to be homeless took a long drink from its upward pointing jet. I followed his lead. The water tasted good, particularly because that gulp was free. A fridge in the kiosk just next to the fountain glistened with rows of water bottles.

If Athens had its own Fontaines Wallaces, would bottled water sales fall in the summer months? Unfortunately, no such studies have been conducted (at least that this researcher has located). Studies of Geneva's and Rome's rich public water bounties could provide valuable data about water drinking behaviours. At least those cities have retained their historic civic fountains, so people there are free to choose whether to trust public water supplies or pay for bottled water. In Spain, such architectural heritage has rapidly declined according to a group of artists based in Madrid. Luzinterruptus claim that 50% of the city's public fountains have desiccated during the last thirty years. To highlight their demise, the collective staged a provocative guerrilla artwork for four hours in January 2012 and called for the restoration of the city's stock of drinking fountains. The temporary protest-cum-artwork *Agua que has de beber* — which translates literally to 'water you must drink'[45] — was mounted during the night for maximum visual effect. Cascades of small recycled glass jars were attached to the spouts and dry bowls of four unused public fountains and illuminated to simulate flowing water.[46] At the base of the objects, more identical jars spread out into a 'pool', seeping into the street. Skilfully, the image simultaneously conveyed both water waste and the unnecessary flow of water bottles into the city, and the waste the latter produces. Photography of the protest preserves the sculptural interventions on the artists' website for further dissemination after the fountains carcasses were restored to their normal state of dysfunction. The artwork's lament for the loss of simple civic amenities more broadly symbolises the decline in the management of public spaces for citizens' benefit. It also reminds us that not all 'progress' is good.

Return to the Thames

Luzinterruptus is unlikely to have received an invite for its members to travel across from Madrid to Barcelona for Zenith International's 9th Global Bottled Water Congress in October 2012. There, The Coca-Cola Company, Danone and Nestlé Waters, amongst others, were scheduled to discuss how to keep on top of the market 'by unlocking more natural value'.[47] In November 2012, Zenith International's tour continued with the UK Bottled Water Industry conference in London, entitled *Green Light for Bottled Water*. Alongside brand development tips, delegates could attend a session on 'improving recycling' with a speaker from the Department of the Environment, Food and Rural Affairs (yes, the government department), or hear how to reduce the environmental impact of plastic packaging with a senior technologist from the Waste and Resources Action Programme (also a U.K. government agency).[48] Positively, credible sustainability advocates are on board the corporate water road show; however their presence is also an admission that bottled water is with us for the foreseeable future. Rather than the 'polluter pays', this policy seems to be 'work with the polluters' because we have no hope of stopping them.

On a website promoting the UK Bottled Water Industry conference, the sole image is a night shot of the London Eye.[49] The photograph shows the illuminated big wheel structure glazed with a neon-pink hue in a tranquil expanse of the Thames. The river itself is not shown in a critical light. In fact, it looks clean, even pristine in a shade of peaceful midnight blue. After my long trawl through London's drinking water history, I cannot help but find the choice of image somewhat ironic. A bottled water conference for London is not advertised with the aid of an image of a rural water wilderness hundreds of miles from the city but with a thoroughly urban representation of the city's water source. Actually, to me, the image is an apt reflection of the parallel drinking water stream that flows wastefully on into the twenty-first century city's second decade.

I remain optimistic that the Water Framework Directive's implementation will improve the quality of London's raw water sources by 2015 and, in doing so, begin to modify the environmental cost of water treatment practices in this century. But I do not believe we should idealise the era of pre-water treatment era. This industrial system has evolved in a large part to pragmatically cope with an industrialised society. Even all being well on the pollution front, we have to consider the impact of natural or industrial disasters on water catchments, for instance those increasingly wrought by climate change, such as flooding. Those freshwater 'gardens of Eden' owned by the bottled water companies presents land ownership and water abstraction licence issues that need further scrutiny, globally. In terms of the

Water Framework Directive, citizens should have free access to information and progress on that monumental project. If raw water intended for drinking is effectively protected from pollution and treatment measures are reduced, the argument that bottled water is superior to tap water will seriously falter.

As an ordinary water consumer, I would have been completely unaware of the radical ambitions of the Water Framework Directive without my foray into the professional, jargon-laden spheres of the Environment Agency and the water industry. Understandably, those organisations are the preserve of engineers and other scientists but water, and particularly drinking water, is too critical a natural resource for consumers not be consulted about very openly. The privatisation of the water industry in England and Wales is unlikely to be reversed any time soon, but the boundaries of that private preserve need to be tested so that more scrutiny and dialogue about how that industry relates to the city and its inhabitants can take place for drinking water and other freshwater uses. Behaviour change alone cannot solve problems that are inherently systemic. In my struggle to find a neat ending to tie up this book, I realise that London's water questions are still far from resolved in the twenty-first century despite incredible progress on some fronts.

London's private and public drinking water is a vital node in the global freshwater conservation challenges of this century. I can only hope that this contribution to those global conversations offers a springboard for others to dive into these questions and to surface with some fresh suggestions for the future of this city, and for other cities.

Notes

Introduction

1. *The right to water (arts. 11 and 12 of the International Covenant on Economic, Social and Cultural Rights)*, General Comment No.15 (Geneva: United Nations, 2002) p. 5.
2. *Metered Charges 2012–2013*, document ref11564E 02/11 (Reading: Thames Water, 2011).
3. *Progress on Drinking Water and Sanitation: 2012 Update* (New York: Unicef and World Health Organisation, 2012) p. 2.
4. *Limits to Growth: The 30-Year Update*, Dennis Meadows, Donella Meadows and Jorgen Randers (Vermont: Chelsea Green Publishing Company) p. xiv.
5. *The right to water.*
6. *Bottled water versus tap water: understanding consumers' preferences*, Miguel F. Doria, Journal of Water and Health 04.2 (London: IWA, 2006) p. 273.
7. *Concrete and Clay: Reworking Nature in New York City*, Matthew Gandy (Massachusetts: MIT Press, 2002) p. 22.
8. *Water and the Search for Public Health in London in the Eighteenth and Nineteenth Centuries*, by Anne Hardy, Medical History, 1984, Vol. 28, p. 250.
9. *Water Politics in Nineteenth-Century London*, Frank Trentmann and Vanessa Taylor, in *The Making of the Consumer: Knowledge, Power and Identity in the Modern World*, Ed. Frank Trentmann (Oxford: Berg, 2006) p. 73.
10. *Liquid Pleasures: A Social History of Drinks in Modern Britain*, John Burnett (London: Routledge, 1999) p. 27.

CHAPTER ONE
Wells, Conduits and Cordial Waters: drinking water sketches A.D. 43–1800

1. *To the honourable assembly of the Commons: The humble petition*

of the whole companie of the poore water-tankerd-bearers of the citie of London, Robert Tardy water-bearer followes this petition, 1621, Guildhall Library.

2. *London before London* gallery, *Dividing the spoils (150–700 BC)*, Museum of London, http://www.museumoflondon.org.uk/ archive/lbl/pages/sectionDetails.asp?sid=5, Accessed 8th August 2012.

3. River god, marble, Mid–2nd century, Museum of London Roman gallery, November 2010.

4. *Excavations in the Middle Walbrook Valley*, Special Paper 13, Tony Wilmott (London: Museum of London and the Middlesex Archaeological Society, 1991) p. 14.

5. Ibid. p. 174.

6. *Water Supply in the Roman City of London*, Tony Wilmott, London Archaeologist vol. 4 no.9, winter 1982, p. 241.

7. *Ten Books on Architecture*, Vitruvius, Eds. Ingrid D. Rowland and Thomas Noble (Cambridge: Cambridge University Press, 1999) p. 96.

8. Ibid. p. 98.

9. Ibid. p. 102.

10. Interview with Jenny Hall, formerly Senior Curator of Roman London collection, 26th November 2010.

11. *Water Supply*, Wilmott, p. 240.

12. *Water Supply* 1st–2nd century, Roman London gallery, case 10, Museum of London, November 2010.

13. *Roman London*, Peter Marsden (London: Thames and Hudson, 1980) p. 62.

14. *Excavations in the Middle Walbrook Valley*, Wilmott, p. 176 / http://www.museumoflondon.org.uk/Collections-Research/ Research/Your-Research/Londinium/analysis/romanlon-doners/population/Estimating+the+population.htm, Accessed 3rd May 2012.

15. *Ten Books on Architecture*, p.101.

16. *Working Water: Roman Technology in Action*, Ian Blair and

Jenny Hall (London: Museum of London, 2003) pp. 16–17.

17. Ibid. p.9.

18. *Roman London's amphitheatre* (London: Guildhall Art Gallery, 2005) p. 2, downloaded from gallery website 3rd May 2012.

19. *Working Water,* p. 42.

20. *Public Baths*: http://www.museumoflondon.org.uk/Collec tions-Research/Research/Your-Research/Londinium /analysis /publiclife/structures/16+baths.htm, Accessed 3rd May 2012.

21. *Aspects of Saxo-Norman London: 2 Finds and Environmental Evidence,* Special Paper 12, Ed. Alan Vince (London: London and Middlesex Archaeological Society, 1991) p. 411.

22. Interview with Jenny Hall, Museum of London.

23. *Food and Drink in Britain: From Stone Age to Recent Times,* C. Anne Wilson (Middlesex: Penguin, 1984) p. 332.

24. *Aspects of Saxo-Norman London,* p. 413.

25. *Our History,* Westminster Abbey, http://www.westminster-abbey.org/our-history/benedictine-monastery, Accessed 3rd May 2012.

26. *The Medieval Household: Medieval Finds from Excavations in London* (London: Museum of London, 1998) p. 242.

27. *The London Encyclopaedia,* Eds. Ben Weinreb and Christopher Hibbert (Oxford: Macmillan, 1995) p. 178.

28. Ibid. p. 630.

29. *A Survey of London,* John Stow, Reprinted from the text of 1603, Volume 1 (Oxford: Clarendon Press, 1908) p. 15.

30. *Holywell Priory and the development of Shoreditch to c1600: archaeology from the London Overground East London Line* (London: MOLA, 2011), Book description of Museum of London website confirms foundation date of the nunnery: http://www.museumoflondonarchaeology.org.uk/Publicatio ns/pubDetails.htm?pid=129, Accessed 25th July 2012 / *The Medieval Nunnery at Clerkenwell,* David Sturdy, The London Archaeologist Winter 1974, Vol.2 No.9, p. 218.

31. *The Reformation of the Landscape: Religion, Identity and Memory in Early Modern Britain and Ireland,* Alexandra Walsham (Oxford: Oxford University Press, 2011) p. 51.

32. Ibid. References in the above text suggest the twin function of external and internal water use, such as on p. 50 and p. 70

33. *Survey of London* p. 18.

34. Ibid. p. 16.

35. *Water Supply of Greater London,* H.W. Dickinson (London: Newcomen Society, 1954) p. 8.

36. Notes on The Great Conduit, Museum of London Archaeological Society website: http://www.molas.org.uk/pages/siteDetails.asp?siteID=ngt00_3, Accessed 3rd May 2012

37. *Survey of London* p. 17.

38. *The London Encyclopaedia,* p. 147.

39. *Water: the book: an illustrated history of water supply and wastewater in the United Kingdom,* Hugh Barty-King (Shrewsbury: Quiller Press, 1992) p. 33.

40. *The Archaeology of Medieval London,* Christopher Thomas (Gloucestershire: Sutton, 2002) pp. 73–4.

41. *A Survey of London* p. 16.

42. Medieval Life, Museum of London pocket histories, http://www.museumoflondon.org.uk/Explore-online/Pocket-histories/Medieval-life/, Accessed 3rd May 2012.

43. *Sweet and Wholesome Water: Five Centuries of Water-Bearers in the City of London,* Ted Flaxman and Ted Jackson (Cottisford: E.W. Flaxman, 2004) p. 32.

44. *Memorials of London Life in the 13th, 14th and 15th centuries: being a series of extracts, local, social, and political, from the early archives of the City of London, A.D. 1276–1419,* Henry T. Riley (London: Longmans, Green for the Corporation of London, 1868), Letter Book F: 1337.

45. *Excavations at Watling Court, Part Two: Late Roman to Modern,* London Archaeologist Autumn 1982, Vol. 4 No. 8.

46. *London Assize of Nuisance 1301–1431: A Calendar,* Edited by Helena M. Chew and William Kellaway (London: London Record Society, 1973) pp. 160, 616.

47. *Chronicles of London,* Edited with introduction and notes by Charles Lethbridge Kingsford (Oxford: Clarendon Press, 1905) p. 108.

48. *A Survey of London* p. 17.

49. *Chronicles of London,* p. 301.

50. *A Survey of London* p. 17.

51. *From conduit community to commercial network? Water in London, 1500–1725,* Mark S.R. Jenner, in *Londonopolis: Essays in the Cultural and Social History of Early Modern London,* Eds. Pauls Griffiths and Mark S.R. Jenner (Manchester: Manchester University Press) p. 250.

52. Ibid. pp. 256, 259.

53. *Sweet and Wholesome Water* p. 17.

54. *The English Spa: A Social History 1560–1815,* Phyllis Hembry (London: Athlone Press, 1990) p. 2.

55. *The Reformation of the Landscape* p. 397.

56. *A compendyous regyment; or, A dyetary of helth made in Mountpyllier compiled by Andrew Boorde of physycke Doctour* (London: Early English Text Society, 1870) pp. 252–253.

57. Ibid. p. 53.

58. *From conduit community to commercial network?* p. 252.

59. Ibid.

60. *A Survey of London* p. 18.

61. *The Givernment of Britain 1509–1714,* Vol.V 42, (London: Her Majesty's Stationer, 1580), State Papers Online: PC 2/13 f.71, British Library.

62. London Bridge Waterworks Company: Corporate Records, Administrative History description for records ACC/2558/LB/01, London Metropolitan Archives.

63. *A Survey of London* p. 18.

64. *Water Supply of Greater London,* pp.16–17.

65. *Copy of New River Charter 1606*, ACC/2558/NR/01/059, London Metropolitan Archives.
66. *Water: the book: an illustrated history of water supply and waste-water in the United Kingdom*, p. 50.
67. *Copy of New River Charter 1606*.
68. *London's New River*, Robert Ward (London: Historical Publications, 2003) p. 57.
69. *To the Honourable Assembly of the Commons. The humble petition of the whole companie of the poore water-tankerd-bearers of the citie of London. Robert Tardy water-bearer followes this petition*, 1621, Guildhall Library archives.
70. *From conduit community to commercial network?* p. 254.
71. Ibid.
72. Testimony from Thomas Duncomb, 1677, COL/SJ/16/021, London Metropolitan Archives.
73. Ibid.
74. *From conduit community to commercial network?* p. 264.
75. *Second Treatise on Civil Government: An Essay concerning the true and original extent and end of civil government*, John Locke, in *Social Contract:* Essays by Locke, Hume and Rousseau (Oxford: Oxford University Press, 1971) pp. 23–24.
76. Ibid.
77. *The Reformation of the Landscape* p. 398.
78. *The English Spa* p. 43.
79. *The Pump Room, Bath: Bath's hot spa water*, (Bath: Bath and North East Somerset Council, 2011) Pamphlet reference: DP 584 06/11 S.
80. *The English Spa* p. 176.
81. Ibid. p. 367.
82. *Spas, Wells and Pleasure Gardens* James Stevens Curl (London: Historical Publications, 2010) p. 92.
83. Ibid. p. 127.
84. *The Compleat Housewife or Accomplished Gentlewoman's Companion*, E. Smith (London: J & J Pemberton, 1737) p. 254.

85. *Cures and Curiosities: Inside the Wellcome Library,* (London: Profile Books/The Wellcome Trust, 2007) pp. 35–37.

86. *The Compleat Housewife or Accomplished Gentlewoman's Companion* pp. 258, 261 and 270–1.

87. *Liquid Pleasures: A Social History of Drinks in Modern Britain,* John Burnett (London: Routledge, 1999) p. 162.

88. Image number p5448722: Collage online gallery, City of London Corporation, http://collage.cityoflondon.gov.uk/coll age, Accessed 23rd November 2011.

89. *Water and the search for public health in London in the Eighteenth and Nineteenth Centuries,* Anne Hardy, Medical History Vol. 28 1984, Wellcome Library, pp. 250–282.

90. *An Essay on Waters in three parts,* C.Lucas M.D. (London: Printed for A. Millar in the Strand, 1756) pp. xxi–xxii.

91. Ibid. p. 138.

92. *Water and the search for public health in London in the Eighteenth and Nineteenth Centuries* p. 256.

93. *The Oxford Companion to the History of Modern Science,* Eds. RC Olby, GN Cantor, JR Christie and MJS Hodge (Oxford: Oxford University Press, 2003) p. 147.

94. *Water: the book: an illustrated history of water supply and waste-water in the United Kingdom* p. 71.

95. *A Short Account of a New Method of Filtration by Ascent,* James Peacock (London: James Peacock of Finsbury Square, 1793) p. 3.

96. Ibid. p. 11.

CHAPTER TWO
Private Water and Public Health 1800–1858

1. *Pollution and Control: a social history of the Thames in the nineteenth century,* Bill Luckin (Bristol: Hilger, 1986) p. 4.

2. Ibid.

3. *Water and the search for public health in London in the Eighteenth and Nineteenth Centuries,* p. 263.

4. *London's Water Wars: The competition for London's water supply in the nineteenth century,* John Graham-Leigh (London: Francis Boutle, 2000) p. 19.
5. *The London Encyclopaedia,* p. 632.
6. *The Peopling of London: Fifteen Thousand Years of Settlement from Overseas,* Ed. Nick Merriman (London: Museum of London, 1993) pp. 118–9.
7. *London's Water Wars,* p. 13.
8. Chelsea Waterworks Company: Corporate Records, Administrative History description ACC/2558/CH/01, London Metropolitan Archives.
9. *London's Water Wars,* p. 33.
10. "The Water Question" *Times* (London, England) 16th January 1828, *The Times Digital Archive.* Web. 24/11/11.
11. *London's Water Wars,* p. 52.
12. *Water Politics in Nineteenth-Century London,* p. 56.
13. Report of the Provisional Committee of the Anti-Water Monopoly Association, 1819, ACC/2558/NR/13/082, London Metropolitan Archives, p. 1.
14. Ibid. p. 6.
15. *Water Politics in Nineteenth-Century London,* p. 56.
16. *Bathroom,* Barbara Penner (London: Reaktion Books, due to be published 2012) Included in draft chapter *The Civilising Bathroom,* page number currently unknown.
17. *To the Gentlemen of the Medical Profession,* T.L. Waterworth, Surgeon, Newport, Isle of Wight, 1813, Drinks Box 1: EPH+7:1, Wellcome Library.
18. *The Dolphin or Grand Junction Nuisance - proving that seven thousand families in Westminster and its suburbs are supplied with water in a state offensive to the sight, disgusting to the imagination and destructive to health,* John Wright (T. Butcher: London, 1827) p. 59.
19. Ibid. p. 7.
20. Ibid. p. 42, p. 32.

21. Ibid. p. 65.
22. "The Water Question" *Times*, 16th January 1828.
23. Ibid.
24. Ibid.
25. "The Water Question" *Times* (London, England) 19th January 1828: 4. *The Times Digital Archive*. Web. 24/11/11.
26. *A Science of Impurity: Water Analysis in Nineteenth Century Britain*, Christopher Hamlin (Bristol: Adam Hilger, 1990) p. 41.
27. "The Water Question" *Times* (London, England) 19th January 1828.
28. *Catalogue of Political and Personal Satires*, Vol. XI 1828–1832, Dorothy George (London: British Library, 1954) p. 44.
29. Ibid.
30. *An Essay on Waters in three parts*, p. 34.
31. *Water: the book: an illustrated history of water supply and wastewater in the United Kingdom*, p. 89.
32. "The Water Question" *Times*, 19th January 1828.
33. Ibid.
34. *By the Crown, which arrived off Liverpool on Sunday evening, we have received advices from Calcutta*, *Times* (London, England) 17th January 1826: 2. *The Times Digital Archive*. Web. 5/5/12.
35. *Cholera*, World Health Organisation website, http://www.who.int/topics/cholera/en, Accessed 5th May 2012.
36. *Symptoms and Treatment of Malignant Diarrhoea, better known as Asiatic or Malignant Cholera as treated in the Royal Free Hospital during the years 1832, 1833, 1834, 1848 and 1854*, William Marsden, (London: Henry Renshaw, 1865) p. 14.
37. Ibid. p. 36.
38. Ibid. p. 15.
39. *Royal Address of Cadwallader ap-Tudor ap-Edwards ap-Vaughan, Water-King of Southwark*, print, London, England, 1832, George Cruikshank, Science Museum, London.
40. *Flora Tristan's London Journal: A Survey of London Life*, A trans-

lation of Promenades dans Londres by Dennis Palmer and Giselle Pincetl (London: George Prior, 1980) p. 17.

41. Ibid. p. 258.
42. Ibid.
43. Ibid.
44. Ibid. pp. 34–35.
45. *The Sanitary Condition of the Labouring Population of Great Britain,* Edwin Chadwick (Edinburgh: Edinburgh University Press, 1964) p. 150.
46. Ibid. pp. 424–425.
47. The Metropolitan Buildings Act, 1844, 7th & 8th Vict. Cap. 84., Schedule H (London: Crown, 1844) pp. 146–147.
48. Towns Improvement Clauses Act, 1847, 10th & 11th Vict. Cap. 34. p. 437 (London: Crown, 1847).
49. Ibid.
50. *The Government of Victorian London 1855–1889: the Metropolitan Board of Works, the Vestries and the City Corporation,* David Owen, edited by Roy MacLeod with contributions by David Reeder, David Olsen, Francis Sheppard (Cambridge, Massachusetts: Belknap Press of Harvard University Press, 1982) p. 29.
51. *On the Mode of Communication of Cholera,* John Snow (London: John Churchill, 1849) EPB/SUPP/P/SNO, Wellcome Library, p. 6.
52. Ibid. p. 9.
53. Ibid. p. 12.
54. Ibid.
55. Ibid. p. 15.
56. Ibid. p. 20.
57. Ibid. p. 23.
58. Ibid. p. 30.
59. Ibid.
60. *Water Politics in Nineteenth-Century London,* pp. 59–60.
61. *A Microscopic Examination of the Water Supplied to the*

Inhabitants of London and the Suburban Districts in 1850,
Arthur Hill-Hassall (London: Samuel Highley, 1850) p. 1.

62. Ibid. p. 2.

63. *A Science of Impurity: Water Analysis in Nineteenth Century
Britain,* p. 104.

64. Ibid. p. 115.

65. House of Commons Debate, 5th June 1851, Vol. 117 468–469

66. Ibid.

67. *The Globe and Traveller* newspaper, 2nd January 1851, British
Library: newspaper collection.

68. *First Report to Parliament,* Royal Commission for the
Exhibition of 1851 Archives: RC/F/3/1/1 p. 150.

69. *The Globe and Traveller* newspaper, 19th August 1851, British
Library: newspaper collection.

70. Pritchard & Collette: an exhibit for purifying water, Royal
Commission for the Exhibition of 1851 Archives:
RC/A/1851/819.

71. *The Globe and Traveller* newspaper, 6th August 1851, British
Library: newspaper collection.

72. House of Commons Debate, 5th June 1851.

73. *Water Supply of Greater London,* H.W. Dickinson (London:
Courier Press, 1954) pp.102–103.

74. Ibid. p. 83.

75. *Microscopical Examinations of the Thames and Other Waters
1852: Reports made to the Directors of the London (Watford)
Spring Water Company,* Edwin Lankester and Peter Redfern p.
ix (London: Printed by Hughes, 1852).

76. Ibid. p. 38.

77. *The Ghost Map,* Steven Johnson (London: Penguin, 2006) p.
160.

78. *On the Mode of Communication of Cholera,* John Snow (London:
John Churchill, 1855) p. 117.

79. Ibid. pp. 41–42.

80. Ibid. p. 43.

81. Ibid. p. 53.
82. *The Ghost Map*, p. 30.
83. *On the Mode of Communication of Cholera*, p. 74.
84. Ibid. p. 79.
85. *The Ghost Map*, p. 204.
86. *An Act for the better Local Management of the Metropolis*, 18th & 19th Victorae, Cap. 120 (Her Majesty's Stationery Office, 1855) LXXXI.
87. *Report on last two Cholera-Epidemics of London as affected by the consumption of impure water; addressed to the Rt. Hon. The President of the General Board of Health by the Medical Officer of the Board* (HMSO, 1856) p. 12.
88. *The Era*, June 20th 1858, June 20th, British Library newspaper collection.
89. *The Morning Chronicle*, June 24th 1858, Issue 28551, British Library newspaper collection.
90. *The Government of Victorian London 1855–1889*, p. 53.
91. *Pollution and Control*, pp. 16–17.
92. Ibid. p. 20.
93. *Local Government Act 1858 and the Acts Incorporated Therewith together with the Public Health Act 1858*, Ed. Tom Taylor (London: Printed by Night & Co., 1859) p. 42, p. 258.
94. *An Act for the better Local Management of the Metropolis*, CXVI.

CHAPTER THREE
Philanthropic Fountains 1852–1875

1. *The Public Fountains of the City of Dijon*, Trans. Patricia Bobeck from the original text in French, Henry Darcy (Iowa: Kendall/Hunt Publishing Company, 2004) p. 42.
2. Liverpool: total population graph 1800–2000 www.visionof-britain.org.uk: University of Portsmouth, 2009, Accessed 15th August 2010.
3. *Nineteenth-century public health: a study of Liverpool, Belfast and Glasgow*, Sally Sheard, PhD Thesis, University of

Liverpool, 1993, p. 189.

4. *Free Water: the Public Drinking Fountain Movement and Victorian London*, Howard Malchow, The London Journal, Vol. 4, No. 2, p. 183.

5. *Nineteenth-century public health*, p. 190.

6. Memoirs of Charles P. Melly, Edward Melly (Coventry: Curtis and Beamish, 1889) p. 6.

7. *A Handbook for Travellers in Switzerland and the Alps of Savoy and Piedmont including the Protestant Valleys of the Waldenses*, John Murray, (London: John Murray and Son, 1838) Reprinted Leicester University Press, 1970 as part of The Victorian Library p. xxxv.

8. *A Paper on Drinking Fountains*, Charles P. Melly, presented at the Health Department of the National Association of the Promotion of Social Science, Liverpool meeting, October 1858, British Library.

9. Ibid.

10. *Fountains: Mirrors of Switzerland*, Pierre Bouffard and René Creux (Paudex: Bonvent & Fontainemore, 1973) p. 22.

11. Ibid. p. 14.

12. *A Paper on Drinking Fountains*, pp. 9–10.

13. Ibid. p.2.

14. Ibid.

15. Ibid.

16. Ibid. p.1.

17. *Free Water: the Public Drinking Fountain Movement and Victorian London*, p.183.

18. pp. 5–6.

19. A. F. Pollard, 'Temple, William Francis Cowper, Baron Mount-Temple (1811–1888), rev. H.C.G. Matthew, *Oxford Dictionary of National Biography*, Oxford University Press, 2004 [http://www.oxforddnb.com/view/article/6515, accessed 15th August 2012].

20. *Business and Religion in Britain*, Ed. David J. Jeremy

(Aldershot: Gower, 1988) p. 165 / *Quaker Businesses in Britain: a historical list*, Library of the Religious Society of Friends.

21. *Family Fortunes: Men and Women and the English Middle Class 1780–1850*, Leonore Davidoff and Catherine Hall (London: Hutchinson, 1987) p. 101, p. 216.

22. *Business and Religion in Britain*, p. 169.

23. *Victorian Quakers*, Elizabeth Isichei (Oxford: Oxford University Press, 1970) p. xxi.

24. *A Water Drinkers Experience*, British Workman's Almanac 1858, viewed at the British Library, Rare Books collection.

25. *Drinking Fountains*, *The Morning Chronicle*, November 6th 1858, Issue 28648, British Library digital nineteenth century newspaper collection.

26. Ibid.

27. Letter from H. Burdett Worthington, *The Standard* (London), November 17th 1858, Issue 10689, British Library nineteenth century digital collection.

28. Daily News, London, January 3rd 1859, Issue 3943, British Library nineteenth century digital collection.

29. *A Plea for Free Drinking Fountains*, E.T. Wakefield (London: Hatchard & Co., 1859) p. 6.

30. Letter from Sidney Herbert to his wife, 6th June 1859, Liberal Democrat History Group, http://www.liberalhistory.org.uk/item_single.php?item_id=20&item=history, Viewed 26th September 2010.

31. *Drinking Fountains in the Metropolis*, Daily News, April 13th 1859, Issue 4029, British Library digital nineteenth century newspaper collection.

32. Ibid.

33. Ibid.

34. The Metropolitan Free Drinking Fountains Association, Annual Report 1865, ACC/3168/018 pp. 7–8.

35. *A Science of Impurity: Water Analysis in Nineteenth Century Britain*, p. 111.

36. *Drinking Fountains, The Lady's Newspaper* (London, England) Saturday 12th March 1859, Issue 637, p. 172, British Library digital nineteenth century newspaper collection.
37. Ibid.
38. *The Opening of the Drinking Fountain, The Lady's Newspaper* (London, England) Saturday 30th April 1859 Issue 664, p. 275, British Library digital nineteenth century newspaper collection.
39. *Drinking Fountains,* Illustrated London News, Saturday 30th April 1859.
40. Minute Book of the Executive Committee 1859–66, Metropolitan Drinking Fountains Association, for example 29th June 1859, 13th July 1859, ACC/3168/001: London Metropolitan Archives.
41. *Drinking Fountains,* Edward Wakefield had defended the high cost of the fountains for several critical reasons in a letter to the editor of *The Times,* (London, England), p.10, col. F, Issue 23287, Issue 23287, 22nd April 1859.
42. For instance, Minute Book of the Executive Committee 1859–66, August p. 50.
43. Ibid. March 1860, p. 113.
44. This concern about the free flowing water disturbing parishioners coming in and out of church had been the reason that St Andrews church rejected a fountain, as reported at least by Edward Wakefield in a letter to The Morning Post, January 14th 1859, Issue 26544.
45. For example, Minute Book of the Executive Committee 1859–66, November 1864 p. 370.
46. The 1865 figures were recorded in the Metropolitan Drinking Fountains Association Annual Report 1867, ACC/3168/19: London Metropolitan Archives, p. 38.
47. *Drinking Fountains in the Metropolis, Daily News* (London, England), 13th April 1859, Issue 4029, p. 3, 19th Century: British Library Newspapers.

48. Metropolitan Drinking Fountains Association 1867 Annual Report, pp. 16–17.
49. Ibid. p. 18.
50. Minute Book of the Executive Committee 1859–66, 1861, p. 169.
51. Metropolitan Drinking Fountains Association 1867 Annual Report, p. 26.
52. Minute Book of the Executive Committee 1866–79, Metropolitan Free Drinking Fountain Association, May 1867, p.35, ACC/3168/002: London Metropolitan Archives.
53. Metropolitan Drinking Fountains Association 1867 Annual Report, p. 26.
54. Ibid. p.27.
55. Minute Book of the Executive Committee 1866–79, June 1868, p. 77.
56. Metropolitan Free Drinking Fountain Association, Annual Report 1873, p. 11, ACC/3168/25: London Metropolitan Archives.
57. Ibid.
58. Minute Book of the Executive Committee 1859–66, November 1859, p.79.
59. Metropolitan Free Drinking Fountain Association Annual Report 1867, p.27.
60. Ibid.
61. Minute Book of the Executive Committee 1859–66, October 1862, pp. 263 – 264.
62. Minute Book of the Executive Committee 1859–66, May 1864 p. 349.
63. Minute Book of the Executive Committee 1866–79, June 1866 p. 9.
64. Metropolitan Drinking Fountains Association 1867 Annual Report, p. 9.
65. Ibid. pp. 20–21.
66. Minute Book of the Executive Committee 1859–66, Vulcan

Temperance Society: April 1860, p. 118, National Temperance League mentioned frequently, for example August 1863 p. 324, Gurney's involvement with the Band of Hope: *The Band of Hope Record*, Rev. G.W. McCree (London: Tweedie & Cawdell, 1862) pp. 341–2.

67. *Brewers, Temperance and the Nineteenth Century Drinking Fountain Movement*, Vanessa Taylor PhD thesis, Birkbeck College, University of London 2006, p. 13. Taylor's extensive research into the involvement of brewers with the Victorian fountain movement is the most in-depth piece of academic research on this organisation on its membership that I located during my research. The Guildhall Library holds a copy of her thesis.

68. Ibid. p. 14.

69. *On Liberty*, John Stuart Mill (London: John W. Parker & Son, 1859) p. 174.

70. *The Advantages of Temperance*, John Robert Taylor (London: James George Taylor, 1864) Letter from Professor Beesly p. 8

71. Minute Book of the Executive Committee 1859–66, August 1863 p. 324.

72. *City Press*, 30th April 1859.

73. *Free Water: the Public Drinking Fountain Movement and Victorian London*, pp. 181–2.

74. *The Victoria Fountain*, The Times (London, England) Monday June 30th, 1862; p. 9, Issue 24285; Col. F.

75. Shoreditch Observer, July 5th 1862.

76. *The Buxton Memorial Drinking-Fountain, Great George Street, Westminster*, Illustrated London News, Saturday 10th March 1866, Issue 1360, p. 242.

77. Ibid.

78. *The Return of the Registrar-General for last week*, The Times (London, England), Thursday 9th August, 1866, p.8, Issue 25572.

79. *London*, *The Times* (London, England), 16th December 1861,

Issue 24117, p.9.

80. Typhoid Fever, World Health Organisation, http://www. who.int/topics/typhoid_fever/en/, Viewed 18th September 2011.

81. Quoted from *The Lancet, The Late Prince Consort, The Times* (London, England), 21st December 1861, Issue 24122, p. 9.

82. Metropolitan Drinking Fountain & Cattle Trough Association Annual Report 1875, fold out map attached to inside of front cover, ACC/3168/27: London Metropolitan Archives.

CHAPTER FOUR
The Birth of Bacteriology and the Death of Corporate Water 1866–1899

1. *The London Water Supply*, Arthur Shadwell (London: Longmans, Green & Co., 1899) p. 66.

2. *Pollution and Control*, p. 28.

3. *Milestones in Microbiology 1546–1940*, Translated and edited by Thomas D. Brock (Washington: American Society for Microbiology, 1999) p. 3.

4. *Bacteriology*, William W. Ford (London: Harpers & Brothers, 1939) p. 63.

5. *Milestones in Microbiology* p. 2.

6. *A Science of Impurity*, p. 47.

7. Ibid. p. 47.

8. *An Act for the better Local Management of the Metropolis* p. 1038 / *Water and the Search for Public Health in London in the Eighteenth and Nineteenth Centuries*, Anne Hardy p. 271.

9. Ibid. p. 155.

10. *On the Mode of Communication of Cholera*, p.119.

11. *Farr, William (1807–1883)*, John M. Eyler, Oxford Dictionary of National Biography, (Oxford: Oxford University Press, 2004) [http://www.oxforddnb.com/view/article/9185, accessed 18th January 2012].

12. *A Science of Impurity*, p. 171.
13. *The Return of the Registrar-General for last week*, *The Times* (London, England), Thursday, 9th August, 1866, p. 8, Issue 25572. Accessed *Times Digital Archive*. Web. 25th July 2012.
14. Ibid.
15. *A Science of Impurity*, p. 162.
16. *Twelfth Report of the Medical Officer of the Privy Council with appendix 1869* (HMSO, 1870) pp. 141–2.
17. Ibid.
18. Ibid. p. 142.
19. Ibid. p. 146.
20. *Lea Bridge Road* sign, Lee Valley Regional Park Authority sign: 'Middlesex Filter Beds Nature Reserve. Once home to the East London Waterworks Company, this 10 acre (4 hectare) oasis...', photographed 15th October, 2011.
21. *Twelfth Report of the Medical Officer of the Privy Council with appendix 1869*, p. 146.
22. Ibid. p. 148.
23. Interview with John Simon, Medical Officer to the Privy Council, *Royal Commission of Water Supply, Report of the Commissioners 1869* (HMSO: 1869) K2.
24. Ibid. A2.
25. Ibid. Q 249.
26. Ibid. N3 212.
27. Ibid. G2 125.
28. Ibid. 249.
29. *Twelfth Report of the Medical Officer of the Privy Council with appendix 1869*, p. 33.
30. The Metropolis Water Act 1871, Public General Act 34 & 35, Victoria 1, Chapter 113 (HMSO: 1871) p. 598.
31. Ibid.
32. Ibid. Clauses 35 & 36, p. 607.
33. *International Congress of Hygiene*, *The Times* (London, England) August 30th, 1884, page 4, Issue 31226, Cl. F &

Sanitary Institute, The Times (London, England) September 28th, 1885, page 7, Issue 31563, col E: *Times Digital Archive.* web, 20th February 2012.

34. *Milestones in Microbiology*, p. 5.
35. *Pure, cool and fresh water obtained by using Maignen's Patent "filtre Rapide"*, Drinks Ephemera: Water. Box 1. EPH107:8, Wellcome Library.
36. Ibid.
37. *Puralis: health: pure distilled aerated water*, The Pure Water Company Ltd, Drinks Ephemera. Water. Box 2. EPH108:23, Wellcome Library.
38. *Wholesome Drinks for Thirsty Millions, Pall Mall Gazette* (London, England) Friday 19th July, 1889, Issue 7593, British Library nineteenth century newspapers: digital collection.
39. Ibid.
40. *Puralis: health: pure distilled aerated water*.
41. *The London County Council, The Times*, Wednesday 18th January, 1893, p. 14, Issue 33851; col. B, *Times Digital Archive*, Accessed 14th January 2012.
42. *The Metropolitan Water Supply, The Times* (London, England), Wednesday, 18th May, 1892, p. 10; Issue 33641; Col. E. *Times Digital Archive.* Web. Accessed 17th August 2011.
43. Ibid.
44. *The London Water Supply, The Times* (London, England) 14th June 1892, The Times Digital Archive. Web. Accessed 20th August 2011.
45. Metropolitan Cattle Trough and Drinking Fountain Association Annual Report 1891, ACC/3168/43: London Metropolitan Archives.
46. Ibid. 1892, ACC/3168/44, pp. vi–vii.
47. *The Metropolitan Water Supply, The Times* (London, England) 14th February 1893, Issue 33874, p. 12. *Times Digital Archive.* Web. Accessed 20th August 2011.
48. Ibid.

49. *Royal Commission to Inquire into the Water Supply of the Metropolis* (HMSO: 1893) p. 143.
50. Ibid. p. 178.
51. Ibid. p. 172.
52. *The Thames Conservancy Act 1894* (HMSO: 1894), printed by Effingham Wilson/Sweet & Maxwell in *The Port of London Act 1908, together with the Thames Conservancy Act 1894*, p. 199.
53. *Micro-Organisms in Water: their significance, identification and removal*, Percy Frankland and Mrs Percy Frankland (London: Longmans and Green, 1894) p. xi.
54. Ibid. p. 89.
55. Ibid. p. 141.
56. Ibid. p. 125.
57. Ibid. p. 181.
58. Ibid.
59. Ibid. pp. 183–4.
60. Ibid. p. 126.
61. *Frankland, Grace Coleridge (1858-1946)*, Susan L. Cohen, Oxford Dictionary of National Biography (Oxford: Oxford University Press, 2004), http://oxforddnb.com/view/article/62321, Accessed 28th June 2011.
62. *The Water Supply in East London (From Our Special Correspondent)*, *The Times*, 29th July, 1895, p. 11, Issue 34641, Col. A, *Times Digital Archive*, Accessed 14th January 2012 / *Liquid Politics: Water and the Politics of Everyday Life in the Modern City*, Vanessa Taylor and Frank Trentmann (University of Greenwich & Birkbeck College, 2011), http://past.oxfordjournals.org/, Accessed 28th December 2011, p. 221, p. 222, p. 234.
63. *The Water Companies and the Public (From a Correspondent)*, *The Times*, 22nd March 1895, p. 13, Issue 34531, Col. C. *Times Digital Archive*. Web. Accessed 14th January 2012.
64. *The Water Companies and the Public (From a Correspondent)*, *The Times*, 8th March, 1895, p. 13, Issue 34519, Col. F. *Times Digital*

Archive, Accessed 14th January 2012.

65. *The Water Supply in East London (From Our Special Correspondent), The Times,* 29th July 1895, p. 11, Issue 34641, Col. A, *Times Digital Archive.* Accessed 14th January 2012.

66. Ibid.

67. East London Water Works Company notice, 21st July 1896 ACC/2558/MW/C/15/25: London Metropolitan Archives.

68. Ibid.

69. Ibid., 2nd notice included for same reference, undated but suggests also 1895-96 water famine period.

70. *East London Water Supply,* Punch, or the London Charivari, 8th August, 1896.

71. East London Water Works Company notice, 26th August 1898.

72. East London Water Works Company notice (in Hebrew).

73. *Water Politics in Nineteenth-Century London,* Frank Trentmann and Vanessa Taylor, in *The Making of the Consumer: Knowledge, Power and Identity in the Modern World,* Ed. Frank Trentmann (Oxford: Berg, 2006) pp. 63–4.

74. Ibid. p. 73.

75. *The Typhoid Epidemic at Maidstone, The Times* (London, England) 18th October, 1897, p. 10, Issue 35337, Col. B, *Times Digital Archive,* Accessed 14th January 2012.

76. Towns Improvement Clauses Act (HMSO: 1847) XVII.

77. *Report on the Means of Deoderising and Utilising the Sewage of Towns, Addressed to the Rt. Hon. President of the General Board of Health,* Henry Austin C.E. (HMSO: 1857) pp. 19–20.

78. *The Typhoid Epidemic at Maidstone, The Times* (London, England) 18th October, 1897.

79. Ibid.

80. *The Typhoid Epidemic at Maidstone, The Times* (London, England) 26th October, 1897, p. 9, Issue 35344, Col. F, *Times Digital Archive,* Accessed 14th January 2012.

81. *London Water Supply, The Times* (London, England) 23rd

November 1897, p. 7, Col. B, Issue 35368, *Times Digital Archive*, 14th January 2012.

82. *The London Water Supply*, Arthur Shadwell, p. 166.

83. Ibid. p. 5.

84. Ibid. p. 2.

85. *Pollution and Control*, Bill Luckin, pp. 27–8.

86. *A Science of Impurity* p. 171, p. 228.

CHAPTER FIVE
ChloriNation 1905–1933

1. *Sir Alexander Cruikshank Houston (1865–1933)*, Obituary Notices of Fellows of the Royal Society, December 1933. Biographies Vol.1 1932–35, p. 335.

2. Search conducted www.google.co.uk, 27th February 2012.

3. Bill Luckin does note his rise as a name in *Pollution and Control* and through this is an important academic text, it is certainly not a mainstream profile of Dr Houston.

4. Search conducted 27th February 2012.

5. Metropolis Water Act (HMSO: 1902) Clause 25.

6. Ibid.

7. Ibid.

8. Ibid. Clause 29.

9. *Fever Swept Town, The Daily Mirror*, 9th February 1905: UK Press Online, Accessed 9th August 2011.

10. *Sir Alexander Cruikshank Houston (1865–1933)*, p. 335.

11. Ibid. p. 343.

12. *The Experimental Bacterial Treatment of London Sewage: Being An Account of the Experiments Carried Out by the London County Council Between the Years 1892 and 1903*, Professor Frank Clowes D.Sc (Lond.) Chemist to the Council and A.C. Houston, M.B. D.Sc. (London: London County Council, 1904) p. 67.

13. Ibid. p. 69.

14. *Sir Alexander Cruikshank Houston (1865–1933)*, p. 337.

15. *Typhoid Fever at Lincoln (From Our Special Correspondent), The Times* (London, England), 25th February 1905, p. 12, Issue 37640, Col. B, The Times Digital Archive, Accessed 15/06/11.
16. *Sir Alexander Cruikshank Houston (1865–1933)*, p. 339.
17. *Chlorination of Water*, Joseph Race (London: Chapman & Hall, 1918) p. 8.
18. *The Early History of Chlorine: papers*, Carl Wilhelm Scheele, C.L. Berthollet, Guyton de Morveau, J.L. Gay-Lussac, L.J. Thenard (Edinburgh: Albemic Club, 1905) pp. 3–4.
19. *Chloride of Lime in Sanitation*, Albert H. Hooker (New York: J. Wiley & Sons, 1913) p. 2.
20. Ibid.
21. *Malignant Cholera, Trial of Various Remedies, Recommendation of Chlorine*, Mr J.G. Lansdown, *The Lancet*, September 1834, no. 578, p. 3.
22. Ibid.
23. *Typhoid Fever at Lincoln, The Times* 25th February 1905.
24. Ibid.
25. *Typhoid Fever at Lincoln (From Our Special Correspondent), The Times* (London, England), 31st March 1905, p. 15, Issue 37669, Col. B, The Times Digital Archive, Accessed 15/06/11.
26. Water Examination Committee Minute Book 1904–08, Metropolitan Water Board, ACC/2558/MW/1/175: London Metropolitan Archives, p. 54.
27. Dr Houston's First Monthly Report on the Water Supply, November 1905, Metropolitan Water Board: ACC/2558 /MW/W/01/009, p. 5.
28. Ibid.
29. Ibid. p. 3.
30. Ibid. p. 24.
31. Fifth Report on Research Work, 1909, Reports of the Director of Water Examination 1908–12, Metropolitan Water Board, ACC/2558/MW/W/010: London Metropolitan Archives, p. 27.

32. *Bathroom,* Barbara Penner (London: Reaktion Books, due to be published 2012) Included in draft chapter *The Civilising Bathroom,* page number in forthcoming unknown.

33. *A Laboratory Handbook of Bacteriology,* Rudolf Abel, M.H. Gordon trans. (Oxford: Oxford Medical Publications, 1907), Translator's Preface.

34. First Report on Research Work, 1908, Reports of the Director of Water Examination 1908–12, Metropolitan Water Board, ACC/2558/MW/W/010: London Metropolitan Archives.

35. Third Report on Research Work, 1909, Reports of the Director of Water Examination 1908–12, Metropolitan Water Board, ACC/2558/MW/W/010: London Metropolitan Archives, p. 1.

36. *A Laboratory Handbook of Bacteriology,* p. 104.

37. First Report on Research Work, 1908, p. 2.

38. Ibid.

39. Ibid. p. 5.

40. Ibid. p. 2.

41. Ibid. p. 9.

42 *Sir Alexander Cruikshank Houston (1865–1933),* p. 343.

43. Fourth Report on Research Work, 1909, Reports of the Director of Water Examination 1908–12, Metropolitan Water Board, ACC/2558/MW/W/010: London Metropolitan Archives, p. 2.

44. *A Laboratory Handbook of Bacteriology,* p. 129.

45. Fifth Report on Research Work, 1909, Reports of the Director of Water Examination 1908–12, Metropolitan Water Board, ACC/2558/MW/W/010: London Metropolitan Archives, Part 3, p. 23.

46. Ibid.

47. *Typhoid Mary,* A Dictionary of Public Health, Ed. John M. Last (Oxford: Oxford University Press, 2007), Oxford Reference Online, Accessed 27th July 2011.

48. Sixth Report on Research Work, 1910, Reports of the Director

of Water Examination 1908–12, Metropolitan Water Board, ACC/2558/MW/W/010: London Metropolitan Archives, p. 18.

49. Eighth Report on Research Work, 1912, Reports of the Director of Water Examination 1908–12, Metropolitan Water Board, ACC/2558/MW/W/010: London Metropolitan Archives, p. 4.

50. Ibid.

51. Ibid. p. 16.

52. Ibid. *Advantages of the "Excess Lime Method"*, p. 16, point 9.

53. Twelfth Report on Research Work, 1916, Reports of the Director of Water Examination 1913–20, Metropolitan Water Board, ACC/2558/MW/W/011: London Metropolitan Archives, p. 11.

54. Ibid.

55. Ibid. p. 15.

56. Ibid. p. 17.

57. Ibid.

58. Ibid. p. 19.

59. Ibid. p. 21.

60. Ibid.

61. *Sterilising Thames Water, The Times* (London, England), 25th November, 1916, p. 6, Issue 41334, Col. B, Times Digital Archive, Accessed 15th July 2011.

62. Ibid. p. 21.

63. *The United Alkali Company Limited, The Manchester Guardian,* 17th April 1919.

64. *Chlorination of Water,* Joseph Race, Preface.

65. *Sir Alexander Cruikshank Houston (1865–1933),* p. 341.

66. *Chlorination of Water,* Joseph Race, p. 63.

67. Ibid. p. 67.

68. *Metropolitan Water Board – Fifty Years Review 1903–53,* W.S. Chevalier (London: Metropolitan Water Board, 1953) p. 256.

69. Fifteenth Annual Report, 1921, Reports of the Director of

Water Examination 1921–24, Metropolitan Water Board, ACC/2558/MW/W/01/004: London Metropolitan Archives, p. 43.

70. Ibid. p. 44.

71. *Some General Notes on the Future of Chlorination*, Sixteenth Annual Report, 1922, Reports of the Director of Water Examination 1921–24, Metropolitan Water Board, ACC/2558/MW/W/01/004: London Metropolitan Archives, p. 17, point a.

72. *Metropolitan Water Board – Fifty Years Review 1903–53*, p. 268.

73. Eighteenth Annual Report, 1924, Reports of the Director of Water Examination 1921–24, Metropolitan Water Board, ACC/2558/MW/W/01/004: London Metropolitan Archives, p. 45.

74. Ibid. p. 46.

75. *The Romance of the New River*, Twentieth Annual Report, 1925–26, Reports of the Director of Water Examination 1921–24, Metropolitan Water Board, ACC/2558/MW/W/01/005: London Metropolitan Archives, see sketches 1–12.

76. Ibid. p. 12.

77. Ibid. p. 15.

78. Ibid.

79. Ibid.

CHAPTER SIX
Blitz on the Board 1937–1945

1. Interview with George Billingham and Arthur Durling, water engineers with the Metropolitan Water Board 1939–45, recorded by Capital Radio, Catalogue number 5370, Reel 2: Imperial War Museum, London.

2. Ibid.

3. *Air Raid Precautions for the Protection of the Board's Undertaking*, Commander G.E. Blackwell, 31st December 1937, ACC/2558/MW/C/05/001 p. 1.

4. Ibid. p. 21.
5. London Government Act 1963, Chapter 33, Part V, 35, Clause 1, Sewerage and Trade Effluents.
6. *Chief Engineer's report on the protection of the Board's undertaking,* Metropolitan Water Board, 1938, ACC/2558/MW/C/05/002: London Metropolitan Archives.
7. Ibid.
8. Ibid.
9. Untitled document within *Air Raid Precautions and Flood Emergency 1940–9* with introductory page statement: 'The following information indicates the steps taken by the Metropolitan Water Board to safeguard their Undertaking against the effects of air raid damage and to ensure as far as practicable a continuous supply of water for domestic, trade and fire fighting purposes.', August 1941, Metropolitan Water Board, ACC/2558/MW/C/05/005: London Metropolitan Archives, p. 6.
10. Copy of the Metropolitan Water Board document, dated 30th June 1939, contained in the Papers of Mrs V.J. Staunton, 92/25/1: Imperial War Museum archives, London.
11. Metropolitan Water Board Emergency Committee Minutes Book, ACC/2558/MW/01/292: London Metropolitan Archives, 31st August 1939, p. 2.
12. BBC radio broadcast recording: http://www.bbc.co.uk/archive/ww2outbreak/7917.shtml, Accessed 27th July 2011.
13. Metropolitan Water Board Emergency Committee Minutes Book, 13th September 1939, p. 8.
14. Ibid.
15. Ibid.
16. Memorandum no.221, *Metropolitan Water Board – Fifty Years Review 1903–53,* pp. 273–4.
17. Metropolitan Water Board Emergency Committee Minutes Book, 13th September 1939, p. 12: Finsbury Council was the local government body for the area where the Metropolitan

Water Board was located.

18. *How To Purify Your Drinking Water,* Statement broadcast by the Director of Water Examination on 13th August 1940, Appendix E to untitled document within *Air Raid Precautions and Flood Emergency 1940–9* (as detailed above).

19. *Pollution of Water Supply,* Metropolitan Borough of Woolwich, 1st August 1941, Water Supply in the City of London 1941–2, COL/TCD/CD/03/035, http://www.nationalarchives.gov.uk/currnency/default0.asp, Accessed 9th March 2012.

20. *In war-time emergencies make your water supply absolutely safe: what to do in emergency,* Milton Proprietary Ltd, EPH470:19, Wellcome Library, London.

21. Appendixes B and C to untitled document within *Air Raid Precautions and Flood Emergency 1940–9* (as detailed above).

22. *Schweppes: The First 200 Years,* Douglas A. Simmons (London: Springwood Books, 1983) p. 80.

23. *Evacuation,* Imperial War Museum website: http://www.iwm.org.uk/history/evacuation#, Accessed 13th March 2012 / BBC website: http://www.bbc.co.uk/history/worldwars /wwtwo/ff3_blitz.shtml, Accessed 14th March 2012.

24. Ibid. BBC website.

25. *Metropolitan Water Board – Fifty Years Review 1903–53,* p. 302

26. Interview with George Billingham and Arthur Durling, Reel 1.

27. Ibid.

28. Untitled document within *Air Raid Precautions and Flood Emergency 1940–9* (as detailed above) p. 11.

29. Interview with George Billingham and Arthur Durling, Reel 1.

30. Ibid.

31. Appendix A, untitled document within *Air Raid Precautions and Flood Emergency 1940–9* (as detailed above).

32. Ibid. p. 17.

33. Interview with George Billingham and Arthur Durling, Reel 1.

34. Ibid.

35. Ibid.
36. Appendix A, untitled document within *Air Raid Precautions and Flood Emergency 1940–9* (as detailed above), p. 22.
37. Ibid. p. 19.
38. Ibid. p. 21.
39. Untitled document within *Air Raid Precautions and Flood Emergency 1940–9* (as detailed above), p. 2.
40. Ibid. p. 3.
41. *How To Purify Your Drinking Water*, Statement broadcast by the Director of Water Examination on 13th August 1940.
42. Untitled document within *Air Raid Precautions and Flood Emergency 1940–9* (as detailed above), p. 14.
43. *Air Raid Precautions and Air Raid Damage*, in *Air Raid Precautions and Flood Emergency 1940–9*, p. 8.
44. Letter from Gerald G. Caney, 29th May 1941, Water Supply papers City of London 1941–2.
45. Letter from the Director of Meyer and Johnson Oriental Carpet Importers to City Sanitary Inspector, 3rd July 1941, Water Supply papers City of London 1941–2, COL/TCD/CD/03/035, London Metropolitan Archives.
46. Ibid. Letter from Dr Charles F. White to the Medical Officer of the Ministry of Health, 11th June 1941.
47. Ibid.
48. Ibid. *Memorandum of the Arrangements made by the War Emergency Water Committee, London Civil Defence Region*, 4th June 1941.
49. *Use of privately owned wells in emergency*, Memorandum of interview with Sir Warren Fisher, 27th February 1942, *Air Raid Precautions and Flood Emergency 1940–9*.
50. *Memorandum from the Chief Engineer of the Chairman of the Board*, 10th October 1941, p.3, *Air Raid Precautions and Flood Emergency 1940–9*.
51. *Blitz Feeding* circular B.80, London County Council, April 1941, Papers of LJ Dillon, 10/2/1: Imperial War Museum

archives, London.

52. *Communal Kitchens connected with Voluntary Organisation in the County of London*, April 1941, Papers of LJ Dillon.

53. *Blitz Stew*, circular B.34, London County Council, Papers of LJ Dillon.

54. *Meals Services: Emergency Water Supplies*, Report of Inter-departmental conference, London County Council, July 1941, point 20, Papers of LJ Dillon.

55. *Blitz Feeding* circular B.80.

56. *Meals Services: Emergency Water Supplies*, Report of Inter-departmental conference, London County Council, July 1941, point 5, Papers of LJ Dillon.

57. *Britain at War*, documentary film directed by Rosie Newman, circa 1946, MGH 3773: Imperial War Museum film archive, London.

58. *The Blitz*, Bruce Robinson: http://www.bbc.co.uk/history/worldwars/wwtwo/ff3_blitz.shtml, Accessed 14th March 2012.

59. *Metropolitan Water Board – Fifty Years Review 1903–53*, pp. 305–6.

60. Cover letter from A.H. King for *Emergency Sources of Water Supply* bulletin, issued to Water Undertakings within the London Region, 7th September 1942, in *Air Raid Precautions and Flood Emergency 1940–9*.

61. Ibid. p. 1.

62. Ibid. diagram showing test for *Emergency Distribution of Water* .

63. Poster no.10, undated, 1939–50, ACC/2558/MW/C/20/01: London Metropolitan Archives.

64. Ibid. *A New Year Resolution*, poster no. 6.

65. *Consolidated Instruction to Invasion Committees in England and Wales* (HMSO, July 1942), p. 8.

66. *London Water Supply – Need for Economy in Use*, The Times (London, England), Saturday 15th January, 1944, p. 2, Issue

49754 / *Call To Save More Water, The Times* (London, England), Saturday 11th March, p. 2, Issue 49802 / *Water Scarcity in London - Flow of Thames Lowest on Record, The Times* (London, England), Saturday 6th May, 1944, p. 4, Issue 49849: *The Times Digital Archive*, Accessed 15th March 2012.

67. *Serious Shortage of Water, The Times* (London, England), 15th August 1944, p. 2, Issue 49935, Col. C: *The Times Digital Archive*, Accessed 15th March 2012.

68. *Emergency Supplies – 63, Edward St*, ACC/2558/MW/C/14/112: London Metropolitan Archives.

69. *Metropolitan Water Board – Fifty Years Review 1903–53*, p. 304

70. *The Watch on London's Water*, in *London's Water Supply – Safeguarding its Purity in Peace and War*, Metropolitan Water Board, 1945, ACC/2558/MW/C/48/055 p. 14.

71. *London in the 20th Century*, Jerry White (London: Vintage, 2008) p. 38.

72. Ibid.

CHAPTER SEVEN
Purity and Poison 1948–1969

1. *Health Minister Urges Compulsory Medication*, London Anti-Fluoridation Campaign pamphlet, publication undated / received by the Metropolitan Water Board 21st October 1966, ACC/2558/MW/C/08/263(6), London Metropolitan Archives, p. 3.

2. *County of London Plan*, Prepared for the London County Council by Patrick Abercrombie and J.H. Forshaw (London: MacMillan, 1943) p. 36.

3. Metropolitan Drinking Fountain and Cattle Trough Association Annual Report 1945, ACC/3168/096, London Metropolitan Archives p. 8.

4. Metropolitan Drinking Fountain and Cattle Trough Association Annual Report 1948, ACC/3168/096, London Metropolitan Archives p. 7.

5. *The National Health Service Act 1946,* Annotated, together with various orders and regulations made thereunder by S.R. Speller (London: H.K. Lewis & Co, 1948) p. 55, Part 3, Section 28.
6. *The Fluoride Wars: How a Modest Public Health Measure Became America's Longest Running Political Melodrama,* (New Jersey: John Wiley & Sons, 2009) p. 1.
7. *Prevention of Dental Caries by Fluoridation,* Report by the Director of Water Examination, Metropolitan Water Board 1952-69, ACC/2558/MW/C/08/265/001, London Metropolitan Archives, p. 3.
8. *The Festival of Britain* (London: Festival of Britain, 1951) p. 4
9. *The Story of the Festival of Britain* (London: Festival of Britain, 1952) p. 25.
10. *Prevention of Dental Caries by Fluoridation,* p. 5.
11. Ibid. p. 2.
12. Ibid. p. 5.
13. Ibid. p. 1.
14. Ibid. p. 5.
15. Ibid.
16. *The Fluoride Wars,* p. 1.
17. *The Fluoridation of Domestic Water Supplies in North America as a means of controlling dental caries,* Report of the United Kingdom Mission (HMSO, 1953) p. 11.
18. Ibid. p. 18.
19. *Housewives Today supporting the policy of the British Housewives League,* 1st January 1953, Fluoridation of water supplies: objections, 1953–68, Metropolitan Water Board, ACC/2558/MW/C/08/263/001, London Metropolitan Archives.
20. Ibid., Response from Metropolitan Water Board to H.F. Marfleet, 23rd January 1953.
21. Ibid. Letter from Housewives Today dated 6th May 1953.
22. *Prevention of Dental Caries by Fluoridation, Report no.2,* p. 3, Fluoridation of water supplies: committee and Board reports

1952–69, Metropolitan Water Board, ACC/2558/MW/C/08/265/001, London Metropolitan Archives.

23. *The Fluoridation of Domestic Water Supplies in North America as a means of controlling dental caries*, p. 21.

24. Ibid.

25. *City Refuses to be 'Guinea-Pig'*, The Manchester Guardian (Manchester, England), 2nd June 1954.

26. Report by the Director of Water Examination, 20th March 1959, p. 1, Fluoridation of water supplies: committee and Board reports 1952–69, ACC/2558/MW/C/08/265/001, London Metropolitan Archives.

27. *The Fluoridation of Water and the Prevention of Dental Decay*, Ministry of Health Reference Note No. 9 (HMSO: 1955).

28. *Fluorides in your water supplies, Picture Post* (London, England), 7th May 1955, Issue 58, Picture Post Historical Archive. Web. Accessed 13th September 2011.

29. *The Fluoridation of Water and the Prevention of Dental Decay*, p. 2.

30. Ibid. p. 4.

31. Ibid. p. 6.

32. Ibid. p. 5.

33. Ibid. p. 4.

34. *The Effect of Purification Procedures on Fluoride Content in Water*, Report by the Director of Water Examination, 20th March 1959, p. 1, Metropolitan Water Board Committee and Board Reports 1952-69, ACC/2558/MW/C/08/265/001, London Metropolitan Archives.

35. *Fluoridation – Why and How To Stop It* (London: The British Housewives League, circa 1959) p. 1, Note pamphlet is undated but was stamped by the British Museum on 1st October 1959. The mention of two recent contemporary anti-fluoridation events in Andover and Darlington also suggests that a late 1958, or early 1959, publication date would be correct.

36. Ibid.
37. *The Effect of Purification Procedures on Fluoride Content in Water*, pp. 2–6.
38. *Fluoridation of Public Water Supplies*, Letter from Clerk of the Board to members, 15th February 1960, Metropolitan Water Board Committee and Board Reports1952–69, ACC/2558/MW/C/08/265/001, London Metropolitan Archives.
39. *A Journey Through Ruins: The Last Days of London* (Oxford: Oxford University Press, 2009) p. 177.
40. *Reports on Public Health and Medical Subjects*, No.105 (HMSO, June 1962).
41. *Report of the Government Steering Committee on the Conduct of the Fluoridation Studies in the United Kingdom and the Results Achieved After Five Years*, Report by the Director of Water Examination, E. Windle Taylor, 16th July 1962, p. 3, Metropolitan Water Board Committee and Board Reports 1952–69, ACC/2558/MW/C/08/265/001, London Metropolitan Archives.
42. Ibid.
43. *British Waterworks Association letter*, October 25th 1962, Metropolitan Water Board Committee and Board Reports 1952–69, ACC/2558/MW/C/08/265/001, London Metropolitan Archives.
44. Ibid.
45. *Fluoridation of Water Supplies*, House of Lords debate, 10th December 1962, vol. 245 cc411–4, quote from Enoch Powell's speech by Lord Newton.
46. Ibid. Lord Douglas of Barloch.
47. *Fluoridation of Water Supplies*, Ministry of Health letter 14th December 1962, Metropolitan Water Board Committee and Board Reports 1952–69.
48. *The Government of London*, Gerald Rhodes (London: Weidenfeld and Nicolson, 1970) p. 140.
49. London Government Act, Chapter 33, Part 1, 1 (HMSO: 1963).

50. Ibid. Section 45, Clause 1.

51. *Fluoridation of Water Supplies*, Report from the Clerk of the Board, May 1963, p. 2, Fluoridation of water supplies: committee and Board reports 1952–69, Metropolitan Water Board ACC/2558/MW/C/08/265/002, London Metropolitan Archives.

52. *Fluoridation*, Statement by E.L. Beers, 29th May 1963, Secretary of the Metropolitan Water, Sewerage and Drainage Board.

53. *Fluoridation of Water Supplies*, Ministry of Health Circular, 25th June 1963, Fluoridation of water supplies: committee and Board reports 1952–69, Metropolitan Water Board ACC/2558/MW/C/08/265/002, London Metropolitan Archives.

54. *Fluoridation*, Ministry of Health (HMSO: 1963) p. 2.

55. Ibid. p. 5.

56. Ibid.

57. Ibid. p. 6.

58. Letter from Marian Reid of London N16 to Metropolitan Water Board, August 1963, *Fluoridation of water supplies: objections*, 1953–68, ACC/2558/MW/C/08/263/002.

59. *Environmental Toxicology: The legacy of 'Silent Spring'*, Volume 19, Wellcome Witnesses to Twentieth Century Medicine, Eds. D.A. Christie and E.M. Tansey, (London: Wellcome Trust/University College London, 2004) p. 8.

60. http://www.rachelcarson.org/, Timeline, Accessed 19th March 2012.

61. *Fluoridation of Public Water Supplies: The Ethical Question is Paramount*, Southern Counties Branch of the National Pure Water Association, undated but included with an array of 1963 materials, Fluoridation of water supplies: committee and Board reports 1952–69, Metropolitan Water Board ACC/2558/MW/C/08/265/002, London Metropolitan Archives.

62. Ibid.

63. Postcard from London anti-fluoridation campaign, undated,

Fluoridation of water supplies: objections 1953–68, ACC/2558/MW/C/08/263/006, London Metropolitan Archives.

64. Ibid. Letter from the Clerk of the Metropolitan Water Board to the London Anti-Fluoridation Campaign, 29th August 1963.

65. *Water Board Wants Cards Stopped, The Times* (London, England), Monday 4th November 1963, p. 6, Issue 55849, Col. F, Times Digital Archive. Web. Accessed 13th September 2011.

66. *A Journey Through Ruins: The Last Days of London*, p. 199.

67. *Fluoridation: A Monstrous Violation of Human Rights*, London Anti-Fluoridation Campaign, undated but likely to be 1963, Introduction, *Fluoridation of water supplies: objections* 1953–68, ACC/2558/MW/C/08/263/006, London Metropolitan Archives.

68. Letter from Lord Douglas of Barloch, 5th July 1963, Letter from Lord Douglas of Barloch, 5th July 1963, Fluoridation of water supplies: committee and Board reports 1952–69, Metropolitan Water Board ACC/2558/MW/C/08/265/002, London Metropolitan Archives.

69. Letter from Miss Marjery Abraham of W2, 4th November 1963, *Fluoridation: supporters* 1962–69, ACC/2558/MW /C/09/200, London Metropolitan Archives.

70. Ibid. Letter from Richard Oliver, 5th November 1963.

71. *Fluoride in Water at Birmingham, The Times* (London, England), Friday 5th June 1964, p. 76, Issue 56030, Col. E, Times Digital Archive. Web. Accessed 13th September 2011.

72. Extract from a speech by the Minister of Health, the Rt. Honourable Kenneth Robinson M.P. to the Annual Conference of the London Boroughs Committee, 1st November 1965, Metropolitan Water Board, *Fluoridation of water supplies: committee and Board reports* 1952–69, ACC/2558/MW/C/08/265/003, London Metropolitan

Archives.

73. Ibid. For example, Letter from the Clerk of the Board to K.F. Lewis Esq., 26th November 1965.

74. Water Examination Department document stamped 26th April 1968, *Fluoridation: correspondence with local authorities*, Metropolitan Water Board, ACC/2558/MW/C/09/201, London Metropolitan Archives.

75. Ibid.

76. Ibid.

77. *Fluoridation of water supplies*, 26th April 1968, extract from Water Examination department document, *Fluoridation of water supplies: committee and Board reports* 1952–69, ACC/2558/MW/C/08/265/003, London Metropolitan Archives.

78. *No Fluoride for Londoners' Teeth*, Leonard Vicars, *Evening News*, (London, England), 23rd May 1968.

79. London Anti-Fluoridation Campaign statement, 1st June 1969, *Fluoridation of water: objectors* 1969–73, Metropolitan Water Board, ACC/2558/MW/C/09/198, London Metropolitan Archives.

80. *Should Fluoride be added to London's Water?* (London: Greater London Authority, 2003), Chair's foreword.

81. Chapter 5: *Drinking Water Guidelines and Standards* (Draft), Sombo Yamamura in collaboration with Jamie Bartram, Mihaly Csanady, Hend Galal Gorchev and Alex Redekopp (Geneva: World Health Organisation, undated) p. 6, Retrieved 29th March 2012, http://www.who.int/water _sanitation_health/dwq/arsenicun5.pdfCrapper Puritas, Catalogue No. 30, p. 50 (London: Thomas Crapper and Co., 1954).

82. *Factories Act*, Clause 41, 1 Edw. 8 & 1, Geo. 6, Ch. 67 (HMSO: 1937).

83. The Drinking Fountain Association Annual Report 1968, pp. 9–10, ACC/3168/119, London Metropolitan Archives.

84. Metropolitan Drinking Fountain and Cattle Trough

Association Annual Report 1960, p. 9, ACC/3168/111, London Metropolitan Archives.

85. Ibid. p. 10.

86. Email from Ron Brooker, 6th October 2011.

87. Email from David Khan, 21st September 2011.

88. Email from Lesley Ramm, 22nd September 2011.

89. Email from Peter Skuse, 22nd September 2011.

90. Telephone interview with Ginnie Smith, recorded 23rd September 2011.

91. Email from Bernard Pellegrinetti, 28th September 2011.

92. Email from Valerie Scott, 4th October 2011.

CHAPTER EIGHT
Maggie Thatcher, Jane Fonda and the Water Cooler
1973–2000

1. *A Journey Through Ruins: The Last Days of London* p. 175 / Interestingly, in Wright's 2009 updated edition of the original book, 1991, the page-long coverage of *Drinking Water in a Toxic State* expanded into a whole chapter, indicating the contemporary resonances of drinking water as a commodity and a representation of the politics of privatisation.

2. Patrick Wright's comment also referred to Perrier's recall of its product following a benzene scandal.

3. *The Politics of London's Water,* A.K. Mukhopadhyay, The London Journal, Vol. 1, No. 2, November 1975, p. 220.

4. The Water Act c.37, Schedule 8, clauses 56 & 57, (HMSO, 1973).

5. Social function to mark end of Board, 1973, ACC/2558/MW/C/09/112, London Metropolitan Archives.

6. *Watershed,* Fred Pearce (London: Junction Books, 1982) p. 4.

7. *A Growing Community,* Europe: Gateway to the European Union 1970–79, http://europa.eu/about-eu/eu-history/1970-79/index_en.htm, Accessed 5th September 2011.

8. The Water Act, 1973, Part1, Clause 1, point 2.

9. Ibid. Part II, Clause 2.

10. *Watershed*, p. 150.

11. Control of Pollution Act, Part II, Clause 31 (HMSO: 1974)

12. *Watershed*, p. 150.

13. Council Directive 75/440/EEC, 16th June 1975 concerning the quality of surface water intended for abstraction of drinking water in Member States, http://eurlex.europa.eu/LexUri Serv.do?uri=CELEX:31975L0440:EN:HTML, Accessed 3rd September 2011.

14. *Watershed*, p. 72.

15. *Environmental Toxicology: The legacy of 'Silent Spring'* p. 20.

16. *Government see no reason to change regulations on drinking water, The Times* (London, England) Friday 2nd April 1976, p. 8, Issue 59669, Col.B, Times Digital Archive. Web. Accessed 1st September 2011.

17. Ibid.

18. *Watershed*, p. 34.

19. *Drought: a contemporary retrospective review*, J.C. Rodda and T.J. Marsh (Oxfordshire: Centre for Ecology and Hydrology, 2011) p. 27.

20. Ibid.

21. *Evening News* (London, England), 14th July 1976, p. 2.

22. *Drought: a contemporary retrospective review*, p. 47.

23. Ibid. p. 32, p. 47.

24. *Troubled Water: Rivers, Politics and Pollution*, David Kinnersley (London: Hillary Shipman, 1988) p. 108.

25. *Watershed*, p. 77.

26. Ibid. p. 79.

27. *London: from Punk to Blair*, John Davis, in *From GLC to GLA: London Politics Then and Now*, Eds. Joe Kerr and Andrew Gibson (London: Reaktion Books, 2003) p. 110.

28. Andrew Marr's *History of Modern Britain*, Episode 4, http://www.bbc.co.uk/programme/b007nn9k, BBC television 2007, viewed 3rd September 2011.

29. *The Penguin Social History of Britain: British Society Since 1945*, Arthur Marwick (London: Penguin, 1982) p. 272.

30. *Implementing European Environmental Policy at the Local Level: The British Experience with Water Quality Directives*, Vol.1, Summary Report, Neil Ward, Henry Buller and Philip Lowe (Newcastle: University of Newcastle, 1995) p. 19.

31. *Council Directive of 15th July 1980 relating to the quality of water intended for human consumption* 80/778/EEC, (Brussels: European Economic Community, 1980).

32. Soda Stream UK, commercial broadcast July 1980: http://www.youtube.com/watch?v=oFeVOCbvHG8&feature =results_video&playnext=1&list=PLF95E6235852D0302, Accessed 20th June 2011.

33. *A Brief History of WRc-NSF* (Reading: WRc-NSF, 2009), published on organisation's website: http://www.wrc nsf.com /history.htm, Accessed 29th March 2012.

34. *Drinking Water Consumption in Great Britain: A survey of drinking habits with special reference to tap-water-based beverages*, Technical Report TR137, (Medmenham: Water Research Centre, 1980), p. 1.

35. The London neighbourhoods included in the survey were Central Croydon, South Newham, Stepney and Poplar (both in the borough of Tower Hamlets), Tooting (Wandsworth), Islington South and Finsbury, South Brent and Hampstead (London Borough of Camden).

36. *Drinking Water Consumption in Great Britain*, p. 7.

37. *The Nutrition of Industrial Workers: Recommended Dietary Allowances* (Revised 1945), Second Report of the Committee on Nutrition of Industrial Workers etc (Washington: National Academy of Sciences, 1945) p. 11.

38. *Drinking Water Consumption in Great Britain*, p. 1.

39. Ibid. p. 8.

40. Ibid. p. 16.

41. *Trace Elements in Water and Cardiovascular Disease – Population*

Exposure to Metals Released from Piping Materials used for Water Distribution in the U.K., Final Report to the Department of the Environment 1977–81, E.J. Bailey (Medmenham: Water Research Centre, 1982) p. 1.

42. *Contamination of Water by Domestic Plumbing Fittings,* R.J. Oliphant (Swindon: Water Research Centre, 1981) p. 41.

43. *Sampling of Drinking Water to Estimate Population Exposure to Lead,* R.J. Bailey (Medmenham: Water Research Centre, 1981) pp. 1–2.

44. *Watershed,* p. 81.

45. *Trace Elements in Water and Cardiovascular Disease,* p. 102.

46. Ibid. p. 42.

47. House of Lords debate, 7th July 1982, Vol. 432, cc790, Accessed Hansard records on www.millbanksystems.com, 5th October 2011.

48. House of Commons debate, 16th November 1982, Vol. 32, cc155, Accessed Hansard records on www.millbank systems.com, 5th October 2011.

49. Ibid., cc202.

50. House of Commons debate, 18th January 1983, Vol. 35 cc245–56, Accessed Hansard records on www.millbank systems.com, 5th October 2011.

51. Verified the identity of the subject in the photograph with News International's syndication department, email from Chris Ball, 29th March 2012.

52. *Standpipes sprout throughout the land, The Times* (London, England), 27th January 1983, p.2, Issue 61441, Col. B, Times Digital Archive. Web. Accessed 5th September 2011.

53. Ibid.

54. Ibid.

55. *6.75m must boil drinking water, The Times* (London, England) 4th February 1983, p. 2, Issue 61448, Col. B, Times Digital Archive. Web. Accessed 5th September 2011.

56. *Londoners told: cut back or else, The Times* (London, England)

14th February 1983, p. 2, Issue 61456, Col. A, Times Digital Archive. Web. Accessed 5th September 2011.

57. Ibid.

58. Inner London population reached a low that year of circa 2.52 million *GLA Demography Update* (London: Greater London Authority, 2008) p. 2 / The 1981 census for Greater London recorded 6,713,165 residents: *The London Encyclopaedia*, p. 632.

59. *'DIY' repairs to the mains, The Times*, (London, England), 15th February 1983, p. 2, Issue 61457, Col. A, Times Digital Archive. Web. Accessed 5th September 2011.

60. House of Commons debate, 15th February 1983, Vol. 37, cc154–8 (UK Parliament).

61. *Number of homes without supply increases, The Times*, (London, England) 18th February 1983, p. 2, Issue 61460, Col. B, Times Digital Archive. Web. Accessed 5th September 2011.

62. House of Commons debate, 14th February 1983, Vol. 37, cc48

63. *Water strike ends, but power struggle begins*, David Felton, Labour Correspondent, *The Times*, (London, England), 23rd February 1983, p. 1, Issue 61464, Col. B.

64. *End of a gentlemanly dispute*, David Felton, Labour Correspondent, *The Times*, (London, England), 23rd February 1983, p. 2, Issue 61464, Col. E, Times Digital Archive. Web. Accessed 5th September 2011.

65. *Bottle firms spring to the rescue*, Richard Evans, *The Times*, (London, England), 25th January 1983, p.2, Issue 61439, Col. E, Times Digital Archive. Web. Accessed 6th October 2011.

66. Ibid.

67. *Bottled water everywhere, The Observer 1901–2004* (England, U.K.), 13th February 1983, p. 19, Accessed 6th October 2011.

68. *Naturally the connoisseur's choice*, Appollinaris Table Water advertisement, *Illustrated London News*, (London, England), 29th June 1974 p. 48. Illustrated London News archive. Web. Retrieved 21st October 2011.

69. *How the British took to sparkling waters,* M. Davie, *The Observer 1901–2004* England, U.K.), 24th July 1983 p. 12.

70. *Physical,* Olivia Newton-John, live performance broadcast on You Tube: http://www.youtube.com/watch?v=tAoDJcFU6iY, Accessed 6th April 2011.

71. *London in the 20th Century,* p. 75.

72. *Bon appetit, The Economist* (London, England), Saturday, 12th January, 1985, p. 22, Issue 7376, The Economist Historical Archive. Web. Accessed 6th April 2011.

73. *The Good Water Guide: The World's Best Bottled Waters,* Maureen and Timothy Green (London: Rosendale Press, 1985) p. 6.

74. Ibid. p. 12.

75. Natural Mineral Water Regulations (HMSO: 1985).

76. *The Good Water Guide,* p. 12.

77. Ibid. p. 123.

78. *Cosmopolitan* (London, England), Summer 1986, *Zest* supplement p. 12.

79. Ibid.

80. *Cosmopolitan* (London, England), Summer 1988, *Zest* supplement p. 13.

81. *Cosmopolitan* (London, England), Summer 1989, pp. 130–31.

82. *Cosmopolitan* (London, England), December 1989, pp. 8–9.

83. Ibid.

84. *Poison on Tap, The Observer* (London, England) *Observer Magazine,* 6th August, 1989, pp. 16–24.

85. *Newswatch, The Observer* (London, England), 7th August 1988, p. 2.

86. *Water supplies monitored after contamination, The Guardian* (Manchester: England), 19th August, 1988, p. 4.

87. *DPP acts on water mishap, The Guardian* (Manchester, England), 24th January, 1989, ProQuest Historical Newspapers: The Guardian (1821–2003) and The Observer (1791–2003), Retrieved 7th October 2011.

88. *Legal cloud over Ridley water sale, The Guardian* (Manchester, England), 30th January 1989, p. 4, ProQuest Historical Newspapers: The Guardian (1821–2003) and The Observer (1791–2003). Web. Retrieved 7th October 2011.

89. *Water Privatisation and the Environment: An Overview of the Issues,* Judith Rees, (London: Friends of the Earth, 1989) p. 50.

90. *Clean up your water now, EC tells Britain, The Observer* (London, England), ProQuest Historical Newspapers: The Guardian (1821–2003) and The Observer (1791–2003). Web. Retrieved 7th October 2011.

91. *Britain's Poisoned Water,* Frances and Phil Craig (London: Penguin, 1989) p. xii.

92. Ibid. p. 31.

93. Ibid. p. 53.

94. Ibid. p. 27.

95. *Water Privatisation and the Environment: An Overview of the Issues,* pp. 52–3.

96. *Poison on Tap,* p. 22.

97. *Tap dancing with the public, The Guardian* (Manchester, England), p. 33, ProQuest Historical Newspapers: The Guardian (1821–2003) and The Observer (1791–2003). Web. Retrieved 7th October 2011.

98. For example *Sick Buildings, The Architects Journal* (London, England), 20th May 1987 pp. 22–3.

99. *Inside the Office, The Architects Journal* (London, England), 19th August 1987, p. 45 and 26th August 1987, p. 47.

100. *Yellow Pages Central London 1986* (Reading: British Telecom), p.1313–17.

101. *Yellow Pages Central London 1985,* p. 1277.

102. *Yellow Pages Central London 1987,* p. 1412.

103. *Yellow Pages Central London 1988,* p. 1746.

104. *Yellow Pages Central London 1989,* pp. 1990–91.

105. *Yellow Pages Central London 1990,* pp. 1990–91.

106. *The Changing Workplace, Buildings Update: Offices 1*, Francis Duffy, *The Architects' Journal* (London, England), 27th September 1989, p. 77.
107. *Yellow Pages Central London 1990*, p. 2100.
108. *Yellow Pages Central London 1993*, pp. 2100–1.
109. *Troubled Water*, p. 127.
110. Ibid. p. 84.
111. Ibid. p. 119.
112. North West Water Authority 1973–6.
113. David Kinnersley's Obituary in *The Guardian* (Manchester, England), Friday, 17th December, 2004, viewed online 7th October 2011 / David Kinnersley's Obituary in *The Independent*, Saturday, 11th December, 2004, viewed online 7th October 2011.
114. 114. *Troubled Water*, p. 139.
115. 115. Ibid. p. 152.
116. 116. *Evening Standard*, 22nd February 1989, p. 7.
117. 117. *The Penguin Social History of Britain: British Society Since 1945*, Arthur Marwick (London: Penguin, 1982) p. 407.
118. *The New Shorter Oxford English Dictionary* (Oxford: Oxford University Press, 1993) p. 3534.
119. *Millions Take the H2O Plunge*, Peter Oborne, *Evening Standard* (London, England), 6th December 1989, p. 2, Col. 6.
120. Drinking Water Inspectorate website homepage description, http://dwi.defra.gov.uk, Accessed 9th April 2012.
121. *Drinking Water to be Checked*, John Hunt, *Financial Times* (London, England) 23rd December 1989, p. 4, Financial Times digital archive. Web, Retrieved 3rd April 2012.
122. *Cosmopolitan*, July 1990, pp. 108–9.
123. 123. *The Good Water Guide*, p. 118.
124. Brita corporate history, http://www.brita.net/uk/history/html?&L=1, Accessed 3rd April 2012.
125. *Eau No. Kay Marles takes a dip into the muddied waters of the filter market. The Observer* (London, England), 7th January

1990, p. A21, ProQuest Historical Newspapers: The Guardian
(1821–2003) and The Observer (1791–2003). Web. Retrieved
7th October 2011.

126. *Drinking Water Quality* leaflet, (Reading: Thames Water),
External relations 2 04 0492, Catalogued 1992 but undated,
Ephemera 470: Water Supply and Sewerage 1, Wellcome
Library.

127. Ibid. Water Filters leaflet, Thames Water Utilities Limited
13010392.

128. *Water Quality Fact Sheet: Bottled Water,* (Reading: Thames
Water, 1992) Reference 25/6/92, Drinks Ephemera EPH109:
Water Box 3, Wellcome Library.

129. *South West Water is fined £10,000 over Camelford, The Times*
(London, England) 9th January 1991, p. 4, The Times Digital
Archive. Web. Accessed 3rd April 2012 / Many Camelford
poisoning victims also received out-of-court settlements
from South West Water in 1994: *Pollution cash, The Times*
(London, England), 19th May 1994, p. 4, The Times Digital
Archive. Web. Accessed 3rd April 2012.

130. *Economics of Lead Pipe Replacement: Final report to the
Department of the Environment* (Swindon: Water Research
Centre, 1992) p. 4.

131. Ibid.

132. *Britain guilty of breaching drinking water standards,* 26th
November 1992, *The Guardian,* ProQuest Historical
Newspapers: The Guardian (1821–2003) and The Observer
(1791–2003). Web. Retrieved 7th October 2011.

133. *EC convicts Britain of poor quality tap water, The Times* (London,
England) 26th November 1992, p. 5, The Times Digital
Archive, Accessed 3rd April 2012.

134. *The Good Water Guide,* 1994 edition, p. 11.

135. Ibid. p. 119.

136. Ibid. p. 120.

137. Ibid. p. 119.

138. *Cosmopolitan Magazine,* June 1996 p. 176.

139. *Drinking Water Consumption in Great Britain,* p. 58.

140. *Tap Water Consumption in England and Wales: Findings from the 1995 National Survey,* (HMSO, 1996) p. v.

141. *A Brief History of Neoliberalism,* David Harvey (Oxford: Oxford University Press, 2005 p. 60.

142. The Drinking Fountain Association Annual Report 1985, p. 2, ACC/3168/137: London Metropolitan Archives.

143. Ibid. 1983–7, ACC/3168/135–39.

144. *London in the 20th Century,* pp. 298–99.

145. Trade Union Congress digital archive: http://www.union-history.info/britainatwork/display.php?irn=978&QueryPage =, Accessed 6th April 2012.

146. *London in the 20th Century,* p. 76.

CHAPTER NINE
Wasteland and Council Pop: tracking the anti-bottled water zeitgeist 2010–2011

1. Natural Hydration Council, Member Brands page, http://www.naturalhydrationcouncil.org.uk/Page/MemberB rands1, Accessed 20th May 2012 / Healthy Hydration Glass page, http://www.naturalhydrationcouncil.org.uk/Page/ HealthyHydrationGlass, Accessed 4th September 2012.

2. 1993 figure: *The Good Water Guide,* 1994 edition / 2003 figure: *The 2010 UK Soft Drinks Report – Investing in Refreshment* (London: British Soft Drinks Association, 2010) p.6.

3. Interview with Jarno Stet, Waste Services Manager, Westminster City Council, conducted and recorded 25th July 2011: all direct quotes in the chapter are from this interview.

4. Additional written responses from Jarno Stet, Westminster City Council, received 11th August 2011.

5. Ibid.

6. *CO$_2$ impacts of transporting the UK's recovered paper and plastic bottles to China,* p. 3, (Banbury: Waste and Resources Action

Programme, 2008), Retrieved from WRAP website, www.wrap.org.uk, 10th April 2012.

7. Ibid. p. 28.

8. Closed Loop Recycling plant website: http://www.closed-looprecycling.co.uk/Home, Accessed 18th November 2011.

9. *Government Review of Waste Policy in England 2011*, p.18, (HMSO, 2011), http://defra.gov.uk/publications/files/pb135 40-waste-policy-review110614.pdf, Retrieved from DEFRA website 18th November 2011.

10. Sustain's strapline is 'the alliance for better food and farming', http://sustainweb.org

11 *Bottled and Sold: the story behind our obsession with bottled water,* Peter H. Gleick (Washington: Island Press, 2010) p. 91.

12. *Have you bottled it? How drinking tap water can help save you and the planet,* Lucia Wanctin, (London: Sustain, 2006) p. 7.

13. All details relating to the Hydrachill project and direct quotes are from an interview recorded with Maria Andrews, former Head of Development for Waste Watch, on 29th March 2010.

14. Recorded in an interview with Christine Haigh and Jackie Schneider of The Children's Food Campaign, Sustain, 10th May 2010.

15. *The Taps Are Turning: Are we ending our love affair with bottled water?* (London: Sustain, 2008) p. 6.

16. *The Clear Choice,* Thames Water press release, 19th February 2008, http://londonontap.org/press/archive/tap/, retrieved 15th November 2011.

17. *Bottled Water: Who Needs It?,* Broadcast BBC One, 19th February 2008.

18. *The Clear Choice.*

19. Ibid.

20. *'Tap Top' is tip top for London's tap water,* 1st December 2008, http://londonontap.org/press/archive/tap/, Accessed 15th November 2011.

21. On sale from The Water Cooler Company at this price, http:www.thewatercoolercompany.com/index.php?id=lond on-on-tap-carafe, Accessed 4th September 2012.

22. Email correspondence with Emma Reynolds of Tsuru Restaurant Group, 19th August 2011.

23. Interview recorded with Sara Lom, Chief Executive of the Royal Parks Foundation, 28th October 2011.

24. *New Drinking-Fountain in Hyde Park, Illustrated London News,* (London, England) Saturday 7th March, 1868, p. 233, Issue 1472.

25. *Freeman Family Fountain,* Annual Report and Accounts 2009–10, (London: The Royal Parks, 2010) p. 37.

26. *The Freeman Family Fountain: New public drinking fountain refreshes Hyde Park,* Press Release September 2009, The Royal Parks and The Royal Parks Foundation, Retrieved 6th October 2010.

27. Interview with Christine Haigh and Jackie Schneider.

28. *Wise up on water!* (London: Water UK), undated.

29. *Thirsty Play,* (London: Sustain, 2010) p. 4, http://sustain web.org/publications/?id=183, Accessed 8th October 2010.

30. Interview with Guy Jeremiah, Director of Aquatina/collabo-rator on Find-A-Fountain recorded 23rd September 2011.

31. Science Museum shop website products: http://www.science museumshop.co.uk/product/312301.html, Accessed 10th April 2012.

32. *Aquatina is...* section on Aquatina website, http://aquatina .com/about?uncompress=1, Accessed 25th September 2011.

33. Title for The City of London Corporation contemporary fountain project 2010.

34. Interview with Victor Callister, Senior Planning Officer, The City of London Corporation, recorded 24th March 2010.

35. *Atlántida,* Santa and Cole website: http://www.santaand cole.com/en/catalogo/fuentes/atlantida, Accessed 10th April 2011.

36. Photographed 21st May, 2010.

37. Recorded at fountain launch, 21st May 2010.

38. Photographed 21st May, 2010.

39. Aquaid Water Coolers, http://www.aquaidwatercoolers .co.uk/what-we-do, Accessed 27th July 2012.

40. Ibid. what-we-do/bottled-water-coolers/freestanding-bottled-water-coolers.

41. *The Freeman Family Fountain*, press release.

42. *Towards A One Planet 2012, 2nd edition* (London: London 2012, 2009), Retrieved from http://www.london2012.com /docu ments/locog-publications/london-2012-sustainability-plan.pdf, Accessed 14th August 2010 p. 25.

43. Ibid.

44. Ibid. p. 37.

45. *Schweppes Abbey Well Gets Off To A Schwimming Start*, Coca Cola press release, http://coca-cola.co.uk/press-centre/ 2009/march/launch_campaign_for_schweppes_abbey_well_ gets_off_to_a_schwimming_start.html, Accessed 17th November 2011.

46. Transcript of Question and Answer Session with the London Organising Committee of the Olympic and Paralympic Games, 21st October 2009, http://legacy.london.gov.uk/asse mbly/assemmtgs/2009/plenaryoct21/minutes/app3-trans criptLOCOG.pdf, Accessed 6th February 2012, p. 2.

47. Ibid.

48. *London 2012 to showcase the best of British food in 2012*, London 2012 press release, 9th December 2009, http://www.london 2012.com/press/media-releases/2009/12/london-2012-to-showcase-the-best-of-british-food-in-2012.php, Accessed 4th August 2011.

49. The event safety guide (second edition), Health and Safety Executive (The Stationery Office, 1999) pp. 75–6.

50. Interview recorded in person with Megan Ashfield, of Populous Architects, Monday 16th May 2011.

51. Telephone interview recorded with James Bulley, Head of Infrastructure, London Organising Committee for the Olympic and Paralympic Games, London 2012, 20th August 2011.

52. Email correspondence with Kath Dalmeny, Policy Director of Sustain, 23rd September 2011.

53. *Food Vision for the London 2012 Olympic and Paralympic Games* (London: London 2012, December 2009) p. 20.

54. Telephone interview recorded with Paul May, Head of Venue Development, London Organising Committee for the Olympic and Paralympic Games, London 2012, 22nd November 2011.

55. MTD website, http://www.mtd.net/drinkwater.php, Accessed 20th April 2012.

56. London 2012 'Facts and Figures', http://www.london 2012.com/about-us/facts-and-figures/, Accessed 20th April 2012.

57. Schweppes Water page, Coca-Cola website (2010), http://www.coca-cola.co.uk/brands/category/schweppes-water.html, Accessed 10th August 2011.

58. Ibid.

59. Inteview with Michael Green, founder of tapwater.org, recorded 15th August 2011.

60. Lifebottle product, tapwater.org/shop/lifebottle, Accessed 16th November 2011.

61. Tapwater.org FAQS, http://www.tapwater.org/faqs, Accessed 19th November 2011.

62. Drinking water, Friends of the Earth website, http://www.foe.co.uk/living/tips/water__filters.html, Accessed 5th June 2012.

63. Tapwater.org FAQS.

CHAPTER TEN
21st Century Tap Water 2011–2012

1. Interview recorded with Professor Jeni Colbourne, Chief Inspector, the Drinking Water Inspectorate, Tuesday 25th October 2011.

2. The Natural Mineral Water, Spring Water and Bottled Drinking Water (England) Regulations 2007, Part 1, Clause 2 (The Stationery Office, 2007).

3. Ibid. Part 2, Clause 6.

4. Ibid. Schedule 1.

5. Email response from Thames Water, Monday 4th July, 2011to enquiry letter sent on Wednesday 11th May 2011 / Email received on 20th September stated that my stated project deadline was too soon for a site visit to be arranged, despite the fact that the initial request was posted in May 2011.

6. Sutton and East Surrey Water PLC education programme, http://www.waterplc.com/pages/community/schools-educa-tional-programme/, Accessed 31st July 2012.

7. *Big Water: Everyday Water: A Sociotechnical Perspective*, Zoe Safoulis, Continuum: Journal of Media and Cultural Studies, Vol. 19, No. 4, December 2005, p. 446.

8. Ibid. p. 452.

9. 'What We Do', Drinking Water Inspectorate website, http://dwi.defra.gov.uk/about/what-we-do/index.htm, Accessed 30th July 2012.

10. Advice Leaflets, Drinking Water Inspectorate website, http://dwi.defra.gov.uk/consumers/advice-leaflets/index.htm, Accessed 27th April 2012.

11. *Drinking Water Inspectorate*, A Hampton Implementation Review Report, (The Stationery Office, 2010) p. 8.

12. *Drinking Water 2011*, A Report by the Chief Inspector of Drinking Water, (Drinking Water Inspectorate/The Stationery Office, July 2012) p. 119.

13. Ibid. p. 85.

14. Email response from Professor Jeni Colbourne to interview follow-up questions, received 25th November 2011.
15. Email response from Steve White, Drinking Water Strategy Manager, to interview follow-up questions, received 1st November 2011.
16. Telephone interview recorded with Steve White, Thames Water, 10th October 2011.
17. *A Compengyous Reyment of a Dietary of Healthe made in Mountpyller by Andrew Boorde.*
18. 'Wholesomeness', Part III, Clause 4, The Water Supply (Water Quality) Regulations 2000 No. 3184 (The Stationery Office, 2000) / On the Quality of Water Intended for Human Consumption Council Directive 98/83/EC (EC: 1998).
19. Ibid. 'Wholesomeness' definition.
20. Walthamstow Reservoirs page, Thames Water website: http://www.thameswater.co.uk/cps/rde/xchg/prod/hs.xsl/62 53.htm, Accessed 27th April 2012.
21. *Edgelands: Journeys Into England's True Wilderness*, Paul Farley and Michael Symmons Roberts (London: Jonathan Cape, 2011) p. 84.
22. Photographed 17th February 2012.
23. *Pesticide Residues in Food and Cancer Risk: A Critical Analysis*, Lois Swirsky Gold, Thomas H. Slone and Bruce N. Ames, in *Handbook of Pesticide Toxicology*, Second Edition, Ed. R. Krieger, (Berkeley: Academic Press, 2001) p. 799.
24. *Pesticides*, Drinking Water Inspectorate consumer advice leaflet, http://dwi.defra.gov.uk/consumers/advice-leaflets/pesticides.pdf, Accessed 27th April 2012.
25. *Guidelines for Drinking-water Quality*, Fourth Edition, (Geneva: World Health Organisation, 2011) p. 1.
26. Table B: Chemical Parameters, Schedule 1: Prescribed Concentrations and Values, The Water Supply (Water Quality) Regulations 2000.
27. Pesticides, 'Drinking water standards explained' page,

Thames Water website, http://www.thameswater.co.uk/
your-water/7503.htm, Accessed 5th September 2012.

28. *Drinking Water 2007*, Thames region, (Drinking Water
Inspectorate/The Stationery Office, 2008) http://dwi.
defra.gov.uk/about/annual-report/2007/Thames.pdf,
Accessed 2nd November 2011, p. 2.

29. *Drinking water 2009*, Thames region of England (Drinking
Water Inspectorate/The Stationery Office, 2010) p. 6.

30. Get Pelletwise! website, http://www.getpelletwise.co.uk,
Accessed 5th December 2011.

31. *Drinking water 2009*, p. 19.

32. *Metaldehyde Slug Pellets* advice sheet (The Voluntary
Initiative Community Interest Company, undated).

33. *Consultation on the implementation of EU pesticides legislation -
Public consultation response from the RSPB*, May 2010,
http://rspb.org.uk/images/RSPB%20responses%20on%20SU
D_tcm9-251411.pdf, Retrieved 5th December 2011, p.1, p. 2.

34. Comment recorded during interview with Jeni Colbourne.

35. 'About Us' page, Our Rivers website http://www.ourrivers
.org.uk/about-us/ and *Diffuse pollution and the White Paper*,
blog post on Our Rivers website, June 14th 2011, retrieved
31st July 2012.

36. *Water Pollution Offences* web page, Law and Your
Environment - The plain guide to environmental law (UK
Environmental Law Association 2008-11), Retrieved 31st July
2012.

37. Fact Sheet: *Material for pest and disease control in organic crops*
(Bristol: Soil Association, 2010).

38. Search conducted 6th November 2011.

39. *Pathogenesis and management of male infertility*, The Lancet
(London, England), Volume 343, Issue 8911, 11th June 1994,
pp.1473–1479.

40. *Tap water link to abnormal sperm*, Liz Hunt, *The Independent*
(London, England), 21st January 1994, Web, retrieved 8th

November 2011.

41. *Oestrogen in Drinking Water* (Drinking Water Inspectorate/ The Stationery Office Limited, 2009).

42. Ibid.

43. *Endocrine Disruptors*, Drinking Water Inspectorate Consumer advice leaflet (The Stationery Office Limited, 2010) p. 2.

44. *Pharmaceuticals*, Drinking Water Inspectorate Consumer advice leaflet (The Stationery Office Limited, 2010).

45. *Thames Corridor Abstraction Management Strategy*, Environment Agency (The Stationery Office Limited, 2004) p. 13.

46. Search conducted 4th November 2011, http://www. environment-agency.gov.uk

47. Glossary of terms related to Urban Waste Water, Environment section of European Commission website, http://ec.europa.eu/environment/water/water-urban waste/info/glossary_en.htm, Retrieved 4th November 2011.

48. Water UK Jargon Buster: http://www.water.org.uk/ home /resources-and-links/jargon-b?s1=five-days&s2=bioche mical, Retrieved 4th November 2011.

49. *Water Quality Planning - prioritised Drinking Water Protected Areas*, Operational instruction 1164_08, Issued 19/12/08, http://www.environment-agency.gov.uk/static/documents /Business/1164_08.pdf, Accessed 23rd April 2012.

50. *Thames Gateway Water Treatment Works - Keeping London on tap*, short film (3'58"), Thames Water, uploaded to You Tube 2010, http://youtube.com/watch?v=oyhXZF_13_s, Viewed 6th November 2011.

51. *The completed acquisition of Thames Water Holdings Plc by Kemble Water Limited*, A consultation paper by Ofwat, February 2007, p. 5.

52. Ibid. The other half includes the Queensland Investment Corporation (Australia) and the Alberta Investment Management Corporation (Canada), amongst others including a pension fund for civil servants in the

Netherlands.

53. *Change in minority shareholders at Thames Water, 12th December 2011*, Macquarie Group Limited, http://www.macquarie.co.uk/mgl/uk/about/news/2011/12122011, Accessed 1st May 2012.

54. *Areas of water stress: final classification*, Reference GEH01207BNOC-E-E (Environment Agency/The Stationery Office, 2007) p. 2, p. 4.

55. *Water desalination plant opens for testing in Beckton, The Guardian*, 28th June 2011 (London, England), http://www.guardian.co.uk/environment/2011/jun/28/water-desalination-plant-beckton-london, Accessed 27th April 2012.

56. *Thames Gateway Water Treatment Works - Keeping London on tap.*

57. *Ensuring future supplies: Thames Gateway Water Treatment Works communications and engagement strategy*, p. 5, Thames Water, undated, http://dwi.defra.gov.uk/stakeholders/conferences-seminars/comms-workshop/6.Thames%20Gateway%20Water%20Treatment%20Works%20Final.pdf, Retrieved from the DWI website 28th April 2012.

58. *Policy & Procedure for Drinking Water Fountains in Public Areas*, Thames Water, November 2009, Unpublished, policy document received by email from Steve White on 11th October 2011.

59. The Water Supply (Water Fittings) Regulations 1999 (The Stationery Office).

60. *Policy & Procedure for Drinking Water Fountains in Public Areas.*

61. Interview with Victor Callister, Senior Planning Officer, The City of London Corporation, recorded 24th March 2010.

62. *Free access to drinking water across London*, Request for a Mayoral decision MD661, Greater London Authority, 2010, p. 3.

Conclusions and Questions

1. *Free access to drinking water across London,* p. 1.
2. *Initiative for free access to drinking water across London,* Mayor's delivery programme, 'Meeting The Vision, Clause 2, Retrieved from www.london.gov.uk 19th October 2011.
3. Interview recorded with John Mills, 2nd June 2010.
4. *Securing London's Water Future: The Mayor's Water Strategy* (London: Greater London Authority, 2011) Executive Summary, p. 15.
5. Ibid. p. 66.
6. *The London Plan: Spatial Development Strategy for Greater London 2011* (London: Greater London Authority, 2011) clause 3.86, p. 103 and Policy 7.5, Public realm p. 215.
7. Telephone interview recorded with Sara Lom, 28th October 2011.
8. *Royal Parks Foundation Drinking Fountain Open International Design Competition* (Competition Brief), The Royal Parks Foundation in partnership with Tiffany and Co. Foundation, June 2010, p. 3.
9. *Two British Designers win International Competition to find 'Ultimate Drinking Fountain',* The Royal Parks Foundation / Tiffany & Co. Foundation, undated, retrieved from Royal Parks Foundation website 14th March 2011.
10. Restored by Julian Harrap architects.
11. Transcribed directly from the fountain.
12. *Royal Parks Foundation Drinking Fountain Open International Design Competition,* p.6.
13. Metropolitan Cattle Trough and Drinking Fountain Association Annual Report, 1949, ACC/3168/100 p. 8.
14. St Pancras was designed by Chapman Taylor and King's Cross by John McAslan + Partners.
15. *HM Prison Service sanitaryware specification,* (Staffordshire: Armitage Shanks, 2003) Use of two drinking fountain types is listed as 'throughout establishment' p. 4.

16. http://www.findafountain.org, data confirmed by Rachel Jeremiah of Find-A-Fountain, by email, 26th January 2012.

17. *Viewpoint: Concord, you can give up bottled water*, BBC News, 30th June 2010 Retrieved 30th April 2012, http://www.bbc.co.uk/news/10444394.

18. *'There's no benefit to drinking bottled water'*, Guardian Environment podcast, Rebecca Smithers, Thursday 21st February 2008, listened 7th September 2010.

19. *How can we reduce the carbon footprint of the city by using drinking water fountains?* Roberto Alejandro Cantu Gomez, MA Urban Design dissertation, University of Westminster, 2011, p. 9.

20. Ibid. p. 43.

21. *'A Paper on Drinking Fountains' read in the Health Department of the National Association for the Promotion of Social Science*, Charles Melly, October 1858 (Geo. Smith, Watts and Co, printers, 1858) pp. 9–10.

22. *The Water Business: Corporations Versus People*, Ann-Christin Sjölander Holland (London: Zed Books, 2005) p.15.

23. *How can we reduce the carbon footprint of the city by using drinking water fountains?* p. 46.

24. Ibid. 58.

25. Thames Water Utilities Limited, Annual report and financial statements for the year ended 31st March 2011 (Reading: Thames Water, 2011), p. 33, downloaded from Thames Water's website 2nd August 2012 / *Thames Water boss awarded large bonus criticised*, BBC News (Business) website, 11th June 2012, retrieved 2nd August 2012.

26. *Big Water: Everyday Water: A Sociotechnical Perspective.*

27. *Liquid Pleasures*, p. 27.

28. *The London Plan: Spatial Development Strategy for Greater London 2011*, pp. 251, 257 and 307.

29. Conversations with Barbara Penner, Alexandra Goddard and Susannah Jordan, August-September 2012 plus my own

attendance of a Wembley Stadium Olympic Games event

30. *A blueprint for change:* London 2012 Sustainability report, April 2012 (London: London 2012) p. 55.

31. *UN 'should take blame for Haiti cholera' - US House members,* Mark Doyle, BBC NEWS website, Latin America and Caribbean, 20th July 2012, retrieved 7th September 2012 / *Health response to the earthquake in Haiti January 2010,* Claude de Ville de Goyet, Juan Pablo Sarmiento and François Grünewald (Washington: Pan American Health Organisation, 2011) Key Findings, No. 5, p. 178.

32. *The Water Manifesto: Arguments for a World Water Contract,* Riccardo Petrella (London: Zed, 2001) p. 93.

33. Ibid. p. 25: 'Dublin Declaration' on *Water in a Perspective of Sustainable Development,* International Conference on Water and Environment, January 1992, See also pp. 65–66.

34. Ibid. p. 93.

35. *The right to water (arts. 11 and 12 of the International Covenant on Economic, Social and Cultural Rights),* General Comment 15, E/C.12/2002/11, 20th January 2003 (Geneva: United Nations 2002) Introduction, clauses 1 and 3.

36. Ibid. clause 1.

37. Ibid. II Normative Content of the Right to Water, clause 12, i) *Physical accessibility.*

38. *Workplace health, safety and welfare: A short guide for managers* (The Stationery Office/Health and Safety Executive, 2011) p. 6.

39. *Viewpoint: Concord, you can give up bottled water,* BBC News.

40. *Bottled and Sold: The Story Behind Our Obsession With Bottled Water,* Peter H. Gleick (Washington: Island Press, 2010) p. 3.

41. Ibid. p. 175.

42. *Bottlemania,* Elizabeth Royte (New York: Bloomsbury, 2008) p.33.

43. *Tapped,* Dir. Stephanie Soechtig, Atlas Films, 2009.

44. Metropolitan Drinking Fountain and Cattle Trough

Association Minute Book, November 1871, ACC/3168/002, London Metropolitan Archives.
45. Translation provided by Sophia Akbar.
46. *Agua que has de beber* blog posting, Luzinterruptus.com, 9th February 2012, Accessed 7th May 2012.
47. 'About the event' page, '9th Global Bottled Water Congress' website information (Barcelona, Spain), Zenith International, www.zenithinternational.com, Accessed 7th July 2012.
48. Ibid. *Green Light for Bottled Water* conference information, planned for Wednesday 7th November 2012, Accessed Zenith International website 17th July 2012.
49. Ibid.

Contemporary culture has eliminated both the concept of the public and the figure of the intellectual. Former public spaces – both physical and cultural – are now either derelict or colonized by advertising. A cretinous anti-intellectualism presides, cheerled by expensively educated hacks in the pay of multinational corporations who reassure their bored readers that there is no need to rouse themselves from their interpassive stupor. The informal censorship internalized and propagated by the cultural workers of late capitalism generates a banal conformity that the propaganda chiefs of Stalinism could only ever have dreamt of imposing. Zer0 Books knows that another kind of discourse – intellectual without being academic, popular without being populist – is not only possible: it is already flourishing, in the regions beyond the striplit malls of so-called mass media and the neurotically bureaucratic halls of the academy. Zer0 is committed to the idea of publishing as a making public of the intellectual. It is convinced that in the unthinking, blandly consensual culture in which we live, critical and engaged theoretical reflection is more important than ever before.